THE YALE GUIDE TO CHILDREN'S NUTRITION

. . . .

William V. Tamborlane, M.D.
EDITOR IN CHIEF

Janet Z. Weiswasser
MANAGING EDITOR

Recipes compiled with cooperation
from the James Beard Foundation

Editors
Teresa Fung, M.S., R.D., C.N.S.D.
Nancy A. Held, M.S., R.D., C.D.E.
Tara Prather Liskov, M.S., R.D.

Foreword by Jane E. Brody

Yale University Press
New Haven and London

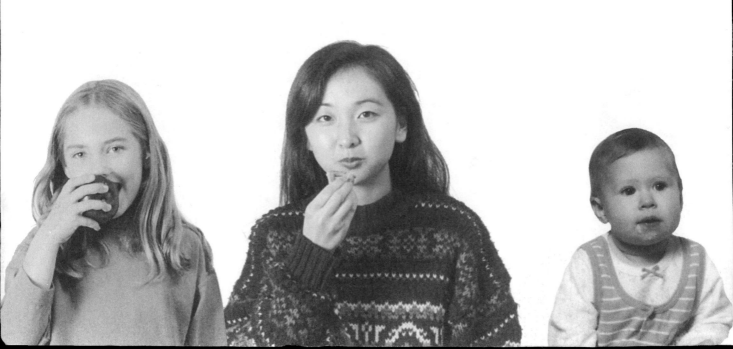

THE YALE GUIDE TO
Children's
Nutrition

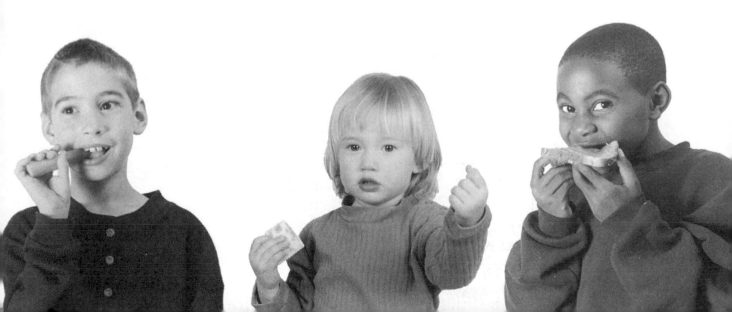

Published with assistance from the foundation established in memory of Calvin Chapin of the Class of 1788, Yale College.

The information and suggestions contained in this book are not intended to replace the services of your physician or caregiver. Because each person and each medical situation is unique, you should consult your own physician to get answers to your personal questions, to evaluate any symptoms you may have, or to receive suggestions on appropriate medications.

The authors have attempted to make this book as accurate and up-to-date as possible, but it may nevertheless contain errors, omissions, or material that is out of date at the time you read it. Neither the authors nor the publisher have any legal responsibility or liability for errors, omissions, out-of-date material, or the reader's application of the medical information or advice contained in this book.

Three recipes by Danny Meyer and Michael Romano, Mashed Yellow Turnips with Crispy Shallots, Sautéed Spinach with Garlic, and Vegetable Lasagna, were adapted from the *Union Square Cafe Cookbook,* by Danny Meyer and Michael Romano. Copyright © 1994 HarperCollins Publishers.

The growth charts in the appendix were reprinted with permission from Ross Products Division, Abbott Laboratories, Columbus, Ohio, 43216. From NCHS Growth Charts. Copyright © 1982 Ross Products Division, Abbott Laboratories.

Babar and the distinctive likeness thereof are trademarks of Laurent de Brunhoff and are used with his permission. Copyright © Laurent de Brunhoff. All rights reserved.

Designed by Nancy Ovedovitz and set in Simoncini Garamond type by Tseng Information Systems. Models on pages ii and iii, from left: Errin Gaulin, Jin Sook Lee, Katherine Richardson, Neil Bacon, Jennifer Gaulin, and Daniel Tilley. Photographs by Bill Grego. Illustrations by David Kiphuth and Laura Margolin. Printed in the United States of America by R.R. Donnelley, Harrisonburg, Virginia.

Library of Congress Cataloging-in-Publication Data
The Yale guide to children's nutrition / William V. Tamborlane, editor in chief ; Janet Z. Weiswasser, managing editor ; editors, Teresa Fung, Nancy A. Held, Tara Prather Liskov ; foreword by Jane E. Brody ; recipes compiled with cooperation from the James Beard Foundation.   p.   cm.
Includes bibliographical references and index.
ISBN: 0-300-06965-0 (cloth), 0-300-07169-8 (pbk.)
1. Children—Nutrition.   I. Tamborlane, William V.
II. Weiswasser, Janet Z.
RJ206.Y35   1997
613.2'083—dc20   96-44774
                CIP

A catalogue record for this book is available from the British Library.

The paper in this book meets the guidelines for permanence and durability of the Committee on Production Guidelines for Book Longevity of the Council on Library Resources.

10 9 8 7 6 5 4 3

This book is dedicated to children everywhere,
and to the memory of Warren H. Weiswasser, M.D.,
champion of children.

CONTENTS

. . . .

Foreword *Jane E. Brody*   ix

Preface *William V. Tamborlane, M.D.*   xiii

Acknowledgments   xv

PART ONE

From Infancy to Adolescence:
Developmental Nutrition

1 Measuring Up: Normal Growth and
Development   3

2 The Digestive Process: What Happens
after You Swallow?   9

3 Taste, Smell, and Food Preferences   16

4 Pyramid Power: A Guide to Healthy
Eating   25

5 Infancy: Eat, Sleep, and Be Happy   30

6 Toddlers and Preschoolers: Emerging
Independence   45

7 School-Age, Preadolescent Children: An Apple a Day   60

8 Adolescence: Life in the Fast Lane   64

PART TWO
Common Concerns

9 Food and the Family   77

10 Not All Vegetarians Are Created Equal   84

11 Feeding the Sick Child   88

12 Too Fat? Too Thin?   92

13 Energizing the Young Athlete   97

14 Acne and Diet: Is There a Connection?   108

15 Alcohol Use and Abuse in Adolescents   112

16 Diet Tips to Keep That Winning Smile   118

PART THREE
Beyond the Basics: Special Challenges in Nutrition

17 Eating Disorders   125

18 Childhood Obesity   133

19 Food Allergies   140

20 High Blood Cholesterol   148

21 Diabetes   161

22 Cystic Fibrosis   170

23 Gastrointestinal Disorders   175

24 PKU and Other Metabolic Disorders   181

25 Feeding the Infant with Cleft Lip and Palate   188

26 Attention Deficit Hyperactivity Disorder   195

PART FOUR
Building Blocks for Good Nutrition

27 Calories: The Key to Energy Balance   201

28 Protein: The Body's Building Blocks   205

29 Cash in on Carbohydrates   209

30 What's the Skinny on Fats and Cholesterol?   215

31 Facts and Myths about Vitamins and Minerals   229

32 Water: Drinking for the Health of It   240

33 Salt: The Spice of Life or the Taste of Doom?   244

34 Fantastic Fiber   252

35 Fresh Facts about Pesticides and Food Additives   257

36 Making Sense of Food Labels   265

PART FIVE
Eating In, Eating Out

37 From the Grocery Store to the Home: Stocking the Kitchen   273

38 What's for Lunch?   277

39 Fast Foods and Restaurants: Are You Speeding Past Good Nutrition?   283

PART SIX
Recipes

Foods for Infants   293
Breakfast Foods   299
Lunch Box Treats   307
Snacks   315
Meat, Poultry, and Fish Entrées   323
Carbohydrate-Dense Dishes   337
Vegetarian Selections   351
Vegetable Side Dishes   363
Desserts   373

Appendixes
Growth Charts   386
Recommended Dietary Allowances   394
Recipe Conversion Table   397

List of Contributors   399
Index   403

FOREWORD

· · · · · · ·

This book can help you develop and execute guidelines that can be readily incorporated into family life, regardless of the structure and circumstances of your family. It contains recipes with child appeal from some of the best chefs in the United States, as well as wisdom from some of the leading scientists in the field of children's health. Not only will your children benefit, but in all likelihood you will too. There is no better time to get yourself on a sensible nutrition track than when your children are learning from your example.

Of the many things I have produced in my life, I am proudest of my twin sons. I should really say "we" because my husband, Richard Engquist, had as much as I did to do with the boys' growing up with common sense as their guide, a healthy respect for the sanctity of their bodies and minds, and sound ideas about the kinds of fuel those bodies need in order to run well.

From the beginning, we were determined as parents not to play games about food and feeding. No "Open Sesame" to shove in spoonfuls of food the boys had little interest in consuming. No "Eat what's on your plate — the children in Poland are starving." I wasn't out of nursery school when I first suggested that my parents send my dinner to Poland because I certainly wasn't going to eat it!

As soon as our sons lost interest in a meal, the food was removed. When a new food or combination of foods was introduced, they had to taste it, but they did not have to eat anything they didn't like. As lunch-box-toting school children, they were asked to bring home whatever they did not eat in school. No comments were made about how little or how much they consumed, although they were sometimes asked if there was a reason they had not eaten a particular item. That reason guided us as to what and how much to stoke their lunch boxes in the days ahead.

We always tried to be adaptable instead of

foisting our own standards and habits on the boys. During the early elementary school grades they were hungriest when they came home from school. So, instead of the traditional after-school snack of cookies and milk (which all too often spoils appetites for supper), they had dinner at half past three. Then they went out to play for two hours and returned hungry enough to eat a light supper with us at seven o'clock. As they got older and ate bigger lunches, after-school snacks were introduced and dinner followed their play-time. While waiting for their meal to be served, the boys downed fistfuls of carrot and celery sticks (one ate only carrots, the other only celery) lightly dipped in a mixture of ketchup and mayo. Because iceberg was the only kind of lettuce they would eat, iceberg was what they got, with sliced tomatoes and cucumbers. Better some kind of salad than none at all, we figured, as we chomped on romaine, redleaf lettuce, and arugula.

At that infamous age when children decide that they do not like most of the things people place between two slices of bread, their lunch sandwiches rotated between turkey breast, sardines, and peanut butter and jelly. Boring, perhaps, but pleasing to them and certainly adequately nutritious. Each lunch box also contained two pieces of fruit, one of which they could trade for someone else's dessert. And during the years they spurned the more sophisticated foods most grownups like, rather than fight with them or restrict ourselves to "kid food," we prepared a separate boys' meal of foods we knew they would enjoy. I could have sworn our boys were made of pasta, cereal, and peanut butter sandwiches, but they seemed none the worse for it, and we figured that eventually this too would pass.

When beset by the hungries, kids will grab whatever is handy. If what was handy was a big bowl of fresh fruit or a fruit salad, homemade muffins, and quick breads (low in fat and loaded with nutritious ingredients) or cut-up vegetables and dip, that's what the boys ate. Chips, cookies, candy, and pop (or what we New Yorkers call soda) were bought only for special occasions and never kept in the house.

Don't misunderstand. The boys liked sweets as much as any other youngsters. In fact, the first phrase I heard them say was "more cookie." But when they did get cookies, they were served two apiece; the box was never brought to the table, and they soon learned there was no point in begging for more.

A child is likely to be irritable and unable to learn properly on an empty or poorly nourished stomach. As the early riser in our family, I made breakfast for our sons every morning, and I made sure they got up and got dressed in time to eat it before dashing off to school. I was eclectic about the contents of breakfast, alternating between cereal (hot and cold), pancakes and French toast with fruit, homemade pita pizzas, toasted cheese sandwiches, spaghetti pancakes, and sometimes soup or some other leftover from the night before. The "boys" are now nearly 28 years old, and I don't think they have once left the house without eating breakfast.

Their breakfast cereals, primarily Cheerios, Wheaties, and Kix, were garnished with granola and raisins and moistened with milk. I say "breakfast cereals" advisedly, because the classic bowl of cereal also served as a between-meal and bedtime snack once they hit that pubescent growth spurt. To this day, a bowl of cereal is supplemental nutrition as well as breakfast for those two still active young men.

When the boys were small, nothing at all was purchased from a vending machine—we told them it was much too expensive and sometimes you lost your money. Not until they were old enough to realize that some vending machines offered milk or apples and until they were wise enough to make that choice did those machines lose their forbidden status.

When the boys spent the night at someone else's house, they could eat all the sugar-coated cereals they wanted. When we dined out and the grownups drank wine or beer, the boys could order sugar-sweetened soda. But because they were unaccustomed to having it, they were 10 years old before they could finish a whole can.

Once a week, we gave each of the boys money to buy a candy bar. At first, they nursed that candy for hours. Then one day I realized I had not seen them with candy for several weeks. When I asked, they said, "Oh, we found out that the store sells knishes, so we pooled our candy money and shared a knish instead." To say the least, I was impressed, not just about their more nutritious selection but also about the benefits that can accrue from giving children choices instead of dicta.

Likewise with fast food dining. We joined the boys from time to time for a burger and shake at a McDonald's or Burger King, although we—and eventually they—preferred pizza. But when it came to eating out on their own money, they quickly realized that it was a lot cheaper to eat at home or take along a homemade sandwich. Thus, at sporting events they spurned the hot dogs and burgers and instead brought sandwiches and drinks from home, even when they spent the entire day watching tennis at the U.S. Open.

I have told you this tale not to set up our family as a paragon of nutritious dining or to establish our approach as an ideal way to bring up children. Rather, I want to persuade you to share my long-standing belief that children come into the world ready and wanting to be guided, and it is up to their parents and caretakers to do the guiding.

Eat well, and may you all live greatly.

Jane E. Brody

PREFACE
·······

People who choose a career in pediatrics do so because they love taking care of children. *The Yale Guide to Children's Nutrition* grew out of this love and out of concern for children's health and welfare. It represents the combined efforts of many talented people at the Yale–New Haven Children's Hospital, including physicians, dietitians, nurses, and social workers. The Children's Hospital is supported by a dedicated group of concerned people who call themselves the Friends of the Children's Hospital at Yale–New Haven. The mission of this group is to improve the health and well-being of children through advocacy, educational programs, and community outreach. And it was the Friends of the Children's Hospital who suggested the unique idea of writing a guide that would present, in understandable language, up-to-date scientific knowledge about the feeding of children, while featuring recipes for dishes that

would taste good and be healthy at the same time. It's not a coincidence that the group of Friends includes world-renowned chefs, such as Jacques Pépin, and other notables in the fields of food and cooking, such as Charles van Over.

The editors, authors, and chefs have contributed their time and talent to this book for a good cause. All royalties from the sale and promotion of *The Yale Guide to Children's Nutrition* will go to child health programs affiliated with the Yale School of Medicine and the Yale–New Haven Children's Hospital, particularly those programs that help economically disadvantaged populations, and to researching treatments and cures for pediatric diseases. With the purchase of this book you benefit not only the children whose lives you directly touch but also the lives of many other children whose physical and psycho-social health is precarious.

Why produce a guide to children's nutrition? To echo a statement made by Charles Dickens over one hundred years ago, these are the best of times and the worst of times with respect to children's nutrition. Parents' awareness of the importance of good nutrition for the future health of their children has never been greater, and the media regularly issue stories related to eating and health. Unfortunately, these short stories and sound bites are often more confusing than informative. In addition, the tempo and pressures of modern living make it difficult to put sound nutritional principles into practice. Reports suggest that in the United States more meals are eaten outside the home than inside it, and that childhood obesity has reached epidemic proportions. Moreover, children and adolescents are consistently bombarded with advertisements for foods without much nutritional value.

In the creation of this book, we were guided by several overriding principles. One was that there is no such thing as a bad food. Foods that are relatively high in fat, for example, provide a dense source of energy that may be especially useful during periods of rapid growth or intense physical activity. It is the balance of different kinds of food that determines the quality of the diet.

Another guiding principle was that the book had to be comprehensive, addressing all the questions adults and children might have about childhood nutrition. For that reason, the book is divided into six parts. Part I starts with basic information regarding normal growth and development, digestion, and taste. The remaining chapters in this part are devoted to the nutritional needs and behaviors of normal children at various stages of childhood and adolescence. Part II provides practical tips for dealing with some common concerns related to children's eating. Part III is intended for families and friends of children with conditions requiring special nutritional attention. Part IV is designed to clarify nutritional terms and provide a good understanding of basic nutritional concepts. Part V supplies information regarding how to ensure that children eat well in contemporary society. Finally, in part VI, the tastiest part of the book, renowned chefs from all regions of the United States present recipes for healthy foods that children will like to eat.

This book will be at home in many rooms in your house: in the kitchen, to be used during meal preparation; in the family room, to be consulted as needed; or on the night table in the bedroom, to be read at leisure. You can read it from cover to cover or jump from one chapter to another. We anticipate that there may be something in each chapter that will make you take special notice because it clarifies something you've always wondered about. Finally, my hope is that you will receive as much satisfaction from using this book as we received from writing it.

William V. Tamborlane, M.D.
New Haven, Connecticut

ACKNOWLEDGMENTS

· · · · · · ·

We have been extremely fortunate to have worked with more than one hundred enthusiastic professionals during the creation of this unique book for today's families. We are grateful to all of them for making this project so exciting and rewarding. In addition to the authors of the chapters, many people deserve special thanks for their ideas, their patience, and their guidance. Francine Farkas Sears and Charles van Over must be recognized first and foremost for providing the inspiration that led to the concept of a nutrition guide for children. Their dedication to the cause of children's health, and that of their colleagues on the Board of Directors of the Friends of the Children's Hospital at Yale–New Haven, have been the driving force behind *The Yale Guide to Children's Nutrition*. We wish to thank Priscilla Martel, for her wise guidance in formulating the shape of the guide, and Georgette Farkas, for her input. Joseph B. War-shaw, M.D., the Chairman of Pediatrics at the Yale University School of Medicine and an innovative leader and advocate for children, gave us the confidence and free rein to pursue this ambitious project. Vincent S. Conti, Senior Vice President of Administration at Yale–New Haven Hospital, has also played an important role in helping us to produce a "user-friendly" nutrition guide. Michele Fairchild, M.A., R.D., F.A.D.A., former Associate Director of Clinical Nutrition at Yale–New Haven Hospital, was active in the planning phase of the book and contributed to the writing of the text. A special thanks to Robert Baltimore, M.D., for his help during the early stages of the book's development. The James Beard Foundation and its Vice President, Caroline Stuart, identified the wonderful chefs across the United States who enthusiastically donated their talents. Jean Thomson Black, our editor at Yale University Press, championed the project, encouraged us, and steadfastly kept us on task. It was a particular joy to work with our extremely gifted recipe tester, Kathy Farrell Kingsley. Kudos to Nancy Canetti for her lightning-speed typing and patience with our multiple rewrites, and a special thanks to Tracy Sotere for her administrative support throughout. Finally, our most heartfelt thanks go to our spouses, Kathy, Ted, Garth, and Russell, who have provided inspiration and support, and to our children, who remind us daily of the importance of this project.

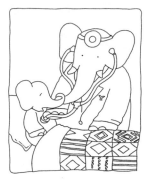

PART ONE

From Infancy to Adolescence:
Developmental Nutrition

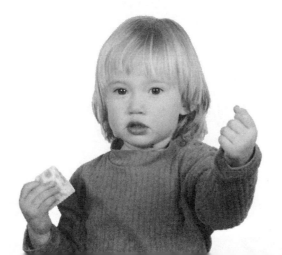

1
· · · · · · · ·

Measuring Up: Normal Growth and Development

Over the course of fifteen to eighteen years, remarkable changes occur in the human body: small, helpless newborn infants are transformed into physically mature young adults. It is particularly important to discuss the normal processes of growth and physical development in children because virtually any disease that a child develops can adversely affect growth and development. Moreover, normal growth and development depend on good nutritional practices, which vary according to the age and developmental stage of the child.

MYTH Coffee will stunt a child's growth.
FACT Although the consumption of coffee is not advisable for children, coffee will not stunt growth. But because caffeine found in coffee may cause irritability and sleeplessness, its use should be limited. Remember that caffeine is found not only in coffee but also in many soft drinks.

· · · · · · · · · · · · · · · · ·

William V. Tamborlane

The term *growth* usually refers to increases in the weight or length of the child as a whole or of a specific body part. *Development,* in contrast, refers to maturational processes that may occur with or without changes in size. The progressive attainment of motor and language skills by an infant or toddler is an example of neurological development, and the changes in body characteristics shown by boys and girls during adolescence are examples of normal pubertal development.

Childhood Growth

In a relative sense, the most dramatic growth in children occurs during the first year or two of life. Most full-term newborn infants weigh between 6 and 10 pounds at birth, and they measure between 18 and 22 inches in length. It takes a few days for the child and mother to establish a good feeding pattern, so it is not uncommon for the baby to lose a few ounces during the first few days of life. But most infants regain their birth weight by 10 days of age, and then their growth rapidly takes off. The healthy infant will usually double his or her birth weight by 4–5 months of age and triple the birth weight by 12 months. The length of the average infant will increase by 50 percent during the first year of life, for example, from 20 to 30 inches. The rate of growth is markedly decreased by the second birthday, but not before the child has picked up an additional 4–5 inches in length and 5–6 pounds in weight. Indeed, average girls reach about half their final adult height by 18 months of age, and boys reach half their adult height by 24 months. The size of the head (usually measured with a measuring tape around the head) also increases by 4–5 inches during the first year, but very little thereafter.

After the first two years of life, the rate of growth settles into a relatively steady pattern averaging about 2½ inches in height (fig. 1.1) and 7 pounds in weight per year during the early school years. Growth speeds up again during adolescence in association with the physical and hormonal changes of puberty. Such hormonal changes then lead to closure of the growth centers in the bones, causing linear growth to stop by 15–16 years of age in girls and 17–18 years in boys. But children whose normal maturational process is delayed may continue to grow beyond these

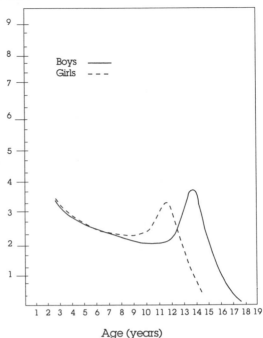

Height increase (in/yr)

FIGURE 1.1
Growth rates of average boys and girls through childhood and adolescence.

ages. Because boys usually start puberty two years later than girls and thus have an extra two years of growth before the start of puberty (at 2½ inches per year), boys end up about 5 inches taller than girls on average.

Childhood Development

The shape and composition of a child's body are also changing during the various phases of childhood growth. Before puberty, these changes are relatively subtle and relate to alterations in the body proportions. Compared with adults, infants have heads that are large in relation to the rest

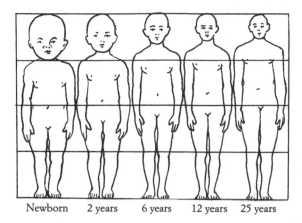

Newborn   2 years   6 years   12 years   25 years

FIGURE 1.2
Changes in body proportions from infancy
to adulthood.

of the body. In addition, the trunk of the infant is longer than the legs. These proportions gradually change throughout childhood, as the length of the legs increases more than the length of the upper body (the trunk and head). At birth the head is about one-quarter the total body length, but it is only one-eighth the body length by the time growth is completed (fig. 1.2). A number of conditions and diseases can interfere with the normal changes in body proportions, so these simple measurements can provide the first clue to a possible problem.

More dramatic changes in physical development occur once boys and girls enter puberty. On average, girls show the first signs of puberty at 10½ years of age, whereas puberty begins in boys at 12½ years. But normal pubertal development in both girls and boys can begin as much as two years earlier or later than these averages. The physical changes that occur during puberty are referred to as the development of secondary sexual characteristics. In this phase the ovaries and testes mature, and the hormones produced by these glands are

responsible for the physical transformation from child to adult.

The first sign of puberty in girls is the beginning of breast development due to increased secretion by the ovaries of the hormone known as estrogen. The small buds of tissue develop into fully mature breasts over the next three to four years. Girls usually begin having their periods about halfway through this process, between 12½ and 13 years of age, but starting two years earlier or later is still normal.

In boys, enlargement of the testes marks the beginning of puberty, and increased secretion of the hormone testosterone by the maturing testes is primarily responsible for the rest of the visible changes. Darker and thicker hair growing around the base of the penis (pubic hair) is usually the first of these changes, followed by the growth of the hair in the armpits (axillary hair) and then facial hair. Boys' voices do not change completely until the end of puberty, three to four years after the first changes occur.

The adrenal glands in girls secrete less-powerful kinds of testosterone-like hormones (also known as androgens), and it is these hormones that are responsible for pubic and axillary hair development in girls. Indeed, in some girls, the appearance of pubic hair precedes breast development. Analogously, boys produce a small amount of estrogen, and this commonly leads to some breast enlargement, especially during early puberty. This breast enlargement usually disappears later in puberty once the testes start producing larger amounts of testosterone, which counteracts the effects of estrogen.

Girls and boys differ with respect to the changes in body composition (the proportion of fat and muscle tissue) that occur during puberty. The total body fat of girls increases from about 15

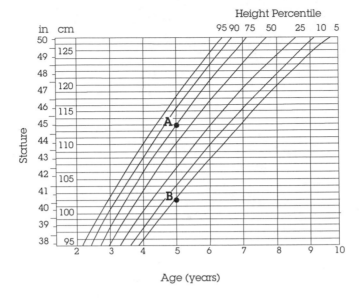

FIGURE 1.3
A growth chart showing the height percentiles in two
normal 5-year-old boys.

percent before puberty to approximately 20–25 percent by the end of puberty. In contrast, boys become more muscular rather than fatter during normal adolescent development.

Assessing Growth in Children

Many factors influence the final height that a person will achieve, and predicting this value in any given child is difficult. The most important factor is usually the heights of the parents: tall parents tend to have tall children, and short parents tend to have short children. It's fairly easy to calculate the height pattern of a family based on the heights of the parents. Add the height of the mother and father (in inches) and divide by two, to find the average height of the parents. Then, if the child is a boy, add 2½ inches; if the child is a girl, subtract 2½ inches. If, for example, the father is 72 inches

tall (6 feet) and the mother is 63 inches (5 feet, 3 inches), their average height is 67½ inches. We would expect boys in this family to end up about 70 inches tall (67½ + 2½ inches), whereas girls should be about 65 inches (67½ − 2½ inches). Men tend to think they're an inch or so taller than they really are, so it's important to make sure that the parents' heights are measured accurately.

Such calculations are just rough estimates. Many other things, including nutritional, metabolic, and hormonal factors, influence whether a person's final height exceeds or falls short of the family pattern. When a child's growth is lagging well behind the family pattern, there may be a physical problem.

One of the first things doctors do during well-baby and well-child checkups is to measure height and weight. This is important because many chronic illnesses and nutritional problems impair

DEVELOPMENTAL NUTRITION

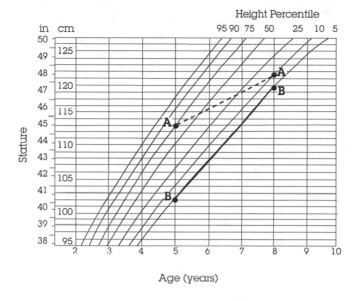

Height Percentile

FIGURE 1.4
Follow-up measurements after three years in the two
boys whose heights are shown in fig. 1.3.

growth. Children should be weighed and measured at least every six months up to 3 years of age and then yearly thereafter. Measurements of the baby's head circumference are especially important during the first two years of life.

The child's health care provider marks each measurement of height and weight on a growth chart (see growth charts appendix). The growth chart is a graph that plots the child's height and weight (the vertical axis) in relation to age (the horizontal axis). The lines that are predrawn on the chart represent the range of heights and weights for normal children of the same age (broken into percentiles); there are separate charts for boys and girls. The heights of two 5-year-old boys are marked in fig. 1.3. Boy A, who is 44 inches tall, falls on the 75th percentile, meaning that 75 percent of boys his age are shorter than he, whereas Boy B, who is 40 inches tall, falls on the 5th per-

centile, meaning that 95 percent of boys his age are taller than he. If only these measurements are taken into account, a doctor is more likely to be concerned about Boy B than Boy A, even though both heights are in the normal range.

Sequential measurements that are plotted on the growth chart over time are more important than any single measurement, because they provide an index of the rate of growth. Because most healthy children maintain a steady rate of growth throughout childhood, their growth chart tends to run on or parallel to one of the percentile lines. Children whose height percentiles progressively decrease are more likely to have a problem. Let's revisit our two boys three years after their first measurements (fig. 1.4). Although Boy B started out shorter, he has grown at a normal rate, maintaining his height at the 5th percentile. In contrast, Boy A's rate of growth has slowed down markedly.

Even though Boy A is still taller than Boy B, Boy A is more likely to have a serious problem.

The relative increases in height and weight can also vary in individual children. In an obese child, for example, the increase in weight exceeds that which would be expected from the normal increase in height (see chapters 12 and 18). In children who have digestive problems or acute nutritional deficiencies, the rate of weight gain decreases before height is affected. Conversely, a falloff in a child's height increase in the face of continued weight gain is suggestive of certain endocrine problems, such as an underactive thyroid. Children with genetic disorders commonly have low birth weights and slow growth in height and weight.

A normal growth chart is reassuring regarding the overall nutritional health of the child. Parents often question whether their child is eating enough or too much. If the child is showing a normal and appropriate gain in height and weight, then the child is eating the right amount of food to support day-to-day energy requirements and to promote normal growth.

Resources

Human Growth Foundation, 7777 Leesburg Pike, P.O. Box 3090, Falls Church, VA 22043. (703) 883-1773.

Phifer, K. *Growing Up Small: A Handbook for Short People.* Middlebury, VT: Paul Eriksson, 1979.

Tanner, J. *Fetus into Man: Physical Growth from Conception to Maturity.* Cambridge: Harvard University Press, 1978.

2

. . . .

The Digestive Process: What Happens after You Swallow?

Food provides the body with all the fuel, nutrients, and raw materials it needs for growth, physical activity, maintenance of tissues, metabolic processes, and fights against infections. But if food is to be of any value to the body, it must first be transformed, mechanically and chemically, by the process of digestion, as the food is propelled along the gastrointestinal (GI) tract. Food must then be transported from the intestine, or bowel, to the bloodstream by the process of absorption. Most nutrients in undigested food, however, are bound in large molecules that are too

MYTH Protein and carbohydrates should not be eaten together, because they can't be digested together.

FACT Foods that are eaten together begin the process of digestion at the same time, so separating foods is unnecessary. In fact, to achieve a balanced diet it is preferable to eat a combination of foods at each meal.

big to pass through the lining of the intestine into the bloodstream. It is the responsibility of the GI tract to break down these large food molecules into smaller nutrient units, which are then readily absorbed. Once nutrients are in the bloodstream, they are delivered to tissues all over the body, where their tasks are finally performed. At the same time, indigestible and nonabsorbable portions of food must be prepared for elimination from the body. The processing of food depends on effective movement, or motility, of the GI tract, and on the presence of various diges-

. . . .

M. Susan Moyer ■ Lisa Devine

tive enzymes and transport systems within the intestine. Thus, in order to nourish the body, the GI tract accomplishes a complicated task that begins with receiving, chopping, and chewing food; lubricating and swallowing it; pushing, churning, and squeezing it; mixing, secreting, absorbing, transporting, and storing it; and finally eliminating the leftovers.

The Anatomy of the Gastrointestinal Tract

In order to understand what happens to food after it is swallowed, it is important to be familiar with the specific structures of the GI tract (fig. 2.1). The GI tract itself is basically a long muscular tube extending from the mouth to the anus. Each segment of the tube has unique anatomic characteristics and performs specialized functions. Accessory organs—the salivary glands, pancreas, liver, and gallbladder—contribute to the digestive process, largely by production of digestive juices and their secretion into the intestine. Finally, nerves, hormones, and blood flow play important roles in regulating the function and maintaining the integrity of the GI tract.

The mouth is the doorway to the digestive tract. The first steps in the digestive process are chewing and swallowing. Saliva, secreted by the salivary glands located below and behind the tongue, lubricates and softens food. In addition, salivary secretions contain an enzyme that begins to digest starches. Food accumulates in the back of the mouth as a mass, or bolus, and is then swallowed. This food bolus passes from the mouth to the stomach by way of the esophagus. The lower esophageal sphincter (LES) is a muscular, ring-like structure at the end of the esophagus that relaxes to allow food to pass from the esophagus to the stomach. No digestive processes occur in the

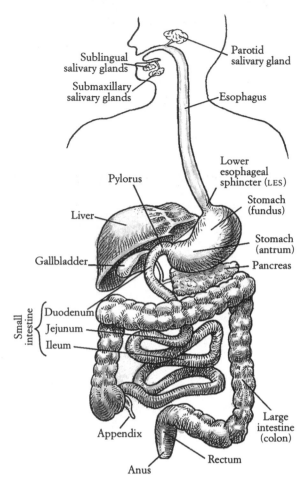

FIGURE 2.1
The anatomy of the GI tract.

esophagus because the food moves quickly from the mouth to the stomach.

The stomach is a pouch-like structure that serves several purposes. First, food is stored temporarily in the upper portion, or fundus, of the stomach. Because of this storage capacity, adults need to eat only two to four times a day. Infants and children have a smaller storage capacity and require refueling of their stomachs more frequently. The lower portion of the stomach, the antrum, is involved in both mechanical and chemical digestion. In the antrum, the food bolus is churned and mixed with potent gastric juices. These gastric secretions are produced by the cells lining the stomach and consist of strong acids and enzymes necessary for breaking down or digesting large carbohydrate and protein molecules. The stomach also produces a mucous layer that protects its lining from these acid and enzymatic secretions. During digestion, the food bolus becomes a semi-liquid, which then passes from the stomach into the small intestine through another muscular "gate" called the pylorus.

The small intestine is responsible for most digestion and absorption. It is called the "small" intestine because its diameter is smaller than the next part of the GI tract, which is called the large intestine. Although its diameter is smaller, the small intestine is much longer than the large intestine. In the adult, the small intestine measures about 22 feet and is miraculously coiled to fit within the abdominal cavity. For comparison, the large intestine is only 4–6 feet long. To approximate the length of the small intestine in children, multiply their height by 3.5. The small intestine consists of three segments: the duodenum, the jejunum, and the ileum. The duodenum comprises approximately the first foot of intestine, and it is here that the digestive process is at its peak. Enzymes that are present on the surface cells of the intestinal lining break down nutrients in preparation for absorption. In addition, the pancreas, liver, and gallbladder deliver crucial digestive enzymes to the small intestine. The pancreas sits behind the stomach. It manufactures several enzymes and usually has one main duct to carry its secretions to the duodenum. The liver, located in the upper right part of the abdomen, is one of the largest and busiest organs of the body. Its role in digestion is to produce bile, which assists in the absorption of fats. Bile flows through ducts to the gallbladder, where it is stored. As food passes

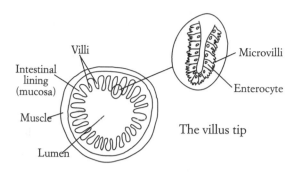

FIGURE 2.2
The anatomy of the small intestine
(cross section).

through the stomach, the gallbladder contracts, and bile is released through the common bile duct into the duodenum. The liver has many additional roles in the handling of nutrients, including control of glucose and cholesterol metabolism, protein synthesis, and regulation of nutrient delivery to the rest of the body.

The jejunum and ileum comprise most of the small intestine. Although digestion continues in the jejunum and ileum, their primary function is absorption of the products of digestion. The inner lining of the small intestine is particularly suited to this role (fig. 2.2). It is folded into millions of tiny finger-like projections called villi. These villi, which line all three segments of the small intestine, increase its surface area and thus its absorptive capacity tremendously. In addition, digestive enzymes, and transport systems for digested nutrients, are found along the villus surface. By the time food has reached the end of the small intestine, almost all of its nutrients have been absorbed.

The final portion of the gastrointestinal tract is the large intestine, or colon. The colon is not only responsible for the absorption of a significant amount of water and electrolytes (sodium, potassium, chloride, and bicarbonate) but also performs the task of collecting, processing, storing, and removing waste. This waste, which enters the colon in a semi-liquid form, consists mainly of undigested food and such nonabsorbable residues as plant fibers. As the waste traverses the colon, water is absorbed and more solid stool, or feces, is formed. Once this solid waste reaches the last part of the colon, the rectum, it is stored before voluntary elimination.

The Motility of the Gastrointestinal Tract

The entire GI tract has powerful muscles within its walls that work to keep food moving in the right direction. These muscles exert strong wave-like contractions, called peristalsis, to propel food down the long muscular tube. Small "housekeeping" waves constantly move fluid secretions and gas along the intestine. In addition, stronger contractions—stimulated by hormones, nerves, or the presence of food in the GI tract—aid in mechanically breaking down a food bolus and propelling the food from one portion of the intestine to the next.

Swallowing is the first major muscle movement in digestion. People swallow voluntarily, but thereafter food is moved along by the involuntary muscles under control of the nervous system. The musculature of the esophagus is so strong that you could eat a meal while standing on your head and food would still be propelled against gravity into the stomach. The lower esophageal sphincter, between the esophagus and stomach, functions as a valve. This ring-like muscle, usually tightly closed to keep stomach acid out of the esophagus, relaxes when a food bolus approaches to allow passage into the stomach. It then closes to prevent the food from coming back into the esophagus. If the LES does not function well, food and stomach acid can regurgitate into the esophagus (this regurgitation is known as gastroesophageal reflux) and cause irritation, or heartburn. At the other end of the stomach, the second muscular gate, the pylorus, keeps food and stomach juices trapped in the stomach for a period of time during digestion.

The stomach performs three mechanical tasks. First, the fundus relaxes to accept and store foods and fluids that have been swallowed. Then, in the antrum, food is mixed with gastric juices by muscular contractions. Finally, the stomach contents are slowly emptied into the small intestine through the pylorus. The stomach empties in one to four hours, depending on several factors, including the nature of the food ingested and the effectiveness of the lower-stomach contractions. Carbohydrates leave the stomach most rapidly, followed by protein and then fat. A stomach that empties too slowly can cause feelings of fullness, or early satiety, and can increase the likelihood of gastroesophageal reflux. If, in contrast, the stomach empties too rapidly into the duodenum, such symptoms as pain, diarrhea, sweating, and light-headedness can occur; this is called dumping syndrome. Infants in the newborn period, and to varying degrees during the first year of life, tend to have relatively slow gastric emptying and relatively relaxed tone in the LES owing to immature function of these muscles. This predisposes infants to gastroesophageal reflux and vomiting during their early development (see chapter 23). In most cases, this reflux is considered normal; it reflects immaturity rather than an underlying physical or functional abnormality. Such simple maneuvers as small, frequent feedings and upright positioning can be helpful for a baby with excessive reflux.

After food enters the duodenum, it is mixed and churned with digestive secretions from the pancreas, liver, and intestine and then pushed forward to allow further digestion and absorption

TABLE 2.1
Digestive Enzymes

Nutrient	Enzyme	Source
Carbohydrates	Amylase	Salivary glands, pancreas
	Sucrase-isomaltase	Small intestine
	Maltase-glucoamylase	Small intestine
	Lactase-phlorizin hydrolase	Small intestine
Protein	Pepsin	Stomach
	Trypsin	Pancreas
	Chymotrypsin	Pancreas
	Peptidases	Pancreas, small intestine
	Peptide hydrolases	Small intestine
Fats	Lipase	Mouth, stomach, pancreas

along the length of the small intestine until the remaining undigested food is deposited in the colon. Peristaltic waves move this waste material forward through the colon to the rectum, a journey that takes approximately one to two days in teenagers and adults. Once stool reaches the rectum, it may be stored for a considerable period of time prior to elimination. As the muscular wall of the rectum is stretched by the accumulation of stool, nerve impulses stimulate relaxation of the innermost muscle of the anus, the internal anal sphincter. Fullness of the rectum automatically triggers the desire to evacuate the stool, but defecation does not occur until the external anal sphincter is voluntarily relaxed. If the urge to have a bowel movement is ignored, it will eventually subside and not return until more stool accumulates in the rectum. Infants and toddlers lack voluntary control and therefore deposit stools in diapers. Toilet training requires that children become aware of their ability to control their bowels. This ability, however, can also lead to voluntary stool withholding and constipation. In general, normal patterns of defecation may vary from several bowel movements a day to one bowel movement a week.

The Digestion and Absorption of Nutrients

Foods must be broken down mechanically and chemically before they can be absorbed. Digestion begins as soon as a person sees, smells, or even thinks or hears about food. How does this happen? As the brain anticipates eating, it sends messages to the digestive tract to start saliva and enzymes flowing in preparation for the incoming food. That's why your mouth waters when you smell or think about food. Enzymes are the workhorses of digestion. They are proteins capable of inducing chemical change in other substances without being changed themselves. Specific enzymes for the digestion of carbohydrates, proteins, and fats are found in various parts of the GI tract (table 2.1). Enzymes split large nutrient molecules into smaller nutrient molecules, which can then be absorbed through the cells lining the intestine and, from there, can travel through the bloodstream to other parts of the body.

CARBOHYDRATES Starches and sugars are carbohydrates that the body can digest, whereas fiber is not digested. In the mouth, salivary amylase is the first digestive enzyme encountered. This enzyme starts the process of carbohydrate digestion. In the duodenum, intestinal enzymes and pancreatic enzymes further process these carbohydrates into smaller molecules. In the final step of carbohydrate digestion, enzymes break down disaccharides (carbohydrates containing two sugar molecules) into simple one-sugar molecules (monosaccharides): glucose, fructose, and galactose (see chapter 29). Only these three simple sugars can be absorbed through the intestinal cells. They are then carried in the bloodstream directly to the liver, where fructose and galactose are converted to glucose, the only simple sugar that can be used by the cells of the body. The liver regulates how much glucose is stored (as glycogen) and how much is sent to other tissues as an energy source for normal cell function.

Deficiencies of the intestinal enzymes that break down sugar result in sugar intolerance and clinical symptoms (see chapter 23). A deficiency in lactase activity (the enzyme that breaks down milk sugar) is relatively common. This deficiency may be the result of a normal decline in enzymatic activity with age, or damage to the lining of the small intestine may cause temporary loss of the enzyme until the bowel recovers. If the amount of lactase is not sufficient to handle the amount of milk sugar ingested, this undigested lactose will travel through the small intestine to the colon, drawing water along with it. Bacteria that are normally present in the colon break down the lactose, producing gas and acidic by-products and resulting in the classic symptoms of lactose intolerance: bloating, gas, pain, and acidy diarrhea.

PROTEINS Proteins are made up of individual amino acids linked together. Just as complex carbohydrates must be broken down into simple sugars, large protein molecules must also be digested before they can be absorbed and used by the body (see chapter 28). Protein digestion begins in the stomach, where the enzyme pepsin breaks down long protein molecules into shorter strings of amino acids called polypeptides. Pepsin needs an extremely acidic environment in order to work, and the stomach provides ideal conditions. As polypeptides reach the duodenum, they are attacked by several intestinal and pancreatic enzymes, which continue protein digestion until either individual amino acids or very small peptides are formed. Intestinal cells are capable of directly absorbing either dipeptides (peptides containing two amino acids) or tripeptides (those containing three amino acids) as well as individual amino acids. Absorption of protein thus differs from that of carbohydrates, which requires sugars to be in their simplest form before they can be taken up by the intestinal cells. Once absorbed, the di- and tripeptides are split into amino acids by peptide hydrolases inside cells. The amino acids then travel to the liver, where they are synthesized into new proteins or released into the circulation to go where they are needed.

FATS The digestion and absorption of fats, or lipids, are more complicated processes than the digestion and absorption of carbohydrates or proteins because fat does not dissolve in water. The digestive tract therefore uses its accessory organs to facilitate the process. Although fat-digesting enzymes (lipases) are present in the mouth and stomach, pancreatic lipase is responsible for breaking down most large fat globules into smaller components in the small intestine. Bile, secreted from the gallbladder, acts as an emulsifier to form water-soluble complexes with the products of fat digestion. These complexes are called micelles. Micelles travel to the villi of the intestine, where they break apart and allow the fat component to enter the intestinal cells. The bile is left behind to form more micelles. When no more fat is present, components of the bile are reabsorbed in the ileum and recycled back to the liver to be used again. Smaller fats can be absorbed intact in the intestine.

VITAMINS Vitamins are generally absorbed unchanged in the small intestine and do not require digestion. They are divided into two classes based on their solubility in water or fat. Water-soluble vitamins include B vitamins and vitamin C. The fat-soluble vitamins are A, D, E, and K. Poor absorption of fat, which occurs if, for example, secretion of bile or pancreatic enzymes is insufficient, may result in deficiency of the fat-soluble vitamins.

WATER AND SALT Water and salt come from the food and liquids people ingest and from the secretions in the GI tract. Water and dissolved salt move across the lining of the small intestine with other nutrients that are being absorbed. In addition, the colon has a remarkable capacity for absorbing water. If the lining of the intestine is damaged, decreasing the absorptive surface area, or if the bowel is moving too quickly, water and salts cannot be efficiently absorbed. Diarrhea and dehydration may result.

This description of the fantastic voyage of food and nutrients through the digestive tract is now complete. Armed with a knowledge of the digestive process, parents can set the stage for good nutritional habits in their children.

Resources

Clayman, C. B. *The American Medical Association Encyclopedia of Medicine.* New York: Random House, 1989.

Gordon, J. *Digestion: Fueling the System.* New York: Torstar Books, 1984.

3
. . . .

Taste, Smell, and Food Preferences

Parents hope their children will have a positive attitude toward eating and will like foods that are healthy. They may wonder why their children like some foods and not others. Children are born liking sweets and disliking bitter tastes. The ability to taste sweetness and bitterness varies genetically, so this may explain some differences in food preferences among children. Learning also plays a large role. Children develop food preferences through positive and negative interactions with their environment. A positive interaction could be regular, relaxed family meals, while negative experiences could include the use of food as a reward or the enforcement of an overly restricted diet. These innate and learned factors blend into a unique template of food preferences that continues to evolve throughout life.

MYTH Newborns like salty food.

FACT The only taste that infants inherently like is sweet. The taste for salt does not develop until several months of age, so newborn infants neither like nor dislike salty foods.

The Role of the Senses in Perception of Food

Food preferences depend on many things, including the flavor of a food, the time of the day, whether one is hungry, and one's mood. Sensory factors—the appearance, the taste, the feel, and even the sound of food in the mouth—also influence whether foods are enjoyable.

Advertisers, food companies, and restaurateurs

. . . .

Valerie B. Duffy ▪ Linda M. Bartoshuk

capitalize on visual characteristics to entice the consumer to purchase certain foods. Looking at attractive food—on a dessert cart at a restaurant, for example—may stimulate people to eat even if they are not hungry. Color can also influence feelings about foods and ability to identify a food. The flavor of oranges, for example, is associated, through learning, with the color orange. If a food is colored orange but flavored with grape, the person will be more likely to identify the food as orange than as grape. Color is also an important determinant of food acceptability. Scrambled eggs are generally yellow, and ham is pink; other colors would make the food seem unappetizing. But children who have read the Dr. Seuss story may be willing to eat green eggs and ham.

The sense of smell serves a dual purpose in how food is perceived (fig. 3.1). By normal breathing and sniffing, odors are taken through the nostrils to the olfactory (smell) neurons at the top of the nasal cavity (behind the bridge of the nose). This is known as orthonasal olfaction. Odors also reach the olfactory receptors from the mouth. Tongue and mouth movements of chewing release the olfactory components of the food and pump them to the olfactory area. This process is known as retronasal olfaction.

Flavor is the combination of retronasal olfaction and true taste. People actually identify foods by retronasal olfaction. The only way to tell root beer from grape soda, for example, is via retronasal olfaction. True taste is the ability to perceive saltiness, sweetness, sourness, and bitterness. You can learn the difference between true taste and smell with a simple experiment. Taste a Lifesaver with eyes closed and nose plugged. It will taste sweet. Then unplug your nose and taste again. You will be able to experience the addition of retronasal olfaction to the sweetness and will thus be able to identify the Lifesaver's flavor. Correct

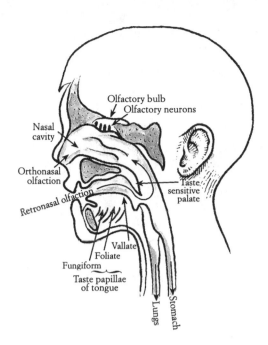

FIGURE 3.1
The paths that odors take in orthonasal and retronasal olfaction.

identification of a smell or flavor, however, depends on more than a functioning sense of smell. It requires the retrieval of the odor name from memory. Even adults with a full range of experiences correctly identify an odor stimulus only about 70 percent of the time.

Infants are born with the ability to perceive sweetness, sourness, and bitterness. The ability to taste salt develops during the first months of life. Pleasurable and displeasurable responses to sweetness, sourness, or bitterness are present at birth and possibly before birth. Babies given sucrose (table sugar), for example, produced what was characterized as a smile-like expression followed by lip smacks and sounds of sucking. In contrast, infants given a bitter substance produced facial expressions suggesting dislike, including a downward arched upper lip, tongue protrusion, and spitting. When given a sour substance, infants puckered their lips, wrinkled their noses, and blinked frequently, much as adults do when thinking about biting into a lemon. Newborn infants neither like nor dislike salty solutions, probably because they are unable to taste salt at birth. By the age of 5 months, infants show a stronger preference for salty water than for plain water.

The ability to smell almost certainly exists prior to birth. The developing fetus may use the olfactory system to detect sensory changes in amniotic fluid that occur with variation of the mother's diet. After birth, the newborn infant may use the sense of smell to differentiate his or her mother's odor from the odor of another female. During breast-feeding, the infant has direct contact with the breast and can learn to recognize its odor. Bottle-fed infants, in contrast, do not develop the ability to recognize the mother's breast.

People have no innate liking or disliking for odors and olfactory flavors. Preferences for odors are acquired through learning. Certain odors seem pleasant because they are associated with such pleasant things as home and family. Likewise, certain odors can become disliked when associated with such unpleasant experiences as illness.

Certain illnesses may modulate the ability to taste or smell and thus influence the sensory quality of foods. The common cold and allergies can cause nasal congestion that can block access of odor molecules to olfactory receptors (see fig. 3.1) and thus impair the ability to perceive the flavor of food. Chronic stuffiness may require evaluation by an ear, nose, and throat specialist to rule out nasal-sinus disease, which is one of the primary causes of loss of olfactory perception.

Otitis media (middle ear infection) may influence the ability to taste. When the middle ear is infected, the nerve that travels from the tongue through the middle ear to the brain can be damaged. Individuals with damage to this nerve have reduced ability to taste from the front of the tongue on the side of the damage. They usually are unaware of any taste loss, however. Other nerves that go to the back of the tongue and throat appear to make up for the loss of perception on the front of the tongue. This maintains taste perception in the whole mouth. But the compensation from the back of the tongue may be too much, especially in response to bitterness. Thus, children who suffer from chronic otitis media may experience enhanced bitterness in some foods and may enjoy them less.

The texture of a food is primarily registered through feeling sensations on the tongue and in the mouth and through hearing the crunch and chewing of the food. Such textural descriptions as creamy, lumpy, smooth, and crisp can help a child identify and compare foods. Texture is the primary cue for fat in food, so fat substitutes and replacements try to mimic the textural properties of fat. Irritation and temperature also contribute to the experience of eating by stimulating receptors in the mouth and nose. Mint, for example, produces a cool feeling in the nasal cavity, and such spices as black pepper, red pepper, ginger, and horseradish produce irritating sensations in the mouth. Many find these sensations enjoyable. Some individuals may experience more irritation than others for genetic reasons.

How to Regulate Food Intake

Scientists who study eating once believed that humans possess the innate ability to regulate all nutrients. According to this "wisdom of the body" theory, if people became depleted of a particular nutrient, their desire to eat foods containing that nutrient would increase. In the 1920s this theory was tested by studying feeding behaviors in infants who had been exclusively breastfed and who were newly weaned. In the experiment, infants were allowed to select foods freely. They were assisted only if food was beyond reach. According to measures of growth, visual assessments of health and energy, and blood and urine tests, the self-selection diet appeared safe, did not cause any digestive problems, and produced the same growth, bone development, vigor, and appearance of health as diets commonly prescribed for infants. It was concluded that young children, without adult direction, could choose the kinds and amounts of "natural foodstuffs" to eat in order to support growth and health.

This pioneering work led nutrition researchers to believe in an instinctive ability of humans to select and consume a healthy diet. But the infants in the study could not fail to select a healthy diet because they were offered only highly nutritious and unsweetened foods. Would the infants have made healthy choices if highly sweetened foods with a low density of nutrients, which are available in grocery stores today, had been offered to them? We now know that most children can maintain a consistent daily caloric intake even though they may vary their intake in successive meals. But external control of feeding can override any innate ability to regulate caloric intake. Mothers who strictly control their children's food intake may have preschool children who are less able to self-regulate their caloric intake.

The sensory characteristics of food may help a child choose a varied diet. During a meal, one's enjoyment of a particular food decreases as it is eaten, whereas the desire for other items increases or does not change. This phenomenon is referred to as sensory-specific satiety. The perfect example of sensory-specific satiety occurs after a complete meal. A person may feel full, but when the dessert cart rolls by, the person feels the desire to eat something sweet. This occurs because the main meal is not sweet.

Sensory-specific satiety also explains several other behaviors. People tend to overeat at a smorgasbord, for example, because this meal offers a large diversity of foods. The opposite example is the monotonous diet that promotes weight loss. Eating the same food over and over satiates a specific sensory quality and may lead to consumption of fewer calories. But the influence of sensory-specific satiety may work only within a single meal and probably does not work to prevent "food jags," or the repeated selection and ingestion of one food, which are often seen in toddlers. (Food jags can be associated with the unwillingness to consume new or unknown foods.) And sensory-specific satiety does not guarantee the quality of the diet—the adequacy of vitamin and mineral intake. A diet may include sensory variety but inadequate nutrient variety.

HUNGERS FOR SUGAR AND SALT The sense of taste provides some guidance in the selection of a healthy diet. When needed, sugar and salt become more pleasant to taste. The body must maintain a normal blood-sugar level to supply the brain with fuel to function. The preference for sweetness can help meet this requirement. Sugar may also trigger the body to produce feel-good chemical messengers called endogenous opiates. Infants who received a concentrated sucrose solution by pacifier before a routine blood test in the doctor's office cried significantly less in response to blood drawing than those given only a pacifier.

The preference for salt (sodium chloride) is also related to bodily need (see chapter 33). Sodium helps the body maintain fluid status and a proper acid-base balance, and aids in the transmission of nerve and muscle impulses. The required intake of sodium for adults (500 milligrams per day) is normally easily met, as sodium is abundant in the food supply, especially in processed foods. But certain medical conditions can lead to serious losses in sodium. A dramatic example was described in the *Journal of the American Medical Association* in 1940. A 3½-year-old boy had been sickly since birth and showed a strong craving for salt that his parents allowed him to indulge. During a hospital stay when he had no access to salt, he died. His doctors discovered that he had suffered from a tumor on his adrenal gland that prevented his body from retaining the salt that he needed to live. His craving for salt had kept him alive. This tragedy had a profound impact on the belief that some cravings are a reflection of biological need.

A less dramatic but nonetheless important example of salt regulation is that of physical exercise, which makes the body lose water and become thirsty. Water is then drunk in response to thirst. The body may also crave salt after exercise. Ingestion of salt again increases thirst, which triggers more fluid intake. The combination of fluid and salt ingestion helps to reestablish hydration after physical exertion and fluid loss. During pregnancy, the craving for sodium may increase. A higher dietary intake of sodium may help to increase the mother's blood volume in order to supply the growing baby with nutrients and oxygen. A specific hunger for salt is biologically wise when the body needs salt, but the more common problem of overconsumption of salt is not wise. Excessive salt intake in susceptible individuals can increase the risk of hypertension.

GENETIC TASTE DIFFERENCES The dislike of bitterness is another example of wisdom of the body, as poisons are often bitter in taste. But a taste for mildly bitter foods can be acquired when the taste is associated with positive consequences. Coffee, for example, is a bitter liquid that many people like because caffeine is a stimulant and because positive social rewards often accompany the sharing of a cup of coffee with a companion.

Humans perceive bitterness differently based on genetic taste differences. The genetic variation in the ability to taste a group of bitter compounds was discovered accidentally by a chemist named A. L. Fox in the 1930s. Fox was synthesizing a compound called phenylthiocarbimide (PTC). Some of it spilled and blew into the air. A colleague tasted bitterness in the air, yet Fox tasted nothing. This observation led geneticists to discover that the ability to taste PTC was genetically determined. Through sophisticated laboratory taste testing, different categories of tasters (nontasters, medium tasters, and supertasters) can be identified. This genetic taste variation is associated with the anatomy of the tongue. The front of the tongue is covered with tiny bumps, or papillae. One kind of these bumps (filiform papillae) is not responsive to tastes. But the larger papillae (fungiform papillae) contain taste buds. Supertasters have more fungiform papillae than nontasters (fig. 3.2). Blue food coloring can help distinguish between fungiform and filiform papillae. The fungiform papillae do not stain as well as the filiform papillae, so they look like pinkish circles against a blue background.

In the laboratory, taste buds can be visualized by staining the tongue with blue food coloring and viewing the tongue under a microscope. Taste buds are buried in the tissue of the fungiform papillae. Taste substances get to the taste buds through a conduit called a taste pore. Blue food coloring stains the taste pores blue. Thus, under a microscope, the taste pores look like dots against

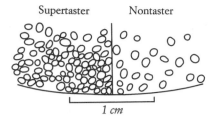

FIGURE 3.2
Density of fungiform papillae on
the tip of the tongue.

the unstained fungiform papillae. In size, the taste pores are to the fungiform as a sesame seed is to a hamburger bun. The number of taste buds can range from as few as 11 per square centimeter in a nontaster to 1,100 per square centimeter in a supertaster.

Differences in tongue anatomy can be demonstrated with a simple test. First, take a piece of wax paper and cut it into 1-inch squares. Using a hole punch, make a hole in the middle of each square. Place a square with a hole on the top of the tongue and paint the hole with blue food coloring. Remove the wax paper and examine the blue circle under a magnifying glass with a flashlight. Count the number of pinkish circles. A nontaster can have less than 20 papillae in the colored area, and the papillae are easily counted. The supertaster typically has three times the number of papillae as a nontaster (60 or more) in the circle. In fact, the papillae in the supertaster are often so tightly packed in the circle that they are difficult to count.

Women are more likely than men to be supertasters. It is not known whether this sex difference exists at birth or if it occurs with maturation. The perception of bitterness is heightened in the first trimester of pregnancy, and taste perception may also vary across the menstrual cycle. It would make evolutionary sense if women became super bitter detectors to protect against ingesting bitter poison, especially during pregnancy. Therefore,

sex hormones are being studied to see if they may play some role in regulating taste perception.

The ability to taste sweetness also varies genetically. Supertasters perceive table sugar (sucrose) and fruit sugar (fructose) as more intense than nontasters. The preference for these sweeteners or sweet foods depends on both genetic taste status and sex. Female supertasters report a "take it or leave it" approach to sweets, whereas female nontasters really love sweet foods. Males seem to like sweets especially if they are supertasters, but female supertasters may find typical desserts too sweet.

Supertasters report more bitterness than nontasters in quinine (found in such substances as tonic water) and calcium chloride (found in milk products, for example). Many green vegetables (especially vegetables from the cabbage family) contain compounds that are more bitter to supertasters than to nontasters. These vegetables are of considerable importance because they are rich in antioxidants, nutrients that may protect the body against chronic diseases. Nutritionists originally thought that the inherent ability of supertasters to taste bitterness might predict a dislike for these vegetables; however, preliminary data do not support this conclusion. In fact, supertasters report higher preferences than nontasters for many vegetables in the cabbage family. Supertasters may experience more intense sweetness as well as bitterness in these vegetables. In addition, such condiments as salt, lemon, or vinegar may blend with the bitterness enough to increase the palatability of the vegetables.

Supertasters perceive more intense burn than nontasters from such oral irritants as black pepper, ginger, chili pepper, and alcohol. This heightened burn sensation is probably due to high numbers of pain fibers on the tongue tip. Taste buds on the tongue tip contain nerve cells for pain as well

Developing Taste in Children: A Culinary Expert's Perspective

I have been in the restaurant and food business for many years, and mothers frequently ask me how to develop taste in their children. A child's earliest tastes are experienced at home, so the development of a taste for nutritious and healthy foods also begins at home. During infancy, and perhaps at no other time in a child's life, parents have the child's full attention. Therefore, infancy is the perfect time to begin introducing a child to nutritious foods.

The premise of the cookbook *Cook Like a Peasant, Live Like a King,* by Jack Denton Scott, is that foods are best when they are simple and flavorful, fresh and seasonal. The peasants of yesteryear ate a healthy diet because, by default, they ate only fresh and seasonal food, as they were unable to obtain foods that were not in season. In the 1990s, most fruits and vegetables are available throughout the year, so the seasonality of fruits and vegetables has, to a large extent, been eliminated. Also, frozen and canned fruits and vegetables are nutritious, when they are included as part of a healthy and varied diet.

Single-parent families, and families with two working parents, are fast outnumbering the traditional two-parent, one-income family. Consequently, people are spending increasingly less time on food preparation. Therefore, although it could be argued that fresh and home-prepared foods are superior to instant and processed foods, busy parents rarely have time to prepare a totally fresh meal. The key then is to balance the use of fresh and seasonal foods with the use of packaged and convenience foods.

Taste development in children is achieved by constantly introducing new and interesting foods. Children should be encouraged, but never forced, to try new foods, even if they are initially turned off by a food's aroma or appearance. Over time, if children grow accustomed to seeing and trying a variety of new and interesting food in the home, they will acquire a taste for a variety of foods.

Charles van Over

---

as taste. People with many taste buds thus would have many pain fibers. This genetic taste variation in the perception of irritation might influence the preference for alcohol. Supertasters find alcohol more bitter and burning to the tongue than nontasters. Some studies suggest that alcoholics are more likely to be nontasters. Perhaps supertasters are protected from alcoholism by the noxious sensations produced by alcohol. Certainly the sensory quality of alcohol is not the only determinant of alcohol ingestion. But genetic taste blindness might be an easily identifiable risk factor for this disease.

LEARNING AND DEVELOPMENT OF FOOD PREFERENCES The idea that nutrient deficiencies would lead to cravings for specific nutrients proved to be true only for salt and sugar. Learning appears to play the strongest role in the selection of the diet.

Infants accept most foods after repeated exposures. The more familiar a food or a flavor becomes, the more likely a child will learn to like it. But children may require as many as ten exposures to a food before they begin to like it. Breastfeeding may set the stage for the ability of children to accept new foods, because the flavor of breast milk varies with the composition of the mother's diet. Even the infant's intake of breast milk varies with flavor changes in the milk. One study, for example, showed that when mothers consumed a diet high in garlic, infants fed longer. Exposure to the maternal diet via breast milk may help to explain how cultural food habits are passed down through generations. Bottle-fed infants do not experience the same diversity of flavors, because the sensory characteristics of formula are constant.

Leann Birch and her colleagues demonstrated that children learn to prefer flavor associated with fat. They gave preschool children novel-flavored yogurt drinks (such as chocolate-orange or pumpkin). The yogurt drinks were either low or high in fat. After eight exposures, the children's preference ratings increased for the flavor that was coupled with the higher fat content. David Booth and colleagues showed a similar preference in college-age students for flavors that were associated with starch.

Aversions (negative conditioning) can occur when a particular flavor is coupled with an unpleasant effect. Foods that are disliked are often associated with a past episode of nausea or vomiting. This is called conditioned aversion. Conditioned aversions are easier to form than conditioned preferences. In particular, flavors paired with nausea can become disliked after a single experience. In one study, children given a novel ice cream flavor just before chemotherapy later showed a dislike for that ice cream. In this case,

the conditioned aversion acted as a scapegoat. That is, the aversion that formed to the novel ice cream appeared to protect the preferences for the rest of the foods that the child normally ate. This is important because many cancer patients suffer from food aversions associated with therapy or with the disease itself. Such simple strategies as providing a scapegoat food (root beer Lifesavers were used in one study) can protect patients from developing food aversions as a side effect of chemotherapy. Conditioned aversions are also common among adolescents who experience nausea and vomiting associated with alcohol abuse. The alcohol-induced conditioned aversions can disappear if the disliked food or beverage is consumed on subsequent occasions when the individual does not become ill.

ENVIRONMENTAL INFLUENCES ON FOOD ACCEPTANCE Children learn to accept foods through repeated exposures within a social context. These social interactions can modify the sensory-based learning experiences. Positive learning occurs when a child observes caregivers, siblings, and peers showing pleasure in consuming a food. But negative learning occurs when a child is coerced into eating. A child can feel anxiety if forced to eat when not hungry. This can also limit the child's ability to respond appropriately to internal cues of hunger and satiety.

Mealtime can be a time of learning and fun. New foods can be introduced slowly and reinforced by the positive responses of other diners to the food. Children can explore such sensory qualities as the color, temperature, texture, and taste of foods. Creating stories about the foods with input from the child can enhance creativity and support the positive experience. Engaging children in food preparation activities can help them develop fine and gross motor control and can contribute to their enjoyment of food. And the ability to enjoy food encourages a child to develop lifetime habits of healthy eating.

Resource

Capaldi, E. D., and T. L. Powley. *Taste, Experience, and Feeding.* Washington, DC: American Psychological Association, 1990.

4

· · · · · · · ·

Pyramid Power: A Guide to Healthy Eating

The first dietary guidelines for Americans were published in the 1890s. Those early guidelines recommended the consumption of adequate protein, fat, carbohydrate, and calories. Through the years the content and emphasis of subsequent guidelines have shifted considerably, as new knowledge was obtained and socioeconomic conditions changed. At one time as many as twelve food groups were identified. In the 1920s and 1930s, as the importance of vitamins and minerals became recognized, dietary guidelines changed from recommending an adequate intake of macronutrients (protein, fat, and carbohy-

> **MYTH** Potato chips count as a vegetable in the Food Guide Pyramid.
>
> **FACT** Although potatoes are found in the vegetable group, potato chips are not. Potato chips are extremely high in fat and therefore should be eaten only occasionally.

drate) to advocating an adequate intake of micronutrients (vitamins and minerals). In 1941, the first Recommended Dietary Allowances were published by the National Research Council, and those recommendations were then also included in subsequent dietary guidelines. Such economic circumstances as the Depression and World War II also influenced dietary guidelines. Through most of the 1940s there were seven basic food groups: (1) milk and milk products; (2) meat, poultry, fish, eggs, dried beans (legumes), peas, and nuts; (3) bread, flour, and cereals; (4) leafy green vegetables and yellow vege-

· · · · · · · · · · · · · · ·

Tara Prather Liskov

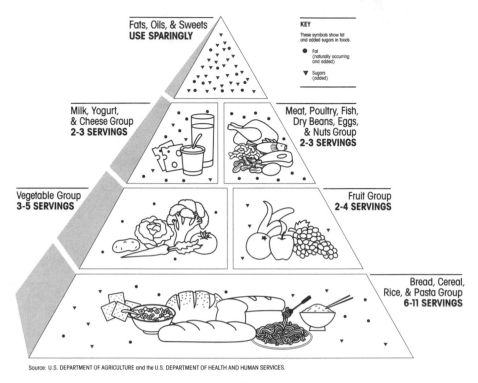

FIGURE 4.1
Food Guide Pyramid.

tables; (5) citrus fruits, tomatoes, cabbage, and salad greens (lettuce); (6) potatoes and other vegetables and fruits; and (7) butter and fortified margarine. As the food supply became more abundant and easily attainable, the emphasis of dietary guidelines shifted from nutrient deficiencies to avoidance of nutrient excesses. The Basic Four (the milk group, the meat group, the bread and cereal group, and the fruit and vegetable group) was the primary guide from the late 1950s through the 1980s.

The Food Guide Pyramid

Many studies of the 1980s and 1990s have shown that dietary practices have an important impact on the risk of developing a variety of diseases and conditions, such as heart disease and cancer. Moreover, obesity in children and adults has been increasing at an alarming rate. In response to this new information and changing conditions, the Food Guide Pyramid (fig. 4.1) was developed in 1992 by the United States Department of Agriculture (USDA). It was designed to represent graphically the 1990 Dietary Guidelines for Americans, which were published jointly by the USDA and the Department of Health and Human Services and updated in 1995:

- Eat a variety of foods.
- Balance the food you eat with physical activity— maintain or improve your weight.
- Choose a diet with plenty of grain products, vegetables, and fruits.

- Choose a diet low in fat, saturated fat, and cholesterol.
- Choose a diet moderate in sugars.
- Choose a diet moderate in salt and sodium.
- If you drink alcoholic beverages, do so in moderation.

Overall, the Food Guide Pyramid is meant to promote variety and moderation. The pyramid is divided into six groups, and the relative size of the groups is meant to represent the relative proportion of the diet that each group should contribute. Therefore, foods from groups at the bottom of the pyramid should contribute the greatest proportion of the diet. Foods from groups toward the top of the pyramid should constitute a relatively small proportion of the diet. The placement of food groups within the pyramid is based on the primary nutrients provided by each group and the relative amount of those nutrients needed by healthy people. For instance, carbohydrates (primarily complex carbohydrates) should compose most of the diet, so foods high in complex carbohydrates are at the base of the pyramid. Protein and fat should provide proportionally fewer calories in the diet, so groups that contain foods high in these nutrients are higher on the pyramid.

The numbers of servings from each group indicated on the pyramid are intended for adults, but they can be used for children in most instances, if portion sizes are adjusted for age (see chapters 5, 6, 7, and 8 for portion sizes for children of different ages). The range in number of servings from each group accounts for differences in caloric (energy) needs of different-sized people. Therefore, normal-weight individuals who need fewer calories should consume the lower number of servings in the range, while normal-weight individuals who need more calories should consume the higher number of servings in the range. Differences in caloric intake are based on both height and activity level.

THE BREAD, CEREAL, RICE, AND PASTA GROUP
Foods from this group provide complex carbohydrates, vitamins, minerals, and fiber. They are relatively low in fat and cholesterol and should compose most of the diet. People should consume 6–11 servings from this group daily. A serving for older children and adults is 1 slice of bread, ½ cup of cooked rice, pasta, or cereal, 4 to 5 crackers, or 1 ounce of ready-to-eat cereal. Some foods in this group are:

Bagels	Popcorn
Bread	Pretzels
Cereal	Rice
Crackers	Rice cakes
English muffins	Rolls
Pasta	

THE VEGETABLE GROUP Vegetables provide carbohydrates, protein, vitamins, minerals, and fiber and are free of cholesterol and fat. In addition, studies have indicated that adequate consumption of vegetables may protect against some forms of cancer. People should consume 3–5 servings from this group daily. A serving for an adult is ½ cup chopped raw or cooked vegetables or 1 cup leafy raw vegetables. Some foods in this group are:

Asparagus	Eggplant
Bell peppers	Green beans
Cabbage	Lettuce
Carrots	Lima beans
Cauliflower	Mushrooms
Celery	Onions
Collard and turnip greens	Peas
	Potatoes
Cucumber	Spinach

Tomatoes	Yellow squash	Cheese	Skim milk
Turnips	Zucchini	Frozen yogurt	Whole milk
Vegetable juice		Low-fat milk	Yogurt

THE FRUIT GROUP Fruits are an important source of calories, fiber, and vitamins, and people should consume 2–4 servings from this group daily. The pyramid separates fruits from vegetables to emphasize the importance of adequate consumption of foods from both groups. A serving for an adult is 1 apple, ⅛ of a melon, ¾ cup juice, ½ cup canned fruit, or ¼ cup dried fruit. Some foods in this group are:

Apples	Grapes
Apricots	Honeydew melon
Bananas	Kiwi
Blueberries	Oranges
Cantaloupe	Peaches
Cherries	Pears
Dried fruits	Plums
Figs	Raisins
Fruit juices	Strawberries
Fruit salad	Tangerines
Grapefruit	Watermelon

THE MILK, YOGURT, AND CHEESE GROUP Foods in this group are an important source of protein, calcium, and other vitamins and minerals. Most people should consume 2–3 servings from this group daily. Adolescents and pregnant and lactating women, however, should consume 4 servings daily. Children under 2 years of age should consume full-fat milk products, because their bodies need fat for energy and for normal growth. After the age of 2, low-fat and nonfat products are appropriate in most instances. A serving for an adult is 1 cup of milk or yogurt or 1½–2 ounces of cheese. Some foods in this group are:

THE MEAT, POULTRY, FISH, DRIED BEANS, EGGS, AND NUTS GROUP Foods in this group provide primarily protein and calories. Most are also good sources of iron, B vitamins, and zinc. Because cholesterol and fat are higher in most foods in this group than in most foods from groups lower on the pyramid, people should consume only 2–3 servings from this group daily. A serving for an adult is 3 ounces of lean meat, fish, or poultry. One ounce of meat is equivalent to ½ cup cooked beans, 1 egg, and 2 tablespoons peanut butter. Some foods included in this group are:

Beef	Lamb
Chicken	Lunch meat (turkey,
Dried beans (kidney,	ham, roast beef,
pinto, navy, black)	bologna)
Eggs	Nuts
Fish	Peanut butter
Hot dogs	Pork

FATS, OILS, AND SWEETS Foods from this group should be consumed only occasionally because they contain many calories but few nutrients. Sugar promotes tooth decay, and foods high in fat can increase the risk of developing heart disease and some forms of cancer. Also, foods from this group can contribute to obesity when eaten excessively. Placement of foods in this section of the pyramid is sometimes difficult, depending on professional philosophy. Most nutritionists have decided to classify potato chips, corn chips, doughnuts, candy, high-fat ice cream, jam, jelly, butter, margarine, oil, sugar, soda, and cookies in this group, as they should be consumed only occasionally. Although there are no "bad" foods, some foods, such as those listed above, should be used only occasionally.

The Food Guide Pyramid should be used to plan an overall healthy diet. Ideally, a child would eat at least the lower number of servings from each food group daily and would eat foods from the top of the pyramid sparingly. The pyramid is, however, a *guide,* so daily fluctuations should not be cause for alarm. An adequate, varied diet will assure proper growth and development in children.

Resources

U.S. Department of Agriculture. *The Food Guide Pyramid.* Home and Garden Bulletin no. 252. Washington, DC, 1992.

U.S. Department of Agriculture and U.S. Department of Health and Human Services. *Nutrition and Your Health: Dietary Guidelines for Americans.* 4th ed. Home and Garden Bulletin no. 232. Washington, DC, 1995.

5
· · · · · · · ·

Infancy: Eat, Sleep, and Be Happy

Infancy (the first 12 months of life) is a time of great change; the changes that take place in both growth and development occur at a rate that will never be equaled in future life. By 4–5 months of age, for example, an infant will have doubled his or her birth weight, and the birth weight will have tripled by 12 months. Newborn infants, who are unable even to hold up their heads without support or to reach out for food, develop into 1-year-olds who can walk and feed themselves. During this first year, the digestive tract and immune system—both of which are important when considering food and nutrition—mature to such an extent that in a 1-year-old child functional abilities are similar to those of an adult. So, before discussing the nutritional needs of infants, we should consider the relation between nutrition and development—how nutrition contributes to an infant's development and how developmental considerations dictate the type of diet that is most appropriate for the growing infant.

MYTH Starting solids early will help your baby sleep through the night.

FACT There is no connection between consumption of solid foods (including cereal in a bottle) and improved sleep patterns in infants. Infants should not be given solid food before 4–6 months of age, because they receive adequate calories from breast milk or formula and are not physiologically ready for solid foods.

· ·

Donna Caseria ▪ Barbara Ackerman ▪ Brian Forsyth

Neurobehavioral Development

A newborn infant has a strong rooting reflex: when touched by an object on the side of the face, the infant will automatically turn to take the object into his or her mouth. This reflex and the sucking that follows, which is also a reflex or automatic action, ensure that the normal process of sucking on a nipple provides the nutrition an infant needs. Solid foods are inappropriate and are handled poorly by an infant in the first few months of life because, for example, touching a spoon to a newborn baby's tongue causes the baby to stick the tongue forward. This also is an automatic response, known as the thrust or protrusion reflex, and it interferes with a baby's ability to get much sustenance from solid foods. This reflex disappears at some point during the first 3 months, making it more appropriate to introduce solid foods later, usually between 4 and 6 months.

From the beginning, feeding is an important interaction between parent and child. The distance at which a baby's vision is most clear, approximately 10 inches, is about the distance between the eyes of the baby and mother when the baby is held in a nursing position.

Even at an early age, infants have a preference for certain foods. They often prefer sweet foods to bitter or salty foods, but it is only in the last few months of infancy that an infant is really able to express preferences. At this time infants start to understand words, can vocalize, and will mimic the actions that adults make when feeding themselves. These changes, along with a newfound sense of independence, can lead infants to assert their own preferences concerning eating.

Physiological Development

Many metabolic changes occur in a baby's body during infancy. Some of the enzymes necessary to break down components of food are produced only in minimal amounts by the newborn infant. Different enzymes are present in the saliva, the intestines, and the pancreas. These increase to sufficient amounts by about 3 months of age. Before then, such foodstuffs as starch are not properly broken down by the immature digestive system. Therefore, food other than breast milk or formula is not an appropriate part of the diet during the first 2-3 months of infancy. Evidence also suggests that during these early months the intestine is more likely to allow whole protein molecules to be absorbed. Normally, protein is broken down and digested before being absorbed. If protein is absorbed without first being broken down, it can cause an allergic reaction (see chapter 19). This is another reason why it is not wise to give an infant too many different types of foodstuffs during the first 3-4 months, particularly if there is a family history of allergies or asthma.

Proportionately, an infant needs more protein and calories than a child or adult, and many different constituents of food—including vitamins and such minerals as iron—are essential for normal growth and development. At the same time, the immaturity of the newborn limits the types of foods that should be given. At the beginning, breast milk or infant formulas are the only foods an infant requires. Later, different types of food are added to the diet, and by the end of the first year, the infant should be receiving a varied diet of table foods.

Thinking about Breastfeeding

For new parents, one of the most important decisions is whether to breastfeed or formula feed. This decision should be based on accurate and current information and should feel comfortable for the parents. Neither choice is right or wrong,

TABLE 5.1
Changes in Breast Milk

Characteristic	Colostrum	Transitional milk	Mature milk
Period of availability	From delivery–day 5	5–14 days after delivery	Usually beginning between the second and third week
Color	Clear at first and then changing to creamy golden or lemony yellow	White	Remains white but is similar to the color of skim milk
Composition	Is high in protein and low in fat, making it easier for the baby to digest; has a laxative effect on the baby's intestine, which helps the baby to get rid of the first stools, known as meconium; is rich in disease-fighting antibodies	Compared with colostrum, is less high in some proteins; is higher in fat, sugar, and calories; is higher in some immunoglobulins and lower in others	Fairly stable in nutrients
Volume	Compared with later milk, less is produced, but the amount will be adequate for a newborn baby	Volume will increase to meet the baby's growing needs; amount will depend on the baby's breastfeeding frequency, duration, and effectiveness	Volume will continue to increase to meet the baby's growing needs; amount will depend on the baby's breast-feeding behavior and frequency

but an informed choice must take into account the baby's nutrition and health. Breast milk and formula are not identical, and they affect the health of babies differently.

THE VALUE OF BREAST MILK The American Academy of Pediatrics, the American Dietetic Association, and the American College of Obstetrics and Gynecology have stated that mother's milk is, under normal circumstances, the best food for a baby. They maintain that breastfeeding alone can provide all the nourishment needed for most babies during the first 4–6 months of life.

Breast milk is a complete, balanced diet that changes to meet a growing baby's nutritional needs. It has more than two hundred constituents and contains all the nutrients needed to support a baby's growth and to enhance the growth and development of the baby's brain and central nervous system. The one exception is fluoride, which may need to be supplemented in exclusively breastfed older infants. Because breast milk is rich in disease-fighting antibodies, early breastfeeding can even be considered a baby's first immunization, which only the mother can provide. During the first several weeks of breastfeeding, a mother's breast milk goes through some unique changes in composition from colostrum to transitional milk and then to mature milk (table 5.1).

Breastfeeding is valuable not only for its nutrient content but also for the nurturing and attachment it affords the mother and her baby. Breastfeeding is convenient and less expensive than using formula; breast milk is easier for the baby to digest, and it provides the baby with some of the mother's infection-fighting antibodies. Research shows long-lasting health benefits for the mother and her baby. Many of these are linked to the duration of breastfeeding: the longer a mother breastfeeds, the stronger the effect. Breastfeeding provides protection against some acute and chronic diseases. Research indicates that infants who are breastfed are less likely to develop gastrointestinal infections, diarrhea, ear infections, and respiratory infections. They are also less likely to develop allergies, especially in the first year. Babies who are breastfed may also have a reduced risk of developing insulin-dependent diabetes. In addition, there is some evidence that in preterm babies, omega-3 long-chain polyunsaturated fatty acids, such as DHA (docosahexaenoic acid), which are found in breast milk, may be beneficial for visual and brain development.

For the mother, breastfeeding helps prevent blood loss after delivery and helps the uterus return more quickly to its prepregnant state. Breastfeeding has also been reported to reduce maternal lower-body fat, specifically hip circumference. Women who breastfeed are at less risk for developing postpartum anemia, premenopausal breast cancer, ovarian cancer, and osteoporosis.

The Mother's Diet

The breastfeeding mother's diet is very important (table 5.2). A woman can obtain all her requirements for a balanced breastfeeding diet by following the American Dietetic Association's general nutrition guidelines (see the accompanying box). Women who are considering the use of vitamins and mineral supplements should check with their health care provider to ensure the need for these additions. If a mother has strict food preferences or requires a special diet such as a vegetarian diet, a lactose-free diet, or a low-fat diet, it is important that she seek appropriate nutritional counseling during breastfeeding. Often special diets do not include the additional nutrients needed during breastfeeding. Such diets may require the addition of mineral or vitamin supplements.

QUESTIONS AND CONCERNS 1. *Is there anything special a woman should do during pregnancy to help prepare for breastfeeding?* A woman should tell her doctor or midwife that she plans to breastfeed and should ask her health care provider to examine her breasts and nipples for any potential problems. She should also ask for recommended books and should inquire about the availability of prenatal breastfeeding classes, such breastfeeding support groups as La Leche League, and local lactation consultants. She should investigate how her body makes milk and how her baby will obtain the milk. A woman should learn as much as she can about breastfeeding during her pregnancy, because as her due date approaches, she will focus on the birthing process and not on breastfeeding. After she has chosen a pediatric practice that is supportive of breastfeeding, she should become familiar with the practice and its routines.

2. *How can a mother tell that her baby is getting enough milk during the first week at home?* When an adequate amount of breast milk is consumed, the baby's appetite will be satisfied for at least two hours and there will be sufficient fluid intake to maintain normal urine and stool output. The following guidelines indicate whether a new baby is breastfeeding well.

- The baby should be nursing at least 8–12 times in 24 hours (every 2–3 hours).

TABLE 5.2
Selected Nutrients Needed by the Breastfeeding Mother

Nutrient	Amount needed per day	Food sources
Protein	65 g for the first 6 months and 62 g from 6 to 12 months	Chicken, beef, turkey, fish, cheese, eggs, milk, yogurt, peas, beans, cottage cheese, nuts and seeds, tofu, whole-grain breads, cereal, peanut butter
Calcium	1,200 mg	Yogurt, milk, cheese, tofu with calcium sulfate or lactate, sardines, figs, spinach, broccoli, bok choy, kale, greens (calcium supplements can also be obtained in tablet and powder form)
Zinc	19 mg	Crab, shrimp, oysters, pork, lamb, beef, legumes, eggs, cheese, yogurt, peanuts, wheat germ, black-eyed peas, whole grains
Magnesium	355 mg	Green vegetables, legumes, nuts, whole grains, oysters, scallops, seeds
Vitamin B_6	2.1 mg	Bananas, soybeans, cauliflower, potatoes, beans, shellfish, eggs, chicken, turkey, other meats
Folic acid	280 μg	Beans, liver, eggs, wheat germ, green leafy vegetables, seeds

- From day 2 to day 4 the baby should have 4–6 wet diapers per day.
- After day 4 the baby should have 6–8 wet diapers of light yellow urine per day.
- By the end of the first week the baby will likely have 4–6 stools per day.
- By day 4 the baby should have stools that are yellow in color.
- The baby should be sleeping for at least 2 hours after a feeding.
- The baby should be latched on to the breast with sucking and swallowing throughout the feeding.
- Feedings should last at least 10 minutes per breast but generally not more than 20 minutes per breast.
- The mother should feel her milk coming in some time between day 2 and day 4 (the mother can usually recognize the change from colostrum to milk by a feeling of fullness in the breasts).
- Once a mother's milk has come in, her breasts should feel full before each feeding and softer after nursing.

3. *What about "appetite spurts"? What are they and when do they occur?* These are fairly specific times when a baby is growing rapidly and therefore requires more breast milk. As the baby goes through these appetite spurts, he or she will breastfeed more frequently than usual to enhance the mother's milk production. The mother should not panic, as these spurts often last only a day or two. As the milk volume increases to meet her baby's nutritional needs, the feedings will once again become less frequent and lengthy. Growth

General Nutrition Guidelines for Breastfeeding Women

Drink plenty of liquids. A minimum of about 8 cups of fluid per day is recommended. Many women enjoy a glass of milk, juice, or water while breastfeeding. Limit coffee, tea, and sodas that contain caffeine. Alcohol passes quickly into breast milk and can harm the baby, so avoid alcoholic beverages, including wine, beer, and liquor.

Eat a variety of foods.

Eat at least three nutritious meals per day, and do not skip breakfast. You will find that you get hungry more quickly while breastfeeding. Start the day with a good breakfast, do not skip meals, and eat nutritious snacks.

Limit foods that are high in sugar and fat and low in nutrients. Candy bars, soda, doughnuts, and chips may fill you up but offer few vitamins and minerals. You should not eat foods that are high in sugar and fats in place of nutritious foods.

Eat about 500 calories more per day than it took to maintain your weight before you were preg- *nant.* The extra calories you need can be in the form of either snacks between meals or slightly larger meals. The following snacks contain about 500 calories:

- A grilled cheese sandwich with a bowl of soup
- A large bowl of cereal with milk, fruit, and fruit juice
- ⅔ cup peanuts
- Corn bread with a bowl of pinto beans
- A large fruit milk shake and 2 graham crackers

Avoid dieting to lose weight rapidly. You should feel good and have energy while returning to your normal weight. A weight loss of 2 to 4 pounds per month will probably not affect your milk supply. Rapid weight loss (more than 4 to 5 pounds per month after the first month) is not advisable for breastfeeding women.

Source: Adapted from "General Nutrition Guidelines for Breastfeeding Women," American Dietetic Association.

---

spurts usually occur around the ages of 10–14 days, 3 weeks, 6 weeks, 3 months, and 6 months.

4. *Can a mother lose weight while breastfeeding?* Crash diets and fad diets are not recommended during breastfeeding. Eating nutritious meals, changing some eating habits, and incorporating a routine of safe exercise is the best approach to gradual weight loss during breastfeeding.

5. *When is a good time to introduce a bottle?* Some mothers introduce breastfed babies to an occasional bottle-feeding to allow for flexibility and convenience. No set rules stipulate when to introduce a bottle, although some recommendations can be made. Bottle-feeding should not be introduced until 3–4 weeks of age because it is most important that breastfeeding be well established before bottles are introduced. The baby

may not be as receptive to bottle-feeding as the mother had anticipated, or the baby may adjust very easily. If the baby has been using a pacifier, parents should consider using a similar kind of nipple. If a pacifier has not been used, parents may wish to try a nipple that resembles the mother's. Parents should not be afraid to experiment with the many different types of nipples. If expressed breast milk is available, the mother should use it for the first bottle-feedings, as the baby is used to the taste and the smell of her breast milk. If breast milk is not available, formula must be used. If unsure of which type of formula to use, parents should check with the baby's health care provider. Some breastfed babies will initially not take a bottle from their mother and may be more receptive to the father, grandmother, or baby-sitter. Be patient; eventually the baby will take a bottle.

6. *How long is fresh breast milk safely kept in the refrigerator, and how long can breast milk be frozen?* Breast milk is a food product, and guidelines for safe storage apply. Milk that the mother has just expressed can be kept safely in a refrigerator for up to 72 hours. If the mother is not planning to use the freshly expressed milk within this period, she should freeze it immediately for future use. Safe storage of breast milk will depend on the kind of freezer compartment used. Breast milk that is stored in a freezer compartment of a refrigerator can be kept safely for up to 2 weeks. If kept in a separate, self-defrosting unit, the milk can be stored safely for up to 6 months. The milk should be placed in the back of the freezer, away from the door and on the top shelf. If a deep freezer (0 degrees or lower) without a defrost cycle is used, the milk can be stored safely for up to 12 months. Breast milk should be stored in clean, tightly covered containers that are clearly labeled with the date of expression. The oldest milk should always be used first.

7. *Can a woman continue to breastfeed when she returns to work?* With thoughtful planning, many women are returning to work and continuing with breastfeeding. The mother's health care provider, lactation consultant, or breastfeeding support group can provide her with helpful information. Women have also found it useful to talk with other women who have combined breastfeeding with working. Some important tips: before the mother returns to work, establish a feeding routine that will fit in with her work schedule; allow enough time for the baby to adjust to the bottle or cup that will be used when the mother is at work; decide whether to use breast milk or formula for the baby's feedings during work time; select and learn how to use a breast pump; investigate whether the mother's work site has a pumping room or a private area for women to express milk; determine where and how to store expressed milk safely; and continue breastfeeding as usual when the mother and her baby are together. With good planning, babies can combine breastfeeding and bottle-feeding quite successfully.

8. *When should the baby be weaned?* Weaning is usually an individual decision made by the mother or the baby, although occasionally other reasons for weaning emerge. No set rules govern when one should wean, however. How long a woman chooses to breastfeed will depend on her personal comfort and situation. Sometimes the baby begins the weaning process when the mother is not ready. This can be a sad time for the mother. In other cases a mother decides it is time to wean. It is then best for the mother and her baby to do so gradually, for example, by replacing one breastfeeding with either a bottle or cup feeding every three to four days.

9. *How can the father help and feel part of the breastfeeding process?* Most fathers want to be involved in the care and nurturing of their baby, but

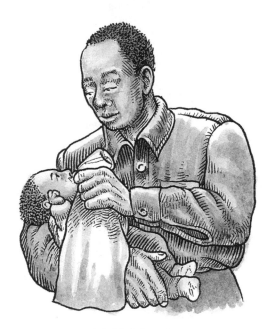

FIGURE 5.1
A position for bottle-feeding.

sometimes they feel left out when the mother is breastfeeding. Fathers can help by supporting and encouraging breastfeeding and by making sure that mothers get enough rest. Fathers can also do many other things to help care for their babies, such as bathing them and getting them ready for a feeding. If desired, once breastfeeding is well established, the father can feed the baby a bottle of expressed breast milk when the mother is unavailable or when he wants to offer her well-deserved time to rest (fig. 5.1).

10. *Can a mother breastfeed if her baby is born prematurely?* If a mother has chosen to breastfeed her baby, there is no reason to abandon this choice because the baby was born prematurely and is unable to nurse right away. In fact, the mother's breast milk offers the baby unique nutritional and health benefits. A woman who is unable to nurse her baby soon after delivery will need to begin stimulating milk production by pumping her breasts to simulate the baby's feeding. The

mother should tell both her own health care provider and her baby's provider that she plans to breastfeed as soon as possible after the delivery. This will enable them to advise her about expressing milk. Each hospital has specific guidelines for the new mother concerning breast milk collection, storage, and transport during the baby's hospitalization. Breast milk that the mother expresses will be fed to the baby when the baby is able to digest the milk. Nursing is usually started as soon as it is safely possible.

11. *What can a new mother do to get breastfeeding off to a good start?* The following basic guidelines and information will help a new mother and her baby. For a more detailed explanation of these recommendations, a new mother should consider purchasing a book or requesting written information specifically about breastfeeding.

- Breastfeeding should begin as soon as possible after delivery.
- The mother should request that her baby room in with her during her hospital stay.
- A new mother should ask for assistance when learning how to position herself and her baby for feeding. She should try different nursing positions and use the ones that are comfortable for her. The three most commonly recommended positions for breastfeeding are the cradle, football, and side-lying positions (fig. 5.2).
- A new mother should ask for assistance to ensure that her baby is latching on and sucking correctly when feeding at the breast (fig. 5.3).
- A new mother should breastfeed frequently (every 2–3 hours, or at least 8 times in a 24-hour period), using both breasts at each feeding with no more than 20 minutes at each breast.
- Parents should avoid the use of pacifiers and bottle-feedings until breastfeeding is well established.

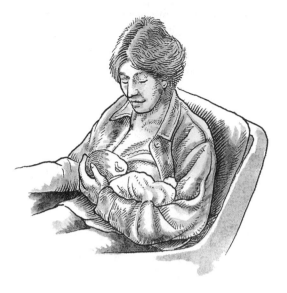

Football

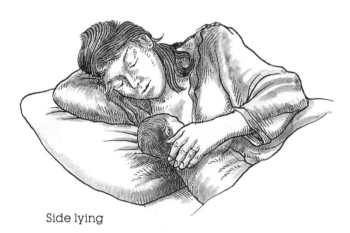

Cradle

Side lying

FIGURE 5.2
Three recommended
positions for
breastfeeding.

- Guidelines that indicate whether the baby is breastfeeding well were presented earlier (see question 2). A new mother should consult her health care provider if she has any concerns that her new baby is not getting enough breast milk.
- The mother should ask her health care professional whom to call for help with breastfeeding.

Formulas

If the parents have chosen not to breastfeed or if breastfeeding is discontinued before the baby is 1 year old, a commercially prepared infant formula should be used. Infant formulas are modeled after breast milk and follow standards set by

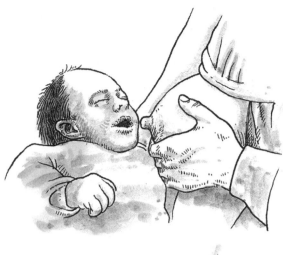

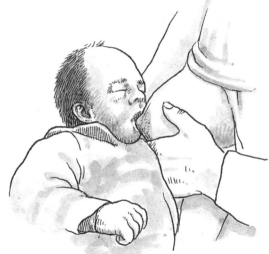

FIGURE 5.3
A mother eliciting the rooting reflex (top)
and a baby latching on to the breast
(bottom).

the Infant Formula Act of 1980, which assure that they contain safe and adequate levels of vitamins and minerals.

Formulas are available in several varieties and forms. Most standard formulas have 20 calories per ounce and are modified from cow's milk. Soy-based formulas are nutritionally equivalent to cow's-milk-based formulas but differ in the types of protein and sugars they contain. Health care providers may change some infants' formulas from one type to another, although there is often little reason for such a change. A change may be necessary, however, when an infant is intolerant of lactose, the type of sugar present in cow's-milk-based formulas. Lactose intolerance is rare in infancy except when an infection (gastroenteritis) is present in the digestive tract. In such cases, a number of days may pass before the infant is able to digest the lactose in cow's-milk-based formulas, and during this time it may be appropriate to change to a soy-based formula, which doesn't contain lactose. When allergies are a concern, an infant's formula may be changed to a hypoallergenic formula. Modified infant formulas are more expensive, and their use should be discussed with the infant's pediatrician.

Once the type of infant formula is selected, the method of preparation must be chosen. Most formulas come in three forms: powder, concentrated liquid, and ready-to-feed. All are appropriate; they differ only in cost and convenience. Powdered versions are usually the least expensive and require the most preparation. Powders must be mixed with water, and directions must be followed to assure correct preparation of the formula. Concentrated liquids are more costly than powder but less expensive than ready-to-feed formulas. Equal parts of water and concentrated liquid are mixed together to prepare a standard (20 calories per ounce) formula. Ready-to-feed formulas are the most convenient but also the most expensive. These formulas are poured directly into the bottle, with no preparation required at all.

Some feeding practices should be avoided:

- Do not warm bottles in the microwave. Microwaves heat unevenly, so the baby could get burned.

- Do not put cereal in a bottle, as the baby could choke.
- Do not put the baby to bed with a bottle. Fluid from the bottle can pool in the baby's mouth and promote tooth decay.
- Do not force the baby to finish a bottle. Such requirements set up poor eating habits.

Because vitamin and mineral contents of formulas are regulated by law, most formula-fed infants do not need routine supplementation. Fluoride is the only exception. In the United States, fluoride is sometimes added to a city's water supply, so if powdered or concentrated liquid formulas are prepared using city water, fluoride supplementation is not required, but if well water is used, a fluoride supplementation may be needed after the baby is 6 months old. Ready-to-feed formulas do not contain fluoride, so fluoride supplementation is necessary.

All formulas are fortified with iron. Both low-iron and high-iron (or "iron-fortified") preparations are available. By far the better choice is the formula with higher amounts of added iron.

Cow's Milk

Regular cow's milk and condensed and evaporated milks made from cow's milk are all inappropriate and should not be fed to infants less than 12 months of age. Cow's milk is too high in protein for the infant to digest. In addition, cow's milk does not contain appropriate amounts of vitamins, iron, and other minerals required by the rapidly growing infant and therefore should not be introduced into the child's diet until after 1 year of age.

Water

If an infant is drinking adequate amounts of breast milk or formula, extra water is not necessary, al-though some parents feel that an extra bottle of water in the summer is a good idea. This is not harmful as long as it does not replace a feeding of milk or formula, which could cause the infant to consume too few calories. For an infant who is 4 months of age or less, the water (including bottled water) should be boiled and cooled prior to feeding to decrease the risk of contamination.

Introducing Solid Foods

The American Academy of Pediatrics recommends that solid foods be introduced sometime between 4 and 6 months of life. In the first 2–3 months, infants' digestive tracts are not developed sufficiently to handle solid foods, and the tongue thrust reflex makes feeding of solids inappropriate. When an infant is ready for solid foods, the tongue thrust reflex will have disappeared, the infant will be able to hold up his or her head, and the infant will show an interest in food (by reaching for food or attentively watching others eat). Recommendations for the introduction of solid foods are listed below:

Age	Foods
0–4 months	Breast milk or formula
4–6 months	Iron-fortified cereals made with rice or barley
6–7 months	Strained fruits and vegetables Fruit juices Teething foods
8–9 months	Pureed meats, potatoes, rice, or pasta
10–12 months	Finger foods (cheese cubes, toast strips), yogurt, and an increased variety of foods

CEREALS The best solid food to feed an infant first is an iron-fortified infant rice or barley cereal. Rice or barley cereals are easily digested, provide an excellent source of iron, and are the least allergenic of the grain foods. Start with 1 tablespoon of cereal mixed with 3 tablespoons of breast milk, formula, or iron-fortified fruit juice. Do not add salt or sugar. Feeding may be very messy at first. Gradually increase the consistency of the cereal and increase the amount of cereal to 3–4 tablespoons once or twice a day. Introduce other single-grain cereals and save mixed-grain cereals until after each of the cereals in the mixture has been introduced separately.

Many parents believe that the introduction of cereal helps babies sleep through the night, which may prompt parents to introduce cereals before 4 months of age. But research has shown that early introduction of cereal does not result in an infant's sleeping through the night sooner. When infants are ready to sleep through the night, they will.

Solid foods should not be put in a baby's bottle. Putting cereal in the bottle adds extra calories, which may contribute to excessive weight gain, and may pose a choking hazard.

FRUITS AND VEGETABLES Fruits and vegetables can be introduced around 6 months of age. Some pediatricians believe that vegetables should be introduced before fruits so the infant doesn't first get used to the sweet taste of fruit. Another option is to alternate between the two. Commercial and homemade baby foods are equally acceptable. Start with 1 tablespoon of a fruit or vegetable and gradually increase the serving size to 4–5 tablespoons twice a day.

Do not introduce several new foods at the same time. Instead, introduce one new food every 3–4 days. If the infant has an allergic reaction, it will then be easy to tell which food is the culprit.

Common signs of an allergic reaction are diarrhea, vomiting, rashes, and excessive irritability. If the infant does show signs of an allergy, avoid that food and then perhaps try a small amount again a few weeks later. Avoid mixed fruits and vegetables until the infant has tolerated all the foods in the mixed dish.

FRUIT JUICE Juice can be introduced around 6 months of age. Try single ingredient juice first, such as apple, pear, or grape. Buy juices enriched with vitamin C. Bottled or frozen juices are fine; there is no need to buy the more expensive infant juices. Juices should be diluted: one-half juice and one-half water. Do not substitute juice for a feeding of breast milk or formula. Four ounces of juice a day is more than sufficient for an infant. Large quantities of juice may prevent the infant from consuming adequate milk.

It is preferable to give juice in a "sippy cup" (a cup with a lid and spout) rather than a bottle. If the infant has difficulty with the cup, keep trying. Don't put the baby to sleep with a bottle of juice or milk; this can promote tooth decay.

TEETHING FOODS Most infants start teething at 6–7 months. It is exciting to see the first teeth erupt, and this is an ideal time to introduce teething foods. Infants will gum such foods as teething crackers, toast, zwiebacks, or frozen bagels. These foods will provide some comfort and help the infant learn to chew. But a baby should never be left unattended when eating these foods because of the risk of choking.

MEATS AND MEAT SUBSTITUTES Meats or meat substitutes can be introduced around 8–9 months of age. Again, introduce only one food at a time. Both commercial baby meats and homemade pureed meats are fine. Try strained beef, poultry, pork, or veal. It's best to avoid jarred baby food dinners, as they have little protein and iron compared to their pure meat counterparts. Mild cheeses, cottage cheese, plain yogurt, and pureed beans are also good choices.

FOODS TO AVOID IN INFANCY Some foods are not appropriate for infants and should be avoided until at least the baby's first birthday. Foods that may cause allergic reactions include egg whites, seafood, chocolate, citrus fruits, and tomatoes (see chapter 19 for more information on allergies). Honey is another food that should be avoided. It may contain botulism spores that, although not harmful to adults, can cause infant botulism, an illness that can be severe. Honey is acceptable, however, as an ingredient in such processed foods as honey graham crackers.

When the infant is still learning to coordinate chewing and swallowing, certain foods pose a risk because of the possibility of choking. For this reason, such foods as raisins, grapes, nuts, peanut butter, pieces of hot dog, and raw carrots should be avoided during this stage.

COMMERCIAL BABY FOODS It is a personal decision whether to use commercial baby foods or to prepare baby food at home. Some parents enjoy making their own baby foods, while others appreciate the convenience of commercial baby food. Commercial baby foods are safe and convenient but more costly than homemade baby foods. Today, baby food manufacturers have responded to the need to avoid excess sugar and salt, and many baby foods do not contain added salt, sugar, or preservatives. But parents should check the ingredient list on the label to avoid added salt or sugar.

HOMEMADE BABY FOODS Many parents make their own baby foods. Listed below are a few simple guidelines for making this alternative safe and economical.

- Use fresh foods, if possible. Remove all pits, seeds, bones, and skin. Cook fruits first. Canned fruits should be packed in juice or water. Prepare foods on a clean working surface and use clean utensils.
- Cook all foods until tender. Do not use any seasonings such as salt or sugar. Steaming is the best cooking technique, because it minimizes vitamin losses. Do not microwave meats before pureeing them, as the meat will become the consistency of sawdust.
- Mash foods to the desired consistency and add some milk, water, or cooking water, if necessary. Baby food grinders, food processors, blenders, or strainers can be helpful.
- Individual portions can be frozen in ice cube trays or on a cookie sheet. Cover the trays before freezing. After freezing, place each portion in a plastic bag, seal it, and return it to the freezer. Label and date all foods and, to be safe, use them within 1 month.
- Thaw individual portions in the refrigerator, double boiler, or microwave (on defrost setting). Do not thaw at room temperature.

TABLE FOODS From 9 to 12 months, the infant will begin to enjoy many new types and textures of food. Foods can be mashed or cut into bite-sized portions. The infant should progress from pureed meats to ground meats, then to finely chopped meats. Many infants like rice, potatoes, and pasta. Cheese slices and grilled cheese sandwiches are also good choices. Diced canned fruits provide a nice snack alternative. Junior commercial baby foods are a convenience, but they are usually lower in protein than home-prepared meals and don't provide much textural variety. Often, the best and easiest food option for an infant of this age is to chop or mash the food that the adults are eating.

Infants know when they are full. If they push food away, do not force them to finish the meal, as this could potentially lead to bad eating habits. Sometimes an infant will show a dislike for a food. Again, it's best not to force it but to try to introduce it again in a few weeks. Breast milk or formula consumption will decrease as the consumption of solid food increases.

By the time a child is 1 year old, his or her meal patterns will have become similar to the family pattern. Keep in mind the Food Guide Pyramid when planning the infant's diet (see chapter 4). In one short year the infant has progressed from a diet solely of breast milk or formula to a varied diet of table foods.

Feeding Problems

It is common, particularly when children are in the first few months of infancy, for parents to be concerned that their baby has some sort of feeding problem or has had an adverse reaction to a particular food. In a study of healthy newborn infants, more than one-third of mothers reported having been concerned that their child had a problem during the first 4 months of infancy. The most common concerns were about excessive crying or colic, spitting up, and feeding difficulties. There was no difference in the frequency of these problems between infants who were breastfed and those who were formula fed, except that spitting up was more commonly reported in formula-fed infants. It is likely that most of these infants were in fact healthy.

These behaviors are common in early infancy and do not necessarily mean there is something wrong. Indeed, the amount of time an infant cries increases during the first few weeks of life, reaching a peak at about 6 weeks. At this age, the average infant cries for about 2¾ hours per day, and one out of four infants cries for more than 3½ hours each day.

About 10 percent of infants have what is commonly called colic: a sudden onset of inconsolable crying. On occasion, colic can be associated with the type of protein in a milk formula or the presence in breast milk of small amounts of something the mother has eaten. But no such connection can be found for most cases of colic. With a colicky infant, it is sometimes worthwhile to try eliminating cow's-milk protein from the diet. But this should be done only with the advice of a pediatrician. For the formula-fed infant, this means changing to a soy or casein hydrolysate formula. For the breastfed infant, it means removing cow's milk and foods made from cow's milk from the mother's diet. Even if these changes appear to have an effect, the baby is not necessarily allergic to cow's milk. Colic resolves by itself at about 3–5 months of age, so it is appropriate to return to a cow's-milk-based formula or for the breastfeeding mother to reintroduce milk products to her diet after the colic resolves.

In the past, other things in the diet have been blamed for causing problems. Most significantly, iron-fortified formulas have been blamed for causing constipation and such behaviors as crying and spitting up. But studies examining this question have found no relation between these behaviors and the iron content of formulas. Therefore, because iron is so important for infants, formula-fed infants should receive an iron-fortified formula.

The overall goal in feeding the infant is the child's proper growth and development. The guidelines for food introduction and feeding will help assure this. Remember that each child is different and that there is no one right way to feed an infant. The process should be enjoyable for both infant and parents and should set the stage for future positive feeding experiences.

Resources

Beham, E. *Eat Well, Lose Weight While Breastfeeding.* New York: Villard Books, 1994.

Breastfeeding National Network. (800) TELL YOU (835-5968).

Huggins, K. *The Nursing Mother's Companion,* 2d ed. Boston: Harvard Common Press, 1990.

Kimmel, M., and D. Kimmel. *Mommy Made and Daddy Too! Home Cooking for a Healthy Baby and Toddler.* New York: Bantam Books, 1990.

La Leche League International. (800) LALECHE (525-3243).

Pryor, K., and G. Pryor. *Nursing Your Baby,* 3d ed. New York: Pocket Books, 1991.

Satter, E. *Child of Mine: Feeding with Love and Good Sense.* Palo Alto, CA: Bull Publishing, 1986.

———. *How to Get Your Kid to Eat . . . but Not Too Much.* Palo Alto, CA: Bull Publishing, 1987.

6

. . . .

Toddlers and Preschoolers: Emerging Independence

Toddlers

PSYCHOLOGICAL DEVELOP-MENT AND FOOD Nutrition and eating concerns are never more prevalent than during the toddler phase of childhood (between 1 and 3 years of age). Babies enter toddlerhood approximately when they celebrate their first birthday or take their first steps. It is generally safe to say that if a child has begun to utter "no" with some regularity or has had a temper tantrum, the child is in the throes of toddlerhood.

The transition from infancy to toddlerhood

> **MYTH** If children eat a snack between lunch and dinner, they won't have room for dinner.
> **FACT** Young children's stomachs have a limited capacity for food, so children frequently need to eat between meals in order to consume an adequate amount of food in a day. Snacks should be healthy and spaced throughout the day.

is often difficult for parents. The once docile, smiling, cooing infant is now an ambulatory, opinionated risk taker with a short attention span. The development of a toddler is characterized by fierce independence and oppositional behavior. In order for children to begin the lengthy process of growing up, they need to achieve some separation from their parents and formulate their own opinions. Some children exhibit toddler-like behavior earlier or later than their peers. And whereas some children have full-blown, frequent tantrums, others exhibit only slight opposition.

. . . .

Elisabeth A. Reilly ▪ Nancy A. Held

But all normal children experience this developmental phase to some degree. Parents should remember that toddlers need to exhibit oppositional behaviors in order to accomplish their developmental tasks. The "terrible twos" are thus normal and necessary.

Eating and feeding can become particularly troublesome for the family of a toddler. Toddlers often exhibit their most fierce independence at mealtime. This is partly because children feel a strong sense of power when they refuse food or demand a favorite snack. They also learn to love the extra attention they receive from their parents when they refuse or demand food. This attention increases when parents become worried that their child will be poorly nourished and thus bargain with the child to eat, give in to the child's demands out of frustration, or otherwise do battle with the child. Such parent-child interactions may lead to continual battles over food, because toddlers by nature will oppose parental demands time and time again.

Toddlers tend to like certain foods for a period of time and then move on to another favorite. These "food fads" may mean that a child one day refuses the food he or she loved the day before. The best way to introduce a new food to a toddler is to serve it along with a favorite food when the child is hungry. The new food may have to be presented numerous times before the toddler agrees to try it. Toddlers can be overwhelmed by large quantities of food, so they should be served small amounts on a small plate with a suction cup on the bottom. Toddlers do not like very cold or very hot food, and hot food also poses serious burn risks. Tepid food or food at room temperature is much preferred. Toddlers particularly enjoy colorful or interesting-looking foods, such as sandwiches cut into shapes with a cookie cutter.

PHYSICAL DEVELOPMENT AND FOOD During toddlerhood the rapid growth of infancy slows and the child's appetite decreases. Often toddlers would much rather play than eat. When they finally want to eat, they may be interested in staying at the table only for 5–10 minutes, and most toddlers will consume meals or snacks in less than 15 minutes. When they are done eating, they will play with or throw their food, begin to make a mess, or otherwise act out to let parents know that they are bored with the meal. Some children will ask to be let down from the table; it is wise to accede to these requests because the children most likely have had enough to eat. In some cases, toddlers will return a bit later to take a few more bites. Dessert may be offered at this time or even during the meal in order to avoid giving children the idea that meals should be eaten in order to earn dessert.

Toddlers' nervous and muscular systems are more developed than infants', so they have better coordination and can begin to feed themselves. Self-feeding is part of being independent, yet toddlers will not achieve neatness and accuracy for some time. At first they will use their hands to pick up food. The textures, colors, and appearance of food are relatively new to them, and they will want to explore. By the preschool years, however, proficiency with small utensils will be achieved. Parents can help toddlers learn to feed themselves by providing foods that are easy to manage and simple to pick up with a spoon or fingers. Waterproof bibs and plastic sheeting or newspapers under the high chair will decrease clean-up time. Cups with safety lids are a must, and offering only a few ounces of beverage at one time is helpful, too.

Chewing becomes easier as the first molars erupt in the second year, and tougher foods can then be managed, as the child can produce a rotary jaw action to grind the foods into pieces small enough for swallowing. Safety is still a concern, however, and parents and caregivers must be vigilant about providing appropriate foods and cutting firm or hard foods into small pieces.

DIVISION OF RESPONSIBILITY Parents are responsible for presenting their children's food, and toddlers are responsible for eating it. Force-feeding is never appropriate for children. When considering a toddler's food intake, parents should think in terms of a 24-hour day rather than in terms of one meal or snack. Children need not eat a large variety of foods at one sitting, but they should have a good variety within a day.

The timing of meals and snacks is important. Although some flexibility is necessary, a consistent routine of eating helps toddlers regulate their appetite. The predictability of mealtime is also emotionally reassuring for young eaters. Having an appropriate chair or booster seat for the child is also advisable, as is using a favorite cup, bowl, or utensil. Make sure that a toddler's little hands can hold and manage the cup or utensils.

Certain rituals of eating may be imperative for children, and toddlers can become extremely dependent on routine. Drinking a cup of milk after eating, for example, may become a routine that cannot be changed without upsetting the toddler. Parents should be sure that they can live with a developing routine before it becomes an important ritual.

Parents of toddlers can often avoid food battles by presenting a child with limited choices. At snack time, for example, it is better to offer such options as crackers and pretzels than to ask toddlers what they want to eat. If parents cannot or do not wish to offer a choice of foods, they can simply state that it is time to eat. The choice for the child then becomes whether or not to eat, and parents need to keep in mind that this is the child's decision, not the parents'. Giving the child the choice between favorite plates or cups may encourage eating or drinking when food and beverage choices are not available. Offering limited choices teaches the child to take some responsibility for eating and shows respect for the child's ability to make decisions.

Because toddlers generally do not serve themselves and often have a small appetite, parents should not insist that their child eat everything on the plate. Children will learn to decide when they have eaten enough only by having control over their intake. An excessively poor appetite, however, may be caused by illness or emotional stress, so parents should consult their child's health care provider if they fear their toddler is not eating enough. Healthy, normal children eat enough food. Often, parents who believe that their child is not eating enough are reasssured to see the gains on the child's growth chart during a routine checkup (see chapter 1).

Taking the time and expending creative energy to encourage good eating habits will pay off. Creating a relaxed atmosphere at meals, remaining flexible and tolerant of toddlers' behavior, and setting gentle, firm limits will ensure that the child's developmental needs are met. The result will be a more cooperative and happy eater, which will set the tone for the child to continue developing an emotionally healthy outlook on nutrition and eating in the years to come.

DEVELOPMENTAL ACHIEVEMENTS The following list summarizes the behavior that toddlers can be expected to exhibit:

- Toddlers show an interest in feeding themselves.
- They will use hands and fingers to pick up foods.

- They like warm foods, not hot or cold ones.
- They begin to chew and grind foods, especially when molars erupt.
- Older toddlers learn to stab food with a dull fork.
- Toddlers can hold a cup to drink.
- They will drink more from a cup with a lid than from a cup with an open top.
- They will spill liquids from a cup, especially before 19 months of age.
- They may frequently refuse certain foods or develop food fads.
- They may prefer nonconventional food combinations.
- They often play with food and create a mess.
- They enjoy mealtime rituals.
- They may tolerate sitting at the table for only 5–10 minutes.
- They will often leave the table and return to eat again, if permitted.
- They have few or no table manners.
- They may throw food when finished eating.
- They need frequent reminders to abide by rules.
- They focus only on their own wishes and desires and are unable to comprehend another's point of view.
- They will imitate parents or siblings.
- They can help with simple meal preparation tasks and limited table setting.
- If given toy plastic dishes or utensils while meal preparation is in progress, they will enjoy imitating the cooking actions of adults.

Preschoolers

DEVELOPMENTAL CONSIDERATIONS AND FOOD Sometime after the terrible twos, children emerge from toddlerhood and enter the imaginary world of the preschooler. From roughly 2½–5 years of age, children go through a busy developmental stage marked by vastly increasing language skills and symbolic play. During this stage, young children are insatiably curious and begin to truly socialize with peers. Often preschoolers spend time in play groups, nursery school, or day care.

For parents, watching the child make the transition from toddler to preschooler is gratifying and fun. It is gratifying to live with a child who is less oppositional, and it is fun to be able to converse in complete sentences with the child. It is a joy to witness the emerging personality of preschoolers, who show their true side during dramatic play. Mealtimes and snacktimes also bring out the pleasantness of preschool children, who are more willing than toddlers to try new foods and want very much to please their parents.

As a result of the changes that occur between toddlerhood and the preschool years, providing a child with a healthy diet becomes easier. Table manners vastly improve as the child seeks to please and imitate adults or older children. The preschooler will be able to sit for longer periods at the table and may even complete an entire meal in one sitting, presuming that the child likes the food and that the meal can be consumed within 15–20 minutes or so. Preschoolers also are gaining skill in using utensils and can feed themselves more neatly and efficiently than before. The child may imaginatively turn the fork into a train and the peas into passengers. Ultimately the bad dinosaur may derail the train and eat all its occupants! Creative parenting may be required to enjoy or at least tolerate such antics, but tolerance will foster a pleasant mealtime environment and produce a well-nourished child.

TODDLERHOOD REVISITED In spite of the preschooler's renewed interest in food, food fads and food refusal frequently recur during this time. Children predictably return to previous developmental stages when tired or under stress. Fortunately, such periods are generally temporary, and the preschooler will continue to make developmental progress in spite of a few setbacks.

When the preschool child exhibits toddler-like behavior or eating habits, it is best to remain flexible. There is no harm in indulging a food fad as long as the desired food is healthy and contributes to a balanced diet. Eating only peanut butter on crackers for lunch instead of a variety of sandwiches is not harmful to the child's health. Soon the child will once again accept a more varied diet. Similarly, the preschooler may occasionally refuse certain foods and ask parents to prepare another meal. In this case, it is wise to encourage the child to try the offending food, but parents should neither demand that the child eat what is offered nor prepare an entirely different meal. The child can be given a simply prepared equivalent such as a sandwich if chicken and rice are refused.

DEVELOPING TASTES As young children develop a heightened interest in new foods, parents can encourage the development of the young palate. It is not unusual for a young child to refuse new foods initially, but he or she generally will accept them after a period of repeated presentations. Food acceptance will be more likely if the preschooler sees other family members and peers eating the new food. A food that a four-year-old hated one day may be eagerly consumed the next day after the child sees friends enjoying it at nursery school.

A calm and enjoyable mealtime environment will encourage children to accept new foods and develop healthy eating habits. Suggestions for making preschoolers' meals pleasurable for the child and family are listed below:

- Serve meals and snacks on a predictable but flexible schedule.
- Prepare relatively simple meals.
- Use the child's favorite plate, bowl, cup, and utensils.
- Present the child with small portions on a small plate.
- Give the child a small amount to drink at one time.
- Allow the child to ask for more food and drink.
- Tolerate mealtime messiness as the child learns to eat independently and neatly.
- Focus attention and conversation on the preschooler to increase the child's interest in staying at the table.
- Give the child 1–2 minutes of uninterrupted time to share the events of the day.
- Allow the child to leave the table when he or she has finished eating (or between courses, if they are long).
- Do not insist that the child finish the meal before having dessert. Consider serving dessert with the meal to deemphasize dessert.
- Praise the child for trying new foods and for exhibiting appropriate behavior at the table.
- Use mealtimes as opportunities to compliment the child for any good behaviors, good deeds, or nice work performed that day.

As preschoolers experience a widening social circle, the outside world increasingly influences their food interests. Television advertising has a dramatic impact on children, and several food producers and restaurants market their products directly to the preschool audience. Once a child realizes that such things as candy and soda exist, the nutritional challenge begins. The child may constantly request sweets. But there are important reasons to control preschoolers' access to sweets, high-fat snacks, and fast foods. The nutritional content of these foods is generally inadequate: they supply a disproportionate amount of sugar and fat compared to other nutrients. Young children have small appetites and will not eat nutritious foods if their intake of sweets and high-fat snacks is high. Sweets and many starchy foods also predispose children to dental caries (cavities).

Sweets, fast foods, and snacks that are high in sugar and fat need not be forbidden, however. It is best not to offer these foods daily, but there is little harm in a treat a few times a week. An excursion to a fast food restaurant (see chapter 39) is fun for the family, and an occasional dessert or chips with a sandwich are tasty. Children will learn through example that moderation is the key ingredient to a successful, healthy diet.

Ultimately, parents have two goals in providing good nutrition to the preschooler: to promote good health and normal growth, and to establish healthy life-long eating habits. Young children who eat well will feel better and will have more energy to play and learn. Moreover, children who learn healthy eating habits early are more likely to make wise food selections as they get older.

DEVELOPMENTAL ACHIEVEMENTS The following list summarizes the behavior that preschool children can be expected to exhibit:

- Preschool children begin to use small spoons and forks well.
- They can use a dull knife awkwardly.
- They need assistance with cutting food.
- They can drink from a cup without a lid.
- They can learn to serve themselves from a platter or dish.
- They can pour a small amount of liquid independently.
- They begin to eat neatly with no help.
- They show increased interest in trying new foods.

- Often they dislike foods mixed together and prefer each food in a separate section of their plate.
- Preschoolers will use simple table manners.
- They can remain at the table for 10–15 minutes.
- They may prefer to sit at a small table with other children if given a choice.
- They enjoy helping to set or clear the table.
- They may demand specific foods.
- Food fads and food strikes may reappear or linger.
- Frequently they may prefer play to eating.
- They may risk being rude to gain attention or to dominate mealtime conversation.

Family Meals and Holidays during Toddler and Preschool Years

As children grow, develop, and reach adulthood, some of their most vivid memories may be of family meals. Some people will fondly remember such events as imitating a waiter and landing spaghetti on the ceiling, or hiding broccoli in their socks. Others will less fondly remember being required to stay at the table until they cleaned their plates. Parents thus have the opportunity to reflect on how best to create a good mealtime and snacktime atmosphere. Mealtimes are often the best opportunity for a family to socialize (see chapter 9). Family meals provide a chance for children to learn good eating habits. But families may not follow traditional meal patterns and yet still be equally well nourished and emotionally intact.

Holidays offer another opportunity for the child to learn about new foods and the social relevance of eating. Parents may find that holiday meals are more pleasant if adults remain flexible about what a young child eats. The child will generally be excited during a holiday and often will have a decreased interest in eating or be more inclined to snack between meals, perhaps at holiday parties. One approach to assuring good nutrition is to offer such healthy snacks as cheese, crackers, and fruit and to serve fruit punch instead of soda. Adults can encourage children to try these snacks and drinks by serving them on paper goods with a popular theme (Disney characters, for example).

Another method of providing optimal nutrition on holidays is to offer the child a good breakfast. Consuming a healthful variety of foods at breakfast will supply the child with important nutrients in the morning, so parents can be less concerned about what the child eats when the holiday celebration begins.

Adventures in Eating

Cooking and preparing food with a child is another way to teach good nutrition and a healthy attitude toward eating. Children are fascinated by the process of creating a particular dish or meal and will love being included in an activity normally performed by adults. Depending on their age, children can help measure, mix, and, of course, taste! Preschoolers, because of their emerging interest in imaginary play, will also enjoy playing the part of a grown-up cook. Another advantage to cooking with children is the opportunity to spend time with them while accomplishing necessary food preparation.

Safety must be the first and most important consideration when cooking with children. Toddlers and preschool children should not be permitted to use the stove or electrical appliances, even under strict supervision. Knives and other sharp utensils must be placed out of reach.

Another food-related task that can be shared with young children is a trip to the grocery store. For most parents, this outing is not enjoyable. Pre-

schoolers may incessantly request items they have seen advertised on television. The children may be fidgety or bored, and may often act out, especially when parents are rushed, bored with the job themselves, and frustrated by the child's behavior. Nonetheless, there is much a parent can do to make this task tolerable and even enjoyable for children and parents. Below are some tips for shopping with young children; see chapter 37 for more information.

- Go shopping when neither parents nor children are hungry or irritable.
- Minimize time spent looking for items by making a list ahead of time.
- Have coupons organized before leaving the house.
- Buckle toddlers securely into the grocery cart seat.
- Pack toys to keep children amused.
- Set up clear rules about behavior during shopping (e.g., no climbing out of the cart, no asking for candy), and praise children for following the rules.
- Enlist children's help in looking for items.
- Play a math or letter game with preschool children: have them look for certain numbers, letters, or colors on food items.
- Talk to children about what is being purchased.
- Do not rush the children. Preschoolers love to look around and discuss what they see.

Eating out at a restaurant may also be an enjoyable family adventure. Children can learn to choose from a menu, try out newly acquired table manners, and have fun socializing with parents who are not preoccupied with meal preparation. To eat out inexpensively, families may choose fast food restaurants or may go out for breakfast or lunch instead of dinner. Toddlers and preschoolers may have difficulty if the wait to eat is long or if too much emphasis is placed on perfect manners in the restaurant. In some cases, particularly pizza establishments, parents can call in their order before leaving home so that the meal is likely to be served shortly after the family arrives. When calling ahead is not possible, it is wise to take along such nutritious snacks as cheese cubes, small carrots, or crackers for the child to eat while waiting for the meal. Many restaurants will provide crackers or bread on request. Another way to amuse a child before food arrives is with crayons and paper.

To avoid spills and embarrassment, parents could ask the server for a plastic cup with a top and a straw for toddlers and preschoolers. Many establishments are happy to comply with this request. In a more formal restaurant such cups are less likely to be available, so plan to take a cup from home.

Another wonderful outing is a visit to a farm, to give young children an idea of where food comes from. At a dairy farm, children will enjoy seeing how cows are milked and how the milk is processed. They might learn about making butter, cheeses, or ice cream. At farms that grow crops, children will learn, for example, that carrots come out of the dirt. Many dairy and vegetable farms sell their products on site, giving children the opportunity to taste the foods they have seen grown or made. And at many orchards, families can pick their own fruit or vegetables.

Nutritional Considerations

In comparison to infancy, physical growth slows tremendously in the toddler and preschooler. Although growth progresses steadily, it can be erratic in some children. Some 2-year-olds still fit into outfits from the previous year, while others experience growth spurts after a period of no growth.

The amount of weight children gain varies, but the following table shows average rates of growth:

Age	Weight gain in lbs (kg) per year	Growth in inches (cm) per year
1–2 years	5–6 (2.7)	4–5 (10.2–12.7)
2–5 years	4–6 (1.8–2.7)	2–3 (3.4–7.6)

Children are more active after the first year as they become more coordinated. By age 2 they are running and even climbing. This physical activity helps straighten and strengthen their legs. Abdominal and back muscles tighten to support an upright toddler. Into the preschool years, arms and legs continue to lengthen and increase in muscle strength.

The growth of children is plotted on growth charts when they are weighed and measured at health care visits (see chapter 1 and growth charts appendix). During the first 2 years of life the growth percentiles of a child may change. For example, the height of an infant at 6 months may be at the 50th percentile, and at 18 months the height may be at the 25th percentile. After about 2 years, established growth patterns normalize and growth generally proceeds along the same percentile. If a 2-year-old is at the 25th percentile for height, at age 4 he or she will probably still be at the 25th percentile.

The Recommended Dietary Allowances (RDAs) are nutrient allowances that include a margin of safety above normal requirements for most healthy children (see the tables in the appendix). If a child is taking in less than the recommended allowance of a particular nutrient, the child's intake is not necessarily inadequate. Although recommendations are stated as amounts to be ingested daily, they really represent averages

TABLE 6.1
Protein and Energy Needs of Toddlers and Preschoolers

Age (years)	Calories needed daily		Calories needed daily	Protein needed	
	per kg	per lb		g/kg	g/day
1–3	102	46	900–1,800	1.2	16
4–6	90	41	1,300–2,300	1.1	24

over a few days or even a week. The child who eats poorly one day will often make up for it the next day. Additionally, children who are the same age and sex can have different nutrient intakes because of their different sizes and levels of physical activity.

CALORIES Parents often wonder what the right amount of food is for their child. The answer varies with the individual child; let the child's appetite dictate intake. During a growth spurt, a child will be hungrier than usual in an effort obtain the extra calories needed for growth (see chapter 27). Toddlers and preschoolers take in more calories than infants because they are bigger, but they need fewer calories per pound because they are growing more slowly. Girls and boys do not require different amounts of calories until age 10. Parents need to remember that a wide range of caloric intake is considered normal (table 6.1).

PROTEIN Protein is essential for normal growth (see chapter 28). Some parents worry about protein intake when their toddler doesn't seem to eat much meat. But it is fairly easy for a young child to obtain enough protein. If a toddler drinks 2 cups of milk and eats 1 ounce of meat per day, he or she is obtaining a sufficient amount of protein. For a preschooler, 2 cups of milk and 2 ounces of meat provide ample protein for one day. Protein defi-

ciency among children is rare in the United States. Many children eat more protein than the minimal requirements. Only extremely picky eaters, strict vegetarians (who eat no eggs or milk), or children with multiple food allergies are at risk for protein deficiency.

FAT Young children need fat in their diets to supply enough calories for growth and to meet their needs for essential fatty acids. It is not appropriate for children under 2 years of age to eat a low-fat diet. Skim or low-fat milk should thus not be given until after age 2. At that point, lowering fat intake to 30 percent of total calories (which is recommended for adults) is acceptable. It is important not to go much lower than that, because fat is necessary for normal growth and development. It is not realistic to expect a toddler to eat a low-fat diet every day. During the toddler years, parents can begin to provide low-fat food choices. By the time a child is 4 or 5 years old, he or she will adjust to and enjoy nutritious low-fat foods if they are consistently served.

MINERALS The mineral that most concerns health care providers of young children is iron. Children need a lot of iron because, as they grow, the amount of hemoglobin in their blood is increasing (iron is one component used to form the hemoglobin molecule). Until age 3, children are

TABLE 6.2
Alternative Foods for Picky Eaters

Alternatives to vegetables
- Sources of vitamin A: apricots, cantaloupe, mangoes, plums, prunes, watermelon
- Sources of vitamin C: grapefruit, oranges, strawberries

Alternatives to milk (foods high in calcium)
- Mozzarella string cheese (part skim), other mild cheese (American, Camembert cubes, mild cheddar), cottage cheese
- Yogurt
- Green leafy vegetables
- Calcium-fortified orange juice

Alternatives to meat (foods high in protein)
- Cooked dried beans
- Peanut butter
- Eggs, mild fish (salmon, flaked tuna, low-fat fish sticks, scallops, shrimp)
- Nuts (including peanuts)
- Milk and cheese

---

at potential risk for iron-deficiency anemia. After their first year, as children eat more table foods, they don't eat iron-fortified baby cereal as much as they previously did. If iron-fortified cereal is not replaced with such iron-rich foods as chicken, ground beef, or fortified breakfast cereals, iron-deficiency anemia can result. Chewable vitamins with iron are available if a child's diet is deficient in iron. These vitamin and iron supplements may be useful for toddlers and preschoolers who have a vegetarian diet.

Calcium, another mineral of importance in children's diets, is essential for building and maintaining growing bone. It is obtained primarily from milk and other dairy products. Children who don't drink milk may not be taking in sufficient calcium. Alternative sources of calcium are shown in table 6.2.

What Should a Child Eat?

The Food Guide Pyramid can be used to help select food for children (see chapter 4). Serving sizes are necessarily small for young children. Generally, 1 tablespoon per year of age or ¼–½ of the adult serving size (use whichever guide seems to work with a particular food) is an appropriate serving for a toddler or preschooler (table 6.3). As a child grows, parents will have a good idea of how much is appropriate.

BREAD, CEREAL, RICE, AND PASTA The group at the base of the pyramid includes such foods as bread, crackers, pasta, cereal, rice, pretzels, English muffins, pancakes, and waffles. Foods in this group provide the bulk of calories and supply carbohydrates, B vitamins, and some iron. Children generally like foods from this food group. Whole

TABLE 6.3
Suggested Portion Sizes and Number of Servings per Day for Toddlers and Preschoolers

Food group	Servings per day	Food	Approximate portion size	
			Toddlers	Preschoolers
Bread, cereal, rice, and pasta	6	Bread	¼–½ slice	½ slice
		Rice or pasta	¼ cup	⅓ cup
		Hot cereal	¼ cup	⅓ cup
		Cold cereal	¼ cup	⅓ cup
Vegetables	3	Cooked vegetables	2 tbsp	¼ cup
		Raw vegetables	2 tbsp	¼ cup
Fruits	2	Fresh fruit	2 tbsp	¼ cup
		Fruit juice	¼ cup	½ cup
		Canned fruit	¼ cup	½ cup
Milk, yogurt, and cheese	3–4	Milk or yogurt	½ cup	¾ cup
		Cheese	1 oz	1½ oz
Meat, poultry, fish, beans, eggs, and nuts	2–3	Meat	1 oz	1½ oz
		Cooked beans	2 tbsp	¼ cup
		Egg	½	1
		Peanut butter	1 tbsp	2 tbsp

grains add fiber and such minerals as zinc and magnesium.

FRUITS AND VEGETABLES The fruit group and vegetable group are on the same level in the Food Guide Pyramid. The foods in these groups are good sources of vitamins A and C, and they contain small amounts of calcium, B vitamins, iron, and trace minerals. Fruits and vegetables are low in calories. The pyramid suggests 3–5 servings of vegetables and 2–4 servings of fruit per day. But fruits and fruit juices can be substituted for vegetables if children do not like them, to ensure that the children take in adequate amounts of vitamins A and C (see table 6.2).

There seems to be no good reason why many children don't like vegetables, which are rich in nutrients and an important component of a healthy diet. To increase the chances a child will eat vegetables, parents should serve vegetables 1–2 times every day, should never force or bribe a child to eat vegetables (or any food), should offer a variety of vegetables (both raw and cooked), and should set an example by eating vegetables themselves. Children will eventually accept that vegetables are a typical part of meals at their house.

Juice, which is included in the fruit group, should be offered only in small amounts, as too much juice may cause a child not to be hungry for meals. A reasonable amount of juice is 4–8 ounces per day. Most juices, even the "natural" ones, do not supply many nutrients. Orange juice and juices fortified with vitamin C and calcium are good choices. Toddlers should be given their first juice in a cup, not a bottle, because juice drunk from a bottle can bathe the teeth in sugar for relatively long periods of time, which contributes to dental caries. Additionally, if a child is accustomed to taking juice in a bottle, it becomes more difficult to discontinue the bottle.

MILK, YOGURT, AND CHEESE All the foods in this group provide protein, calcium, vitamin D, and riboflavin. Calcium is provided primarily by this food group. Toddlers and preschoolers should consume approximately 2–3 cups (16–24 ounces) of milk or the equivalent each day. The serving size for toddlers is 4 ounces of milk or yogurt and 1 ounce of cheese. It is unrealistic to expect a 2-year-old to drink 8 ounces of milk (which is the adult portion) at one time, although some children do. Combination foods, such as pizza, provide both protein and calcium from cheese.

Some children prefer juice to milk. And some toddlers will drink milk only from a bottle. Parents of these children often continue bottle-feeding long past the time the child is able to manage a cup. This is not necessarily the best approach. Milk should be an integral part of structured meals and snacks. One suggestion is to serve milk in a cup with every meal, and juice at one or two snacks. Children will then expect to see milk at meals. For those who follow kosher dietary practices, a routine of offering milk with meatless snacks can be established.

Many parents discontinue bottle- or breast-feeding at around 1 year, when babies begin to eat an increasing amount of table food and become less interested in milk feedings (see chapter 5). There is no "right" time to wean a child, however. If toddlers are still drinking from a bottle or breast, they should be offered the bottle or breast for snacks or before bedtime only, because a bottle with meals (before or after) will decrease the toddler's food intake at meals. During the weaning process, parents may see an overall reduction in milk consumption, because a child initially does not drink as much milk from a cup as she or he had from the bottle or breast. But this is not a reason to discontinue weaning. Milk intake will increase gradually if milk is offered regularly in a cup.

Most children eventually drink cow's milk from a cup if they are not pressured. For those children who are learning to manage a cup or those who have milk allergies, alternative foods that are high in calcium are appropriate (see table 6.2). Some yogurts, however, now contain added products—such as chocolate chips, or granola in a small package attached to the yogurt container—that supply extra sugar and fat. As an alternative, parents can try putting fresh fruit in plain yogurt.

Prolonged or excessive milk feeding is not desirable. Overconsumption (like overconsumption of juice) can replace other nutrients and interfere with a child's normal developmental progression. If a child is very picky at meals, evaluate how much juice and milk the child is drinking. If a toddler sips a bottle while falling asleep, the sugar in the milk can promote dental caries (see chapter 16). Breast- or bottle-feeding is fine for a before-bed snack but should not be used to put a child to sleep, because the toddler may associate the bottle or breast with sleep and may ultimately develop sleep problems.

MEAT, POULTRY, FISH, BEANS, EGGS, AND NUTS The foods in this group are good sources of protein, iron, B vitamins, and such trace minerals as zinc. A serving for a toddler is about 1 ounce of meat, 2 tablespoons of cooked beans, ½ egg, or 1 tablespoon of peanut butter. For preschoolers, a serving is 1½ ounces of meat, ¼ cup of beans, 1 egg, or 2 tablespoons peanut butter. Many young children like such processed meats as hot dogs, chicken nuggets, and lunch meats because they are tender and easy to chew. Unfortunately, they are usually high in fat and sodium. These foods are acceptable to serve occasionally (1–2 times a week), if they are balanced on other days with such lower-fat choices as low-fat hot dogs and turkey meats. Lean ground beef or ground turkey are well accepted in the form of meatloaf or hamburgers. Although parents should be sure not to overcook chicken or other meats because they become tough and difficult to chew, undercooking meat and eggs is dangerous because of the risk of food-borne illness. Cut meat into small pieces, especially for toddlers. If toddlers and preschoolers do not like meat or poultry, acceptable alternatives are available (see table 6.2).

Remember, portions for little people are little. Don't expect your toddler to eat a 4-ounce hamburger on a bun, French fries, carrots, and a glass of milk. Preschoolers and especially kindergarteners can be extremely active and certainly may eat this meal. A 2- or 3-year-old will do better with a hamburger cut into bite-sized pieces and bread or a bun on the side.

FATS, OILS, AND SWEETS The top section of the Food Guide Pyramid includes such items as oil, margarine, butter, jelly, salad dressing, candy, doughnuts, chips, and soft drinks. Fruit snacks and whipped topping also belong in this section. These foods primarily contribute fat or sugar to the diet. Items in this group are acceptable but should be used only occasionally. Remember, foods in other food groups may also contain fat and sugar.

Snacking

Well-chosen snacks between meals help meet caloric needs. Young children have a limited stom-

ach capacity and cannot eat enough in three meals to meet their caloric requirements. Generally, they need to eat every 3–4 hours. Snacking too often, however, prevents a child from developing an appetite and eating well at meals. At least 1½–2 hours should pass between meals and snacks. Otherwise, whatever eating schedule works for each family is right for them.

Snack time can easily turn into a free-for-all, particularly with older preschoolers. It is important for parents and caregivers to control when, what, and how snacks are offered. Snacks may provide about ¼ of a child's total caloric intake in a day. They can be from any food group or combination of food groups (see the box "Suggestions for Nutritious Snacks"). The type of snack offered should depend on when the next meal will be eaten. If a meal is in 1½ hours, a piece of fruit is probably enough. But if the next meal is 3 hours away, a snack of crackers and low-fat milk may be more appropriate. By the same token, if a preschooler has been playing outside all afternoon, a more substantial snack may be needed. Children given no guidelines may request "empty calorie" snacks. Offering two to three items allows a child choice (and some control) and also enables parents to set a standard for appropriate (nutritious) snacks.

Snacks should be an integral part of the daily eating schedule. Children should sit in the kitchen or designated eating area, just as they do for meals. A snack should not consist of cookies in front of the television, or a gooey doughnut consumed in the supermarket to make shopping easier. Snack time should have a beginning and an end. Just as at mealtime, when the child is finished eating or sitting, snack time is completed. Allowing children to walk around the house with food is not only messy but also promotes poor eating behaviors. When a snack on the run is unavoidable, parents

Suggestions for Nutritious Snacks

Fresh fruit
Apple slices
Banana slices
Grapes (sliced)
Orange or grapefruit sections
Peach, nectarine, and pear slices
Plums (pitted)
Strawberries

Dried fruit
Apples
Apricots
Dates (pitted)
Peaches
Pears
Prunes (pitted)
Raisins*

Milk group
Cheese sticks and cubes
Cottage cheese
Frozen yogurt
Milk
Sherbet
Yogurt

Bread group
Bagels
Bread
Cookies
Crackers (saltines, whole-grain crackers,
    graham crackers, animal crackers)
Dry cereals
Popcorn*
Pretzels
Rice cakes

Vegetable group
Baby carrots*
Broccoli florets
Cauliflower
Celery*
Cucumber slices
Green beans*
Zucchini
(All vegetables can be served plain or with dip)

Meat group
Hard-boiled egg
Peanut butter

*Not appropriate for toddlers

---

should try to make the snack nutritious and limited to a specified amount (pretzels in a sandwich bag, not the family-sized bag of potato chips).

Food and Safety

Food served to children must be developmentally appropriate to assure safety. Foods that are small, hard, and not easily dissolved are potential choking hazards. Toddlers should not eat the following foods:

Big pieces of hot dog	Raw carrots
Jelly beans	Seeds
Nuts	Small hard candies
Popcorn	Tough meat
Raisins	Whole grapes

To help prevent choking, parents can quarter grapes, slice hot dogs, and cook carrots to make them tender. A number of mealtime rules promote safety and comfort for all ages. Mealtime should be pleasant and calm. Children should sit while eating. Jumping, running, screaming, or laughing can cause a child to inhale food and choke. An adult should be present while young children are eating.

Eating contaminated food can cause fever, vomiting, diarrhea, and dehydration. Routine sanitary precautions are generally common sense. Children should wash their hands before and after meals, after using the toilet, and after handling pets or other animals, to prevent the spread of bacteria.

Proper handling of raw meats is important, particularly because children are more vulnerable than adults to bacterial infection from contaminated food. Safe-handling labels appear on all raw and partially precooked meat and poultry. At the supermarket, raw meats should not be put in the same bag as fresh produce. Raw meat should be frozen or refrigerated quickly after shopping. Don't thaw frozen food on the countertop for more than two hours, even during the winter months. Separate cutting boards should be used for raw meats and raw produce; plastic or glass cutting boards are preferable to wood. By establishing safe habits of food preparation, parents will reduce the risk of contamination while teaching their children to handle food safely.

Resources

Fraiberg, S. H. *The Magic Years.* New York: Charles Scribner's Sons, 1959.

Leach, P. *Your Baby and Child: From Birth to Age Five.* New York: Alfred A. Knopf, 1993.

Nissenberg, N. K., M. L. Bogle, E. P. Langholz, and A. C. Wright. *How Should I Feed My Child?* Minneapolis, MN: Chronimed Publishing, 1993.

Satter, E. *Child of Mine: Feeding with Love and Good Sense.* Palo Alto, CA: Bull Publishing, 1986.

———. *How to Get Your Kid to Eat . . . but Not Too Much.* Palo Alto, CA: Bull Publishing, 1986.

7

. . . .

School-Age, Preadolescent Children:
An Apple a Day

The school-age child presents new nutritional challenges for parents. According to a national survey, most school-age children in the United States eat at least five times a day, and almost all eat at least three times daily. The challenge, then, is for parents to influence their school-age child's food choices even though the parents are no longer able to control the choices directly. Parents must ensure that their children eat a balanced diet at home and at school, and also avoid battles over food selection and mealtimes. In many ways, the school-age preadolescent child is the ideal child to parent. The tantrums of the toddler stage are left behind, and the rebellion of adolescence

MYTH Fish is brain food.

FACT Fish provides many essential nutrients and is an excellent food choice, but it does not have any special effects on brain development or learning.

has yet to come. School-age preadolescents are interested and inquisitive and often will listen to and believe what their parents tell them. But this period is not without its conflicts. Mealtime problems can and do occur at every age, but once a child attends school, issues can become more complicated. Lunch or breakfast may be provided by the school or taken to school, and parents often do not know whether their child eats these meals. Some common food-related clashes between school-age children and their parents involve eating breakfast, composing school lunches (and deciding whether lunches are taken to school or purchased there), eating vegetables, and select-

. . . .

Ronald Angoff ▪ Kathy French

ing beverages. The best way for parents to approach such conflicts is to choose one or two problem areas they would most like to address.

Caloric Requirements

The school-age, preadolescent child grows at a slower pace than either the infant or the teenager. Considerable individual variation in growth patterns is determined by both genetic and environmental factors. Periods of relatively rapid growth and periods without growth require a respective increase or decrease in the energy requirements for a particular child. The activity level of a child also affects caloric requirements. There are even differences in caloric needs among children who are at rest or performing the same task. The health of a child may affect caloric requirements, as well. A chronically ill child requires additional energy for basic metabolic processes and for fighting the illness itself. Guidelines for caloric intake are based on standard growth patterns and provide sufficient calories for all but the very active or very ill child (see chapter 27).

Meals and Snacks

Ideally, a child should eat a well-balanced breakfast, lunch, and dinner, and two or three small snacks a day.

BREAKFAST Breakfast is essential for school-age children, and it is important to allot adequate time in the morning routine for a good breakfast. Studies consistently indicate that children who skip a morning meal have difficulty concentrating in the classroom. Children who say that they don't feel like eating when they first get up because their stomachs do not feel right should take food along with them to eat on the way to school. Sandwiches or low-fat granola bars with juice boxes are examples of nutritious portable breakfasts. To make breakfast time go smoothly, parents can prepare breakfast food in the evening, or before the child wakes up in the morning.

LUNCH Lunchtime is a perfect opportunity to provide a child with a balanced meal. A typical lunch of a protein-rich sandwich with fresh fruit and milk combines all the food groups (see chapter 4) in a compact package. But the pressure of the school lunchroom may interfere with the best eating habits.

Ideally, lunch should provide a fruit or vegetable, milk or another dairy product, meat or a meat substitute, and bread. The U.S. Department of Agriculture is working on making school lunches and breakfasts healthier and better tasting. The increasing awareness of the dangers of excess salt and fat in children's diets has led to the inclusion of lower-fat entrées in school menus. When children are given brief explanations of the benefits of these changes, they choose low-fat offerings with surprising frequency.

Concerns have been raised regarding the increased availability of vending-machine snacks in the lunchroom. Schools and parents need to evaluate carefully the nutritional value of items offered in these vending machines (see chapter 38).

A child who buys a school lunch may actually eat more balanced noon meals than a child who takes lunch to school, if the brown-bag lunch consistently contains foods that are high in fat or sugar, such as cold cuts, chips, and snack cakes. Children who take their lunches to school should be involved in food selection. Be creative. Leftover chicken breast or yogurt with fresh fruit may be a welcome change, especially if the child has chosen his or her own food.

SNACKS Small, quick snacks are advisable in the mid-morning and mid-afternoon to prevent hunger pangs and provide energy. After-school snacks are often a source of excess calories, fat, salt, or sugar in the form of chips, doughnuts, cupcakes, and candy. Having such foods as pretzels, crackers, fresh fruit, and yogurt readily available will promote healthier snacking.

DINNER Much writing about the trends in family dining has focused on the family dinner, or lack thereof. Two working parents or a single parent are not likely to have the time to prepare a three-course dinner midweek. But keeping pre-cut fresh vegetables, fruits, and pasta on hand can help parents avoid the fast food dinner trend. Other strategies include making extra servings to ensure leftovers, cooking some weekday meals on weekends, setting up a Crock-Pot in the morning for a fast evening meal. The goal is for dinner to provide a combination of vegetables, milk products, meat or a meat substitute, fruit, and bread.

These are guidelines for meal composition, so parents should not worry if they are not followed at every meal. If a child consistently avoids an entire food group, parents should make up missing nutrients from other sources. For instance, if a child avoids meat, cheese and milk could supply added protein.

Vitamins and Minerals

The Recommended Dietary Allowances (RDAs) suggest a safe level for each vitamin and mineral, which takes into consideration not only the age and growth requirements of a child but also the incremental increase in needs when a child experiences a growth spurt (see growth charts appendix). Any child who consumes foods from all food groups on a daily basis will meet the RDA's requirements for vitamins and minerals. The fruit and vegetable groups are the main source of ascorbic acid (vitamin C); the milk, yogurt, and cheese group is essential for riboflavin, vitamin B_{12}, niacin, and calcium; the meat, poultry, fish, beans, eggs, and nuts group contains iron-rich foods; and the bread, cereal, rice, and pasta group is a good source of thiamine, pantothenic acid, and pyridoxine (vitamin B_6). Surveys have shown that the nutrients most likely to be lacking in children's diets are calcium, iron, ascorbic acid, vitamin A, folic acid, and pyridoxine.

Approximately one-quarter of school-age children take vitamin or mineral supplements. This practice may provide a false sense of security for the parents of a child who does not eat a balanced diet. Not all commercial children's vitamins are equal, and they may not provide calcium and iron, two of the minerals that are often deficient in children's diets. Moreover, a supplement is an unnecessary expense for a well-nourished child.

Exercise

Exercise is beneficial for the school-age child for several reasons. Active children are more likely to be hungry at mealtime, thus lessening the possibility that they will refuse meals. Exercise also promotes weight control, an important consideration because the risk of developing obesity increases at this preadolescent stage.

Once children enter school, their playtime may be limited to recess (which can be further limited by climate) and physical education classes. It is essential, therefore, to encourage children to ride bicycles, skip rope, skate, or hike for pure enjoyment. Children are far more likely to exercise on a regular basis if their parents exercise as well.

Organized sports provide opportunities to exercise and to learn concepts of team play. Some activities, such as dance, skating, and gymnastics, require leanness, which may lead a child to diet unhealthily to maintain or lose weight. Changes in eating habits or weight should be monitored closely to prevent potentially dangerous practices.

Physiological Problems

Any problem involving a child's health, nutrition, or eating should be discussed with the child's health care provider. One of the most common physiological disturbances in the school-age child is constipation, which can occur after a gastrointestinal virus or from lack of exercise, fiber, or fluid in the diet. A quick, safe remedy is to increase the child's intake of fluids and soluble fiber. Apple juice or almost any other juice is a good fluid, and oat bran is an excellent source of soluble fiber. Children who like hot cereal will consume oat bran readily if it is topped with jelly or cinnamon. Bran cereal can also be used in muffins or cookies to increase the fiber content of the diet (see chapter 34).

When children develop vomiting or diarrhea that is not associated with an obvious acute illness, it is wise to keep a detailed log of the symptom. Such a log helps the child's health care provider identify any allergic, infectious, physical, or emotional factors that may have caused the symptom.

Strategies for Successful Negotiation

Negotiating with a child over food-related issues can require as much skill as diplomatic negotiations at the U.S. State Department. Children must be made to feel as though they have some choice in food selection. Involve the child in developing the weekly or monthly menu. Use the Food Guide Pyramid to illustrate the need for an appropriate balance of foods (see chapter 4). Some children will eat only a severely limited diet. To expand a child's options, take the picky eater to the grocery store once or twice a month to pick out a new vegetable or meat to taste; the child should also decide how to prepare or flavor it. A child who likes Russian dressing, for example, could choose red pepper or cheddar cheese or even turkey breast to dip in the dressing.

A parent should not be a short-order cook, preparing several different entrées in the hope of pleasing the difficult eater. Instead, parents should have on hand a supply of the most nutritious foods their child likes, to be prepared quickly in case the child rejects the dinner menu. In every meal, include one or two foods the child likes. Some experts advocate serving the dessert with the entrée to avoid making it a special reward.

It is not necessary to provide a balanced diet every day, but over the course of a few weeks it should be possible to do so. The key is to empower the child and decrease conflicts. As with all aspects of a child's development, the parent supplies a model for the child's behavior. Good eating habits in a parent is a predictor of good habits in the child.

Resources

Ronamiello, C., N. Van Domelen, and L. H. Tobler. *Off to a Good Start,* 3d ed. Englewood, CA: Wildwood Resources, 1992.

Satter, E. *How to Get Your Kid to Eat . . . but Not Too Much.* Palo Alto, CA: Bull Publishing, 1987.

8

· · · · · · · ·

Adolescence: Life in the Fast Lane

Diversity characterizes the growth patterns, the sequence of sexual maturation, and the nutritional requirements and choices of adolescents. At no other point in their lives are two people of the same age likely to be so different. The most consistent difference among adolescents is that girls' growth spurts begin about two years before those of boys. The growth spurt of adolescent boys and girls can occur at an average age or as much as two years earlier or later than average. Such a growth spurt occurs in no other phase of life and is closely linked to the process of sexual maturation. Both transform a child into an adult,

> **MYTH** Teens are too old for milk.
> **FACT** The teenage years are critical for the deposit of calcium in bones, and milk is the best source of calcium in the diet. Adolescents need 1,200 milligrams of calcium per day, which can be obtained by drinking 4 cups of milk.

and coincidentally involve substantial changes in nutritional requirements.

The Growth Spurt and Sexual Maturation

A speeded-up growth rate of the body, or of any of its parts, is called a growth spurt. On average, girls reach their peak growth rate at about 11½ years, and boys reach theirs at about 13½ years (fig. 8.1). Some girls reach their peak growth rates when they are as young as 9½ years, and some boys have peak growth rates when they are as young as 11½ years. In addition to having higher peak growth

· ·

Teresa Fung ▪ Walter R. Anyan, Jr.

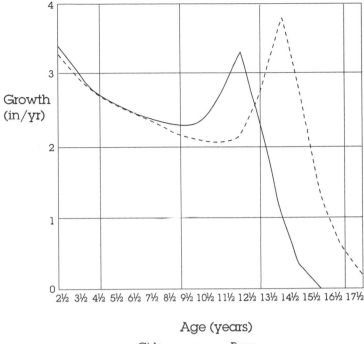

Growth (in/yr) vs **Age (years)**

Girls ———   Boys - - - -

FIGURE 8.1
Average yearly increases in height in
boys and girls.

rates, girls and boys who have early growth spurts also grow at faster rates during childhood than peers who mature later, but those who mature early stop growing sooner. Conversely, girls and boys who have their growth spurts toward the older end of the normal range have lower peak growth rates but continue to grow longer.

The initial phase of the growth spurt is generated, to a great extent, by lengthening of the legs, and this phase is also associated with clear signs of the onset of sexual maturation. Girls usually experience some growth acceleration before they develop their first physical signs of sexual maturation. Slightly before 11 years of age, those who mature at average rates notice some breast development, which begins as the appearance of firm breast tissue beneath the surface of the overlying

areola (the part of the breast visible throughout childhood). In most of these girls, growth of pubic hair follows when they are slightly older than 11; however, it is quite normal for breast and pubic hair development to be simultaneous, or for pubic hair growth to be the first sign of sexual maturation.

The onset of menses is also closely linked to the growth process and will have a lasting impact on the adolescent girl's nutritional requirements. About three years pass between the onset of the growth spurt and the first menstrual period. At an average age of 12½ years, after the peak growth rates have passed and at a time when the growth rates have slowed substantially, girls have their first menstrual periods. Nearly mature breast development and pubic hair growth are present when the first menstrual period, also known as menarche, occurs. The most important nutritional implication of the start of menstruation is that the blood lost during each menstrual period contains iron that must be replenished by the diet.

The first evidence that puberty has begun in boys is a somewhat subtle change, consisting only of growth of the testes. In boys who mature at an average pace, the testes start to enlarge when they are 11½, and at about the same age their growth spurts begin. Noticeable enlargement of the penis and development of pubic hair usually follow a year later, and by that time, further testicular growth will have occurred. Like girls, boys complete the process of sexual maturation as their growth rates are decreasing.

BODY SIZE Before the onset of puberty, boys and girls who are the same age are similar in size. Two years after the onset of puberty, average girls will have reached their peak growth rates and will be 1½ inches taller than average boys. Then the boys start their growth spurts. On average, boys catch up with girls in height by about 14 years of age, and they end up about 5 inches taller than girls.

As the growth spurt in height progresses, body weight increases. Increases in weight are proportionately greater than the changes in height: the weight of average boys and girls at the onset of the growth spurt is only 53–54 percent of the weight of average 18-year-olds.

A practical method of evaluating nutritional adequacy is by monitoring growth. Growth patterns can be tracked on the height and weight growth charts developed by the National Center for Health Statistics (see growth charts appendix). These charts make it possible to compare the progress of an adolescent with others of the same age and sex via percentile rankings (see chapter 1). By using these growth charts, parents and

boys and girls can monitor the growth trend over many years.

BONE GROWTH As bones grow, their dimensions change and alter the shape and size of the maturing body. One noticeable change involves the relation between the widths of the shoulders and the pelvis. As each measurement increases during the growth spurt, boys' shoulder width increases more than their pelvic width, and girls' pelvic width increases more than their shoulder width. Each change contributes to the acquisition of a typical mature shape.

A major increase in the mineral content of the bones also occurs as they grow, and 40–45 percent of the bone mass of young adults is usually acquired during adolescence. When girls are about 10 years old, the mineral content of their bones begins to increase at a much faster rate than it did during childhood, and the accelerated rate continues until girls are about 15. Boys, in keeping with their tendency to develop later than girls, acquire bone mineral most rapidly between 13 and 17 years of age. The crucial mineral involved in this aspect of bone growth is calcium, and optimal intake of calcium must be achieved to assure that bone development is not compromised by an inadequate supply of building material. Bone mineral content is also enhanced by physical activity and vitamin D.

GROWTH IN MUSCLES AND RED BLOOD CELLS In order to grow, muscles require dietary protein and adequate supplies of minerals, particularly iron and zinc. As the body grows, the amount of blood it contains must increase to keep pace with its increasing demands for oxygen. The ability to produce enough red blood cells depends on a good supply of iron. Red blood cells possess the highest concentration of iron of any tissue in the body: 2.2 pounds (1 kilogram) of red blood cells contain 1 gram of iron. The same quantity of muscle contains 1 one-hundredth of a gram of iron. During mid- and late adolescence several of the standard blood counts that measure red blood cells, or hemoglobin, show somewhat higher levels in boys than in girls.

TIMING THE GROWTH SPURT The timing of the growth spurt is influenced by many genetic and environmental factors. First of all, if family members have had growth spurts and sexual maturation relatively early or late, those in subsequent generations generally will follow the same pattern. Good health and good nutrition during childhood are strong positive influences on the rate of growth before and during adolescence and have been responsible for the increasingly early average ages at which growth spurts and sexual maturation have occurred. Menarche, for example, occurred at an average age of 16½ years in the mid-nineteenth century, whereas in the 1990s it occurs at an average age of 12½ years. Although the impact of good health and nutrition seems to have leveled off in children born since 1950 in the United States and many other countries, it is still true that children who weigh more than the average for their height tend to mature early, while those who weigh less than the average for their height mature later. Further, stature tends to increase most rapidly during the spring and summer, while weight either increases at a fairly steady rate over the entire year or undergoes a more rapid increase during the autumn. Growth and development also tend to be somewhat delayed and somewhat slower among children who live at high altitudes.

ENERGY NEEDS For adolescents, as for children and infants, food provides energy, vitamins, and minerals for three main purposes (see chapter 27).

The first purpose is to operate the body while it is at rest. Adolescents of the same age, size, maturity, and sex expend a similar amount of energy while resting. The second purpose is to enable physical activity. The energy required for physical activity varies widely among adolescents, ranging from less than half the energy in an adolescent's diet to a majority of the energy, depending on the intensity and duration of the activity. Generally, the daily energy requirement for physical activity among adolescents is about 1.6–1.7 times the resting energy expenditure. The third purpose of food is to enable growth. But because the other two purposes of energy take priority, growth and the sexual maturation that accompanies it both suffer when nutritional intake falls short of the body's demand. In adolescence, nutritional requirements for growth are highest when growth rates are most rapid. Adolescents who have early growth spurts require more energy to support them than later-maturing adolescents, whose growth spurts are slower. Regardless of when the growth spurt occurs, growth consumes the smallest piece of the nutritional pie, about 100 calories per day.

Cognitive Changes

During adolescence, the child who used to look at teenagers and be unable to comprehend the possibility of having a similarly mature body learns that the process is under way. That realization brings with it a mixture of fascination, delight, and dismay, as the adolescent surveys the changes in body size and shape, compares them with the physical attributes of others, and forms opinions about any apparent differences. For a time, particularly in early and mid-adolescence, girls and boys can be very self-conscious. Adolescents may be especially distressed when they discover features that they believe others will notice and consider unattractive. Weight, because it is thought to be amenable to intervention, often becomes the target of such attention. In general, adolescent girls are likely to think that they weigh more than they do, or to express a desire to weigh less. Boys, in contrast, often overestimate their weight or wish to gain weight.

Such thought processes are not restricted to the contemplation of weight but are part of the acquisition, typically during adolescence, of a new way of thinking. According to the developmental psychologist Jean Piaget, it is usually during adolescence that the ability to think in abstract terms supersedes the ability to think in concrete terms. This development means that a young person considers the body not just as it is but also as it might be. Similarly, adolescents' thoughts about nutrition can easily shift from past and current patterns to an array of possibilities that are not attached to any previous experiences. Adolescents can contemplate the nutritional and aesthetic properties of foods and think about new ways of using them to make meals or snacks, they can anticipate the results that might be obtained by using various combinations, and they can decide which combinations are worth trying. New cognitive skills also make it easier for adolescents to conceptualize such constituents of foods as cholesterol and fiber, to manipulate dietary intake of them skillfully, and to poke fun at others whose diets strike them as less than ideal. Some dietary diversions of adolescents may horrify or amuse parents just as much as changes in other areas of their children's lives do. An adolescent's family may be astonished to discover a nutritional rebel in their midst. The adolescent's peers also exhibit such "deviant" behavior, and parents and younger siblings often believe that the dietary practices of a friend are largely responsible for all the trouble. From time to time, teenagers will discover new diets and wish to try them. As they gain experience, they will decide whether these diets meet their expectations.

Nutritional Requirements

CALORIES (ENERGY) Optimal growth requires an adequate supply of calories (see chapter 27). But it is difficult to determine the exact caloric needs of a teenager, as individual teenagers differ so much in size, activity levels, and growth rates. A growing teenager who competes in sports every day is apt to require many more calories during a week than one who spends a couple of hours each afternoon working as a cashier in a grocery store. The Recommended Dietary Allowance (RDA) of calories during adolescence is 2,500–3,000 calories per day for boys and 2,200 calories per day for girls. These estimates are based on the average caloric intakes of adolescents with average body weights and light activity levels. The recommended calorie intake, then, is best used as a guide, rather than a rigid rule. The best way to judge whether an adolescent is eating the right amount is to monitor the teenager's height and weight gain.

MACRONUTRIENTS Macronutrients include protein, carbohydrates, and fats. Protein is essential for growth, development, and maintenance of the body, and it also provides energy (see chapter 28). One gram of protein yields 4 calories, and protein should constitute a minimum of 7–8 percent of total caloric intake. The RDA for protein varies with body weight, age, and sex (table 8.1).

Fortunately, inadequate protein intake is rarely a problem in developed countries. A 14-year-old who weighs 110 pounds (50 kilograms), for example, needs 50 grams of protein daily. This translates into two 8-ounce glasses of milk (any kind), 3 ounces of meat (a serving that looks about the

TABLE 8.1

Protein Requirements in Adolescence

Age (in years)	Protein requirement (in g) per 2.2 lb (1 kg) of body weight
Boys	
11–14	1.0
15–18	0.9
Girls	
11–14	1.0
15–18	0.8

size of a deck of cards), 2 slices of bread, 1 table-spoon of peanut butter, and a handful of crackers. A typical adolescent would usually eat more than that amount of protein in a day, and 12–14 percent of the calories in most adolescents' diets comes from protein.

Carbohydrates include all starchy foods, which are also called complex carbohydrates, and simple sugars (see chapter 29). Soft drinks and candy provide simple carbohydrates, and pasta, cereals, rice, and potatoes yield complex carbohydrates. In one day, about 46 percent of the energy intake of a typical American's diet comes from a combination of simple and complex carbohydrates.

Fats and oils are the macronutrients that are most dense in caloric value, as each gram of fat provides 9 calories (see chapter 30). Sources of fat include butter, margarine, oils, fried foods, egg yolks, mayonnaise, salad dressings, ice cream, cream cheese, hard cheeses, nuts, fatty meats, doughnuts, and chips. The National Health and Nutrition Examination Survey of 1988–1991 showed that fat contributed an average of 33–34 percent of the caloric intake of adolescents aged 12–19 years. Although fat is a valuable source of energy, excess fat intake is linked to many chronic diseases that appear later in life. Therefore, moderate intake is recommended during adolescence.

VITAMINS AND MINERALS During the adolescent years, the amount of vitamins and minerals that the body requires for growth and development increases. A well-balanced diet provides a good supply of vitamins and minerals, making supplements unnecessary. Many adolescents, however, have marginal or inadequate intake of calcium and iron because they consume inadequate amounts of vegetables, meat, and dairy products (see chapter 31).

Calcium is essential for bone growth; boys need more calcium than girls. Ninety-nine percent of the body's calcium is found in its bones and teeth, and 40–45 percent of the adult's skeleton is built in the adolescent years. The RDA for calcium is 1,200 milligrams for adolescents. This translates into 2 glasses of any kind of milk (each glass contains about 300 milligrams of calcium), 6 ounces of yogurt (totaling about 300 milligrams of calcium), and 2 ounces of cheese (with about 150 milligrams of calcium in each ounce). Since about 1980, consumption of dairy products has decreased. The best source of calcium is found in dairy products, but other good sources include shellfish, sardines, almonds, broccoli, and tofu. Adolescents with lactose intolerance can use reduced-lactose milk, like Lactaid, or lactase supplements. The degree of lactose intolerance is often mild enough that adolescents can tolerate dairy products as long as small amounts are consumed at one time. Yogurt, which has less lactose than milk, may be well tolerated. Calcium-fortified juices are widely available.

Iron is essential for the expansion of blood volume during adolescence, and with the onset of menses is especially important for girls. Iron is classified as "heme" or "non-heme" iron. Heme iron is obtained from animal sources and is more readily absorbed by the body than non-heme iron, which is provided by plants. Good sources of iron are meat, fish, poultry, dark-green vegetables, dried fruits, and fortified cereals and breads. On average, people absorb 10 percent of ingested iron. Vitamin C enhances the absorption of non-heme iron. Therefore, drinking fresh orange juice with meals that contain iron will increase iron absorption. In contrast, such substances as phytate and tannins, which are common in teas and coffees, may decrease iron absorption by as much as 50 percent. The RDA for iron is 12 milligrams for adolescent boys and 15 milligrams for adolescent girls. Many professionals believe that female athletes should obtain 30 milligrams of iron daily.

Folate, one of the B vitamins, is involved in cell division. Folate deficiency can cause one form of anemia. It is not surprising to find a low folate intake in many adolescents, as the best sources are green leafy vegetables, which are not often favored foods of teenagers. Other sources of folate include seeds, beans and peas, asparagus, and broccoli.

Obtaining Adequate Nutrients and a Balanced Diet

The keys to a healthy diet are variety, balance, and moderation. A diet that includes many different foods usually does a good job of supplying all the necessary nutrients. A diet with adequate portions from each food group further ensures that adequate amounts of each nutrient are obtained. The Food Guide Pyramid illustrates the basics of healthy eating. It divides foods into six groups (the bread, cereal, rice, and pasta group; the vegetable group; the fruit group; the milk, yogurt, and cheese group; the meat, poultry, fish, beans, eggs, and nuts group; and the fats, oils, and sweets group) and provides the recommended daily number of servings of each group. Serving sizes for adolescents are the same as those for adults (see chapter 4).

A high or low intake of a particular food can be related to a chronic disease. A high sodium intake is associated with hypertension, and a high fat intake is linked to coronary heart disease, obesity, and cancers of the colon and breast. A low intake of fiber is associated with an increased risk of colon cancer. To help prevent chronic diseases, it's important that good eating habits, established earlier, be maintained during adolescence.

Smoking

Adolescents shouldn't smoke, and those who do should quit! Those adolescents who do smoke tobacco, however, should be aware of the impact that smoking can have on nutrition and the effect that quitting smoking can have on weight.

Smoking has a unique effect on the amount of vitamin C a person needs. The recommended daily intake of vitamin C for both girls and boys during adolescence is 50 milligrams for those who are 11–14 years old and 60 milligrams for those who are 15 years and older. This requirement is increased during pregnancy and lactation. Smokers, however, use vitamin C at a faster rate than nonsmokers. Consequently, smokers are advised to increase their daily intake of vitamin C to at least 100 milligrams, an amount easily obtained by drinking 8 ounces of fresh orange juice.

Smokers burn extra energy in small, short bursts following each use of nicotine, so people who quit smoking may experience weight gain in the absence of the nicotine. Former smokers may also eat more after quitting. An adolescent who is still growing and who quits smoking is likely to experience an increase in the rate of weight gain. If, upon quitting, an adolescent wants to avoid extra weight gain, then weight should be checked once a week, and small reductions, such as 10 percent, in total daily energy intake can be made until the desired control is achieved. An alternate approach that appeals to many adolescents involves adding 20–30 minutes of daily physical activity, the amount of which can be increased gradually, if necessary.

Food Choices and Customs

By the time they reach adolescence, children have developed a set of attitudes, preferences, values, and habits regarding food. If parents enjoy trying new foods, their children may also be adventurous. When parents encourage children to consume some foods and discourage them from eating others, they influence the formation of children's food preferences. The use of ethnic foods, for example, is important to many families. Such mealtime rituals as how the table is set, how the seating is determined, how the use of certain foods is associated with special occasions or specific people, and how the time for meals is determined, are all learned. Whereas adolescents often disagree with their parents, what they have learned about food stays with them as they move toward adulthood. The amount of time that family members allocate for food preparation and mealtime also influences teenagers' exposure to foods, as some families rely heavily on convenience foods or take-out products and others prepare food from scratch. The activities and schedules of teenagers often conflict with family customs, and parents may need to make an effort to continue these traditions. Furthermore, if teenagers are so busy that they are always eating on the run, togetherness and communication within their family are compromised.

In early and mid-adolescence relationships with peers become stronger, and peers can exert considerable influence on food choices. Adolescents usually will make changes in their lifestyles to achieve the approval of their peers. Meals offer opportunities for new social activity, and they can be challenging situations for those who need to follow a special diet but don't want to be different from their friends. In such cases, it is important for teenagers to educate their peers about the special diet.

Adolescents are active consumers, and advertisers recognize the importance of their purchasing power. Among all types of media, television has the greatest impact on adolescents, and almost 50 percent of television commercials attempt to sell food. Commercials during children's programs often focus on sweetened cereals, fast foods, snacks, and candies. Sports heroes, famous models, movie stars, and rock musicians appear in commercials with themes of good looks, fun, sex appeal, and other characteristics of importance to adolescents. Advertisers create an association between certain foods and desirable physical and personal characteristics. A commercial that shows everyone at a party drinking the same soda, for example, conveys the message that the soda helps the adolescent fit in and have fun. Many commercials suggest that certain foods be used for a purpose other than satisfying hunger, such as looking good.

Although many advertisements and commercials are attractive and clever, they seldom encourage healthy nutrition. Frequently in an advertisement or commercial, a person reaches for a beer or a soft drink, not juice or milk, to quench a thirst. And although many teen magazines offer nutritional advice, one survey found that the nutritional information in those magazines was often not reliable or accurate.

Eating Out, Eating Late, and Cooking

Many adolescents are busy with such after-school activities as sports, theater and music rehearsals, or part-time jobs. During weekends and vacations, adolescents like to spend time with their peers. They are not at home as much as they used to be, and when they do go home, it's often late. Eating out and eating late become the norm, and nutritional nightmares can be avoided if teenagers know how to choose healthy food when they eat away from home. When they come home late, a kitchen stocked with nutritious food that requires little or no preparation can be helpful. Meals that are simple and quick to prepare can also be very nutritious. A sandwich, yogurt, a piece of fruit, and a glass of juice make an easy, healthy meal. As parents are usually the primary grocery shoppers in the family, they select the foods that adolescents have to choose among at home. Parents can help adolescents meet their increased nutritional requirements by stocking the kitchen so that teenagers can eat, snack, or prepare a meal without relying on inappropriate foods. Many adolescents, especially those who are old enough to drive or who live close to supermarkets, begin to take some responsibility for shopping for the family. They can bring back what they were asked to buy, have an opportunity to familiarize themselves with a wide array of foods, make some personal selections, and acquire some experience in making choices that involve consideration of the cost of food.

Diet and Body Image

Adolescents are very aware of their bodies and are often willing to modify their diets in order to look attractive. Many are afraid of becoming over-weight and thus restrict the amount they eat or the frequency of eating, or use weight-loss products. Excessive control of weight is inappropriate in a growing adolescent, and severe restrictions can diminish growth. Some weight-loss products tend to cause water loss rather than loss of fat, and stringent food restriction prevents adequate intake of vitamins and minerals. Excessive concern about body size and shape and stringent control of eating accompany such eating disorders as anorexia nervosa and bulimia nervosa (see chapter 17).

Many boys try nutritional supplements that they hope will enhance muscle development. These muscle-building products are ineffective when adequate protein and calories are being consumed in their regular diet.

Eating Behaviors

Adolescents' meal schedules can be irregular, and meals are often skipped. Although most adolescents know the importance of breakfast, it is the most commonly skipped meal, usually because of lack of time in the morning. Dinner is the most regularly eaten meal. Missed meals are usually compensated for by snacks that can make up as much as 25 percent of daily caloric intake. Snacking is often deemed undesirable by parents who worry that snacks between meals are unhealthy or will ruin the appetite for the next meal. But snacking is one way to obtain calories and other nutrients in a healthy fashion. Snacks can be low in fat and high in vitamins and minerals. Some suggestions for snacks include fresh fruits, low-fat crackers, plain popcorn, pretzels, cut-up vegetables (broccoli, celery, or carrots) with low-fat dip, low-fat yogurt, milk, fruit juice, seltzer water, frozen yogurt, fruited gelatin, pudding, and angel food cake.

As adolescents learn more about nutrition, they

tend to have more independent opinions about food. They still believe that eating with their family is important, but they may disagree about various details. Some foods adolescents commonly like are soft drinks, hamburgers, pizza, spaghetti, chicken, French fries, and ice cream. Vegetables are generally not too popular, although raw ones are better accepted than cooked ones, and such sweet ones as corn are preferred to bland or bitter ones. Some consider milk a baby's drink and therefore choose soft drinks.

CAFFEINE Caffeine consumption increases during adolescence with greater intake of coffee, tea, and soft drinks. Caffeine is the most widely used central nervous system stimulant. Its effects vary among individuals, depending on body weight, amount of caffeine ingested, and personal tolerance. Caffeine tends to reduce the sense of fatigue and decrease drowsiness. Too much can upset the stomach, cause insomnia, provoke anxiety, and set off palpitations. Coffee, tea, and cola-type soft drinks contain a substantial amount of caffeine, and chocolate and cocoa-containing foods and beverages contain smaller amounts of caffeine:

Food	Caffeine (mg)
Brewed coffee, 6 oz	105
Instant coffee, 6 oz	55
Mountain Dew, 12 oz	55
Regular cola, 12 oz	45
Diet cola, 12 oz	35
Brewed tea, 6 oz	35
Milk chocolate, 1 oz	10
Cocoa mix, 1 packet	5
Instant chocolate pudding, 4 oz	5

Mild withdrawal symptoms, such as headaches and a craving for a beverage containing caffeine, may occur if someone who has consumed caffeine regularly suddenly stops using it.

FAST FOODS Fast food plays an important role in the lives of teenagers. Its convenience, speed, and accessibility, and the lack of cleanup involved, number among its biggest attractions. When parents work and teenagers are responsible for some of their own meals, fast food seems to be the simplest answer. Fast food restaurants are affordable to many adolescents and serve as social gathering places, as well. Many fast foods are high in fat (especially saturated fats), calories, and sodium and low in vitamins and minerals. Fat can account for 40–50 percent of the calories in fast food. But some fast food establishments offer healthy choices that are not inherently high in fat and not prepared with large quantities of fat (see chapter 39).

PART TWO

Common Concerns

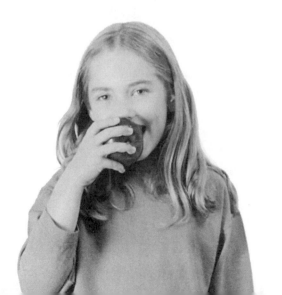

9

. . . .

Food and the Family

Children begin to develop a relationship to food in early infancy, and many of the patterns children establish will remain with them throughout their lives. Parents need to remember that children grow at different rates and that all are capable of regulating their food intake. When parents understand this, they can maximize the possibility that their children will develop a healthy, positive relationship with food.

The family table should be a place for communication and comfort, a place for socialization as well as enjoyment of tastes. A happy table is often indicative of a happy family. It is important for parents to agree on issues of food and eating, since children tend to do better with eating, as well as with other aspects of their lives, when their parents agree with each other. And with food, as with other aspects of childrearing, parents must provide love and nurturing as well as limits. A myriad of challenges and influences affect parents' ability to establish a positive food culture at home. This chapter explores some of them.

> **MYTH** Children should be taught to clean their plates.
>
> **FACT** Forcing children to "clean their plates" does not establish healthy eating habits and may promote obesity. Generally speaking, children regulate their own intake appropriately.

. . . .

Sylvia J. Lavietes ▪ Mary E. McDonnell ▪ William V. Tamborlane

Developmental Considerations

Parents are responsible for preparing and presenting nutritious meals and children are responsible for how much and even whether they eat. This division of responsibility begins in infancy and continues through adolescence. In infancy, parents must be aware of and learn to trust the cues their infants give them to indicate satiety, such as turning away from the breast or bottle, playing with the nipple, pushing away the spoon, or becoming irritable or distracted (see chapter 5).

During the toddler years, parents may find that fostering the child's positive relationship with food has become more challenging. Toddlers take pride in the independence they are developing, and any interference with their autonomy is likely to create a battle. If a toddler does not want to eat a certain food, or a certain amount of food, do not force the issue. With toddlers it is important to choose one's battles and to think about the long term. Problems that seem monumental at the moment will recede in importance with the passage of time. For instance, when toddlers are learning to eat, they may be very messy and prone to spill things. But, rest assured, as they grow older, their coordination and tidiness will improve. Keep in mind that toddlers, as well as school-age children and adolescents, may show a substantial day-to-day variation in the amount of food that is eaten. When averages are taken over 3 or 4 days, however, the amounts are remarkably consistent. So, if toddlers do not seem interested in eating today, do not worry; they will make up for it tomorrow. Toddlers may also develop certain rituals connected with food: eating all of their potatoes before they eat their meat, for example. As long as these rituals do not interfere with a healthy diet, children should be allowed to exercise their autonomy and to make these choices.

School-age children develop more consistent appetites. They are sometimes more willing to try new foods, but certain foods will probably remain their favorites. During these years they may be swayed by television advertising, which may encourage them to eat foods that are high in simple sugars and fats. If this happens, use the opportunity to discuss the manipulative effects of advertising with your children and to explain that the goal of advertising is to persuade them to buy the product, whether it is healthy to eat or not. Children in this age group may also be susceptible to the influence of their peers: if your child's friends are taking chocolate cookies to school for lunch, your child may wish to do so as well. The parents' role is to ensure that their school-age children are being offered a variety of nutritious foods, both for regular meals and for snacks.

Adolescents are also influenced by television advertising, and as their lives become busier, fast food restaurants and snacking may become a way of life for them. Peer pressure is, of course, another significant factor in their lives. Because parents have less influence on foods that are eaten outside of the home, there is an even greater need to provide nutritious, healthy foods at home. Many adolescents may seem insatiable at times, and again, parents should remember that their children are generally able to regulate their food intake themselves. On the day after a big game or a long practice session, adolescents may need to eat a lot to make up for the extra energy burned during the previous day's intense period of exercise (see chapter 13). Other teens, concerned about being overweight, may experiment with potentially harmful fad diets. Parents must educate themselves about proper nutrition and maintain an awareness of their child's eating behaviors in order to determine whether such attempts at weight reduction should be an issue of

TABLE 9.1
Parental Role in Children's Nutrition during Different Stages of Development

Stage of development	Characteristics	Parental role
Infancy	Self-regulating Learning to suck and swallow Growing rapidly	Provide an enjoyable and nurturing environment during feeding Trust the infant's ability to self-regulate Provide appropriate foods
Preschool	Developing food rituals May be willing to try new foods Developing strong food preferences Developing independence	Respect food preferences and rituals Provide a variety of nourishing foods
School-age	Developing hearty appetites Becoming susceptible to peer pressure Being influenced by television advertising	Set regular meal and snack times Prepare healthy, nourishing meals Help children understand television advertising for high-sugar, high-fat, low-nutrient-dense foods
Adolescence	Becoming concerned about appearance Being influenced by television advertising, especially for fast foods Becoming very susceptible to peer pressure May be experimenting with fad diets Growing rapidly	Provide nutritious foods at home Become informed about and be aware of the problem of fad diets Provide guidance Set a good example

concern (see chapter 12). The role of the parent in establishing healthy eating habits in relation to the child's stage of development is summarized in table 9.1.

Parental Roles in Feeding

Parents can begin to encourage their children to develop a healthy approach to eating in early infancy. With many women choosing to breastfeed, the first parent to feed the new baby is usually the mother (see chapter 5). Because the mother's feelings and emotions are easily transmitted to the child during breastfeeding, efforts should be made to make this experience pleasurable for both mother and child. Fathers can contribute to this process by helping with other aspects of care (diapering, bathing) and by providing bottle-feedings of formula or breast milk when needed. It is not unusual for mothers to be anxious or tense (as well as exhausted from the rigors of childbirth) when they begin breastfeeding for the first time. If given enough time, information, and encouragement, however, most will become very comfortable and confident in feeding their infants.

Feeding problems often result when parents become anxious about how much the child is eating or when they insist that certain foods or amounts be consumed. One of the main reasons for well child checkups with the pediatrician is to make sure that children are eating enough to grow and develop normally. Too much confusion at mealtime, too much or too little time for eating, and hastily prepared and unattractively presented food can also lead to feeding problems.

One of the most important ways that parents can teach good eating habits is by setting good examples in their own eating behaviors. Such good examples are especially important for school-age children and for adolescents. If children are to be encouraged to reduce or eliminate candy, snack cakes, chips, and doughnuts from their diets, then parents should be making similar adjustments in their diets. One mother became discouraged because her daughter refused to eat hearty, well-balanced meals and sought nutritional counseling. The counselor discovered that the mother's own constant dieting gave her daughter the message that food was the enemy, not a source of pleasure and sustenance. Parents should also not let television and newspapers interfere with mealtimes; meals are social as well as nutritional events for a family, and mealtime conversation may well be as important as the food.

In a busy family where both parents work and where the children are involved in numerous extracurricular and recreational activities, family meals may be few and far between, especially during the school and work week. When this happens, family meals during weekends and holidays take on special importance and deserve to be given priority. Such family meals should be pleasurable experiences, not battle zones where discipline is meted out. A calm and supportive atmosphere at the table fosters both communication and digestion; save negativity and confrontation for another venue.

Parents may be tempted to use food as a reward or to punish by depriving the child of certain foods. Using food in this way establishes a role for food that far exceeds its rightful limits. The food involved might become tainted by virtue of the circumstances: "If you don't eat your spinach, you won't get dessert." "If you don't eat your dinner, you can't watch television tonight." Food, and the meal, in this case have become associated with punishment, not pleasure.

Using food—specifically dessert foods or treats—as a reward for good behavior or for eating more nutritious foods may achieve quick results, but in the long run may do more harm than good. If children are constantly being rewarded with ice cream for eating their green beans, they will begin to perceive the ice cream as being more important and better than the green beans. It is important to remember that parents are trying to help children develop a healthy relationship with all foods without forcing them to eat. Using food as a reward is a form of force-feeding, against which children may eventually rebel.

Power struggles over food create havoc at the table as well as within the family in general. Friction generated by fights over food, whether the fights are overt or subtle, interferes with usual family interactions. Tension at the table creates an atmosphere that is not conducive to eating or socializing. The reasons for such struggles are complex: they may reflect an acting out of feelings about something totally unrelated to food, but reflective of the relationship between the sparring family members. It is important to maintain awareness of the real causes of such struggles and keep them isolated from mealtimes. As with parenting generally, it is important to attempt to be reasonably flexible and to permit the child to grow naturally within established limits. For families that can do this, the rewards will be more pleasant mealtimes and greater enjoyment of the food as well as of each other.

Societal Influences

Over the past few decades, the family unit and the family environment have changed dramatically. In two-parent families, both parents often work outside the home; single-parent families are more common, as is shared custody for the children of divorced parents. For all of these families, the responsibility for a good deal of child care may rest with baby-sitters or day care providers. Parents must make sure that nutritious foods are available in the home for meals provided by baby-sitters, and it is the parents' responsibility to monitor what foods are eaten and how the meals are presented. Similarly, the types of foods and the mealtime environment should be an important consideration in selecting a day care center. Paradoxically, in the quest to ensure their children's financial security, many parents are left too exhausted to provide the level of daily food and meal preparation that they would prefer. By default, children and adolescents may be expected to be more independent and self-reliant than ever before.

Other challenges posed by our modern society can adversely affect the feeding of children and their development of healthy eating habits as well. To the child watching television, sugar-coated breakfast cereal is a far more appealing breakfast than an egg and toast or a bowl of oatmeal. Children often nag, whine, and negotiate to persuade their parents to purchase less healthy foods as treats. Parents may relent, purchase less healthy foods, and make them available for snacks at home or include them in lunches carried to school. Of course, as far as lunch is concerned, it is always possible that the child will trade the healthy and lovingly prepared brown-bag lunch for a less nourishing, but better advertised, substitute. As children grow older, the influence the media and their peers exercise upon their food choices becomes more substantial. In addition, teenagers are enticed by the convenience, taste, and cost of fast foods. Teens also like the autonomy of buying their own food out of the home.

The Picky Eater

Some children love food and eat many foods with enthusiasm, whereas others are much choosier about what they put into their mouths. Most children vary in what they like: one day they love peas and the next day they spit them into their napkin. One day they love canned ravioli, but as soon as the parent buys a case to have on hand, the passion for ravioli has abated. Normal childhood eating habits provide challenges for responsible adults; picky eaters provide the consummate challenge.

One might question whether the picky eater was born that way or made that way through experience. Some children may indeed have a negative physiological reaction to certain tastes and have a sensitive palate (see chapter 3).

Behaviorally, it seems that all children eat best when parents provide food in a supportive, comfortable, emotionally satisfying fashion and when they observe their parents enjoying meals. Parents need to agree on appropriate limits and then abide by them. Children who recognize the family cook's tremendous investment in providing appetizing meals can garner attention by refusing to eat what has been prepared. This often heralds the introduction of the short-order cook, the person who leaps to the stove when the child rejects what is on the table and has a special request. Some parents may feel perfectly comfortable providing this service, but others may find it manipulative and disruptive. For some families the short-order format may work for lunch but not for dinner, or it may work if requests are made in advance, but not after everyone has sat down at the table. For instance, for lunch one day a child was presented with one of her favorite meals—macaroni and cheese. It did not appeal to her that day, so she asked for a grilled cheese sandwich. Her parents agreed to provide the sandwich. For dessert the child was given chocolate pudding, a usual favorite. In a whining voice, she asked for an alternate dessert. At this point the parents felt that their daughter was being manipulative and decided that, since she did not *need* to eat dessert at all, she could decide whether to eat the chocolate pudding, but no other dessert would be offered. By intervening in this way, the parents gave the child the message that they were responsive to her needs, but that there were limits to their indulgence.

Finicky eaters set up the expectation that they are likely to be dissatisfied with what has been prepared. If the parents are anxious about whether the child will eat the meal, the child may react to their anxiety and become even pickier, exacerbating the already tense family mealtime. Providing choices during each meal may be a way of minimizing a child's pickiness.

It is easy to say that eating should not be an issue in a child's or a family's life. As much as parents of picky eaters would love to feel relaxed and ignore the problem, it is often difficult, if not impossible, to do so. A parent needs to evaluate whether the child truly does not like certain foods, or whether the child is using food to manipulate the parents. In either case, but especially in the latter, parents must remain aware of their feelings and of the message they are sending to the child. Is the child regarded as bothersome or provocative or "just like your sister"? How are the parents managing the situation? Is their tone of voice caustic, accusing, or angry? Is their attention, negative though it may be, perceived as a reward by the child?

Problems with eating largely depend on the relationship between the parents and the child. To find solutions to problems at mealtimes, each challenging situation needs to be evaluated as it occurs. Children need to know that a certain structure exists regarding meals and that certain standards of behavior are expected. They need to know that they are expected to join the family at meals and that they can choose from the variety of food available. They do not have the right to make mealtimes unpleasant for other people at the table.

Parents need to approach food and eating in as neutral and casual a fashion as possible. When parents exert too much pressure on children to try new foods, the children may react by refusing to eat. They need to allow the child to consider the new food without feeling pressured. Saying, "It's delicious; eat some," or even surreptitiously scrutinizing the child, anticipating his ingestion of the food, will surely backfire with a picky eater. One way to maximize the possibility that the child will accept a new food is to introduce it with another food that the child enjoys.

When possible, involve the child in planning menus for the family, and be sure to include at least one food that the child likes in every meal. Many children also enjoy assisting in preparing the meal or setting the table. If children feel like participants in the process rather than simply the recipients of the final product, they may feel that the meal is "theirs" and be more willing to eat what has been served.

What happens if the child opts to eat nothing at a given meal? Under usual circumstances this de-

TABLE 9.2

The Picky Eater

Common feeding problems	Solutions and helpful hints
Child won't eat vegetables.	Present the vegetables with a nutritious dip. Let the child choose the vegetables. Offer a variety of vegetables with different colors and textures. Try raw instead of cooked vegetables.
Child insists on eating the same foods.	Allow the child to eat his or her favorite foods, but offer small amounts of new foods along with them. Continue to offer a variety of nutritious foods. Remind yourself that this phase will eventually end.
Child appears to have a small appetite.	Be mindful of age-appropriate portion sizes. Offer nutritious foods before the child gets too tired or hungry. Remember that the child's intake will vary from meal to meal and from day to day.
Child won't drink milk.	Try other sources of calcium: yogurt, cheese, pudding, calcium-enriched orange juice. Add nonfat dry milk powder to casseroles or soups. Try blending yogurt, fruit, and frozen banana slices for a nutritious treat.

cision will not have serious consequences. Usually, there is, in fact, something that the child will eat, such as bread, potatoes, or rice. The lost nutrients will usually be consumed at another meal.

In regard to children's tantrums over food, it is advisable to ignore them as much as possible, while assuring the child's safety. That might involve employing a calm, soft, assured tone of voice, and continuing with whatever activities were previously under way. Set the limit that it is all right to be angry, but it is not all right to interfere with the rest of the family's pleasant mealtime. Picky eaters challenge parental patience. They provoke a plethora of feelings in parents about their own childhood experience with nurturing; their adequacy as nurturers; relationship issues between parents, between parent and child, within the family; and the child's ability to function socially. It is important to have confidence that the picky child will one day explore food and even enjoy it. Until then, like it or not, you have a picky eater. Some helpful hints regarding possible responses to specific problems of the picky eater are summarized in table 9.2.

Resources

Berman, C., and J. Former. *Meals without Squeals*. Palo Alto, CA: Bull Publishing, 1991.

Brazelton, T. B. *Toddlers and Parents: A Declaration of Independence*. New York: Delacorte Press, 1975.

Brody, J. *Jane Brody's Nutrition Book*. New York: Norton, 1981.

Satter, E. *How to Get Your Kid to Eat . . . But Not Too Much*. Palo Alto, CA: Bull Publishing, 1987.

10

· · · · · · · ·

Not All Vegetarians Are Created Equal

Vegetarian is a general term used to describe people who exclude meat, fish, poultry, or animal-derived foods from their diets. Vegetarian diets have become increasingly popular in recent years. The increase in popularity may be due to philosophical, religious, ecological, or health-related concerns, or to some combination of these. Both vegetarian and meat-containing diets can be beneficial, if they are well planned and combined with a healthy lifestyle. But both kinds of diets can also lead to nutritional problems if a balanced combination of foods is not eaten.

Just as there is diversity in people's reasons for becoming vegetarians, there are different views

> **MYTH** Vegetarians are unhealthy.
> **FACT** If foods are chosen wisely, vegetarian diets are healthful. A variety of foods helps ensure an adequate intake of nutrients.

about what constitutes a vegetarian diet. Four major categories exist: semi-vegetarian, lacto-ovo-vegetarian, lacto-vegetarian, and vegan.

Semi-vegetarians are people who omit some but not all groups of animal foods from their diets. They usually exclude red meat but may occasionally consume chicken or fish. Semi-vegetarians are also called quasi or partial vegetarians and may be further divided into pesco-vegetarians (include fish, but no chicken or red meat) or pollo-vegetarians (include chicken, but no fish or red meat). Semi-vegetarians usually follow this diet because they believe it is healthier to exclude red meats. Lacto-ovo-vegetarians in-

· · · · · · · ·

Linda Gay

clude dairy products and eggs, in addition to the fruits, vegetables, and grains in their diets, but they do not eat any meat, poultry, or fish. Lacto-vegetarians include dairy products, fruits, vegetables, and grains in their diets. Vegans exclude all animal-derived foods, including dairy products and eggs, and are also called pure vegetarians or total vegetarians.

In addition to the exclusion of some or all animal-derived foods, vegetarians sometimes adopt other dietary practices such as a preference for foods grown organically using crop rotation or natural fertilizers in place of artificial fertilizers and pesticides. Other vegetarians may eat only raw plant foods. Some prefer to avoid sugar and processed foods. One group, fruitarians, eat only fruit, nuts, seeds, olive oil, honey, and whole grains. The more restrictive the diet, the greater the likelihood of nutritional deficiencies.

Some vegetarians may choose to follow a macrobiotic diet. The Zen macrobiotic diet has ten stages. As a person advances through the ten stages, progressively more foods are eliminated and replaced with grain products. Lower-level macrobiotic diets, if carefully planned, can meet nutritional needs, but strict adherence to higher levels of the diet can result in serious malnutrition, growth retardation, or even death. These diets are especially hazardous to growing children, since it is difficult to obtain adequate calories, vitamins, and minerals while adhering to such a strict regime.

Healthy Aspects of a Vegetarian Diet

There are many positive health aspects associated with vegetarian diets, since the diets are usually high in fiber and can be low in fat. In general, vegetarians tend to be closer to a healthy body weight than meat eaters. Vegetarians also have a lower incidence of high blood pressure, even though their salt intake is similar to meat eaters. Plant-based diets tend to be low in total fat, saturated fat, and cholesterol. It is not surprising, therefore, that vegetarians tend to have lower blood cholesterol levels than meat eaters. Since high levels of cholesterol in the blood are associated with cardiovascular disease, the vegetarian diet can help protect against this disease.

Constipation and diverticular disease are also less common among vegetarians than in the general population. The high fiber content of the diet helps to produce stools that are softer, bulkier, and pass through the intestine more quickly. In general, lower cancer rates correlate with a low intake of meat and a high intake of grains and vegetables. The cancer rate for Seventh-Day Adventists, who are primarily lacto-ovo-vegetarians, is one-half to two-thirds that of the general population. This is true even when cancers related to smoking and alcohol are excluded. This lower risk may be due to a decreased meat intake, a larger intake of vegetables and cereal grains, or to other lifestyle factors.

Possible Problems with a Vegetarian Diet

Lacto-vegetarians or lacto-ovo-vegetarians generally do not have to worry about nutritional deficiencies. By including eggs or dairy products or both in the diet, the vegetarian is assured an adequate intake of calcium, vitamin D (found in fortified dairy products), vitamin B_{12} (found only in animal products or fortified vegetable products), and high-quality protein. Lacto- and lacto-ovo-vegetarians may have a diet that is high in cholesterol and saturated fat, however, if they choose full-fat dairy products over low-fat ones.

PROTEIN Protein is used by the body to build and maintain tissues. The building blocks of protein are called amino acids, and there are 22 amino acids found in protein. Although the body is able to manufacture some amino acids (nonessential), there are others which it cannot manufacture (essential). These essential amino acids must be obtained from food. A high-quality protein is one that contains all of the essential amino acids in the correct proportions. Animal foods, including eggs and milk, are rich in high-quality protein, whereas plants usually contain insufficient amounts of one or more of the essential amino acids. Plant foods can be combined to obtain adequate amounts of essential amino acids. This combining of plant foods is called protein complementation. Major plant sources of protein include breads, grains, nuts, seeds, dried beans, peas, and legumes. It was previously thought that amino acid complementation was necessary at each meal. However, now it is known that eating a variety of plant foods daily will assure adequate protein complementation. Other vegetables and fruits provide calories, vitamins, and minerals, but very little protein.

VITAMIN B_{12} Our bodies require only a small amount of vitamin B_{12}, but this vitamin is found only in animal foods, including eggs and milk products. Vitamin B_{12} is not produced, stored, or used by plants, so vegans will receive no B_{12} in their diets. The only exception is the B_{12} found in algae, spirulina, or fermented products, but these forms of B_{12} are not bioavailable for humans. For a plant food to contain this vitamin, it must be contaminated with B_{12} synthesizing bacteria. In countries with good sanitation, such as the United States, bacterial contamination is unlikely. Therefore, leaving fresh fruits and vegetables un-

washed will not provide adequate vitamin B_{12} for the vegan's diet. Since vegans rely solely on plant foods, they must consume foods fortified with B_{12} such as milk substitutes, cereals, nutritional yeasts, or meat analogs, or they need to take a supplement of B_{12}.

ZINC Approximately one-half of the zinc in the average diet comes from meat, fish, and poultry. The zinc present in plant sources such as cereals, legumes, and soy products used as meat alternatives is not well absorbed. In addition, soy products can interfere with zinc absorption. Vegetarian diets, therefore, are often limited in the quantity or quality of zinc. To help combat this limitation, vegetarians should eat meat alternatives such as black-eyed peas, pinto beans, or kidney beans more often than soy products. Pesco-vegetarians could include oysters, crab meat, and shrimp, which are high in zinc.

CALCIUM AND VITAMIN D For those vegetarians who exclude milk products, calcium-fortified foods are necessary. Not all milk substitutes are fortified with calcium and vitamin D, so careful label reading is important. Tofu, if it has been processed with calcium, can be a good source. Although adequate vitamin D will be produced when the skin is exposed to sunlight, this is not always possible in winter months, especially in northern climates. Vitamin D deficiency can lead to the development of rickets (a bone disease) in children.

IRON Iron is another limiting nutrient in vegetarian diets. Iron is found in animal foods such as red meat, chicken, eggs, dark leafy vegetables, iron-fortified cereals, and whole-grain breads. Although the iron found in plant foods is not as easily absorbed as the iron found in animal foods, eating foods high in vitamin C at each meal will improve the absorption of iron from plant foods.

Special Considerations

PREGNANCY AND LACTATION Nutrient needs increase during pregnancy and lactation, and women who follow any type of vegetarian diet need to be especially attentive to nutritional requirements. Iron levels should be monitored during pregnancy and a daily supplement of 30 milligrams of ferrous iron should be taken during the second and third trimester. Vegan women need to be certain that they consume foods fortified with vitamin B_{12}, calcium, and vitamin D.

GROWTH IN CHILDREN Lacto-vegetarian and lacto-ovo-vegetarian diets can adequately support growth in children. Lacto-ovo-vegetarian children experience the same growth patterns as children who eat meat. Vegan children usually grow within the normal range, although they tend to be shorter and weigh less than children who consume animal foods.

Obtaining adequate energy and nutrients may be more difficult for vegan children. Parents who want their infants to avoid cow's milk need to use a suitable commercial formula, such as fortified soy milk, to avoid any nutritional risk for their child. Since plant foods are bulkier and generally contain less energy per ounce than animal foods, vegan diets usually fail to provide sufficient energy and nutrients within a volume that is small enough for a child. Children may feel full before they have consumed enough food to meet their nutritional needs. The plant foods best suited to provide protein and energy in small volumes are legumes, cereals, and nuts. These foods should be emphasized in the diet of the vegan child. For the young child, smooth nut butters should be used in place of chunky nut butters or whole nuts because of the risk of aspirating pieces of nuts into the lungs.

Adolescents require a varied and calorically adequate diet. Since calcium is important in attaining peak bone mass, adolescents must obtain adequate calcium. At least three servings of dairy foods or fortified alternatives should be consumed daily. Dairy alternatives should be fortified with both vitamin D and calcium (250 to 300 milligrams of calcium per cup).

Carefully planned vegetarian diets can provide adequate nutrition throughout the life cycle. The more restrictive the diet, the greater the likelihood that nutritional deficiencies will occur. Careful attention must be paid to certain limiting nutrients, especially calcium, vitamin D, vitamin B_{12}, iron, and zinc. Amino acid intake is usually adequate when the diet includes a complementary variety of foods sufficient to meet caloric needs. For vegan children, it is important to provide dense and nutritious foods such as legumes, nuts, cereals, and fortified milk substitutes. The principles of variety, balance, and moderation apply equally to vegetarian and traditional diets.

Resources

Lappé, Frances Moore. *Diet for a Small Planet.* Rev. ed. Westminster, MD: Ballantine, 1992.

The Vegetarian Resource Group. P.O. Box 1463, Baltimore, MD 21203. (301) 366-8343.

Vegetarian Times. P.O. Box 446, Mount Morris, IL 61054-8081.

11

. . . .

Feeding the Sick Child

Most childhood ailments are accompanied by a loss of appetite and therefore a decreased intake of fluids and solid foods. There are no hard and fast dietary rules regarding these illnesses. Instead, feed children as much as they want without forcing food or forcing the issue.

MYTH "Starve a fever; feed a cold," or is it "Feed a fever; starve a cold"?

FACT Neither! Fevers and colds both require adequate nutrition. Although sick children may not have an appetite for many foods, it is still important to encourage frequent food and fluid intake.

a day. If vomiting and diarrhea persist, extra liquids should be offered to compensate for these additional lost fluids.

The choice of fluids depends on the child's age as well as individual preference. Infants who are having problems with continuous vomiting or diarrhea may require a commercial oral hydration solution (see table 11.2). These formulas provide extra sodium and potassium to replace important electrolytes (salts) that are being lost but supply only a small amount of calories in the form of carbohydrates. Apple juice and soda have more calories, but fewer electrolytes.

Fluid Requirements

Fluid intake must be maintained in a child who is nauseous or vomiting, has diarrhea, or is refusing to eat. Basic fluid requirements are given in table 11.1; every attempt should be made to get the child to drink at least this amount of liquid in

. . . .

Kathy French ▪ John M. Leventhal

TABLE 11.1
Daily Fluid Requirements

Weight	Fluid requirements
≤22 lb	1.5 oz/lb
23–45 lb	33 oz plus 0.67 oz for every lb > 22 lb
45+ lb	50 oz plus 0.33 oz for every lb > 45 lb
Examples:	
18-lb infant	18 lb × 1.5 oz/lb = 27 oz
31-lb child	33 oz + (9 × 0.67 oz) = 39 oz
70-lb child	50 oz + (25 × 0.33 oz) = 58 oz

TABLE 11.2
Oral Hydration Formulas and
Clear Liquids (per oz)

	Calories	Sodium (mg)	Potassium (mg)
Pedialyte*	3	30	23
Infalyte*	4	35	29
Apple juice	15	1	37
Ginger ale	12	2	1
Cola	13	Trace	Trace

*Oral hydration formulas

Parents should closely monitor the amount that the sick child is drinking. One way to do this is to measure the amount of fluids the child is drinking by using a measured bottle, cup, or spoon. Another approach is to keep track of urine output, which indirectly monitors intake. A six-month-old infant, for example, should have five to six wet diapers a day. Medical treatment should be sought if an infant does not wet a diaper for eight hours.

Older children will also require fluid replacement for vomiting and diarrhea. If food is not tolerated, clear liquids (fluids that you can see through) such as apple juice, cranberry juice, carbonated beverages, gelatin, and popsicles will usually be sufficient to maintain fluid intake.

Calorie Requirements

Children tend to eat less when ill, even if the symptoms of nausea and vomiting are not present. Their lack of appetite may be due to a general feeling of malaise, but it may also be due to a lack of activity. Bed rest, or even a day spent on the couch, does not require much energy expenditure; caloric requirements decrease substantially.

The exception to this rule would be any illness accompanied by fever. A temperature of 1°F or more above normal (98.6°F) will increase caloric needs. A child who has a fever for several days and suffers from loss of appetite may experience weight loss.

Upper Respiratory Illnesses

From sniffles to sore throats, from sneezing to a lingering cough, a cold may interfere with a child's usual meal pattern. Nevertheless, children should be encouraged to eat as regular a diet as possible. When children have a cold, they should be encouraged to drink more than usual. Sneezing, coughing, and "drippy" noses lead to extra fluid losses. Warm soothing liquids such as broth, weak tea with milk and sugar or honey (for the older child), and hot cereal thinned with warm milk are well tolerated. Chicken noodle soup has been found to have possible medicinal properties, validating childhood memories of "mom's" chicken soup.

A sore throat, although short-lived, may make swallowing particularly painful. Small amounts of fluids and soft foods should be offered often, but never forced. Cold drinks such as apple juice and "flat" ginger ale, as well as popsicles, gelatin, pudding, yogurt, and ice cream, may help soothe the throat as well as provide calories.

As symptoms subside, mildly seasoned foods should be more readily accepted. Lightly buttered toast cut in interesting shapes (strips or triangles), whipped potatoes, rice, and canned fruits should be introduced, followed by a gradual return to family meals.

Infants with upper respiratory illnesses may have difficulty nursing or taking a bottle; smaller, more frequent feedings may become necessary to compensate. Clearing the nose of mucus with a special suction device just before the feeding may also help.

Nausea and Vomiting

Vomiting in infants and children will obviously interfere with their normal intake of foods and fluids; children may be hesitant to eat or drink for fear of vomiting again.

Infants suffering from vomiting may benefit from commercial hydration formulas (see table 11.2) to replace lost fluids. Feedings should be small (1 to 2 ounces initially) and given as often as every hour. Since these formulas provide little other than fluid and electrolytes, these hydration formulas should not be used for more than 2 to 3 days. Short periods of nursing or small amounts of formula (given as one-half formula and one-half water to begin with) should be initiated as soon as possible.

Children should be offered sips of clear fluids hourly in measured amounts. Once symptoms have subsided, amounts should be increased with the goal of attaining the daily fluid requirement (see table 11.1). Medical advice should be sought if the child cannot meet these basic fluid requirements. Once fluids are tolerated, dry toast and crackers should be introduced. A gradual progression to soup with rice or noodles, puddings, and applesauce, all in small amounts, should be

TABLE 11.3
Commercial Children's Formulas
(per 8-oz serving)

	Calories	Protein (g)	Percent RDA (ages 1–10 years)
Pediasure	240	7	19
Kindercal	240	8	25

attempted. Commercial children's formulas, such as Pediasure or Kindercal, may be beneficial if a child resists solid foods. Although nutritionally complete if taken in large quantities (see table 11.3), these formulas should be used on a short-term basis only.

Diarrhea

There are an estimated 21 to 37 million episodes of diarrheal illnesses each year in the United States, and children between the ages of 1 and 3 are most frequently affected. The nutritional goal is to avoid dehydration. Diarrhea can lead to a dehydrated state quickly, especially in infants who are also experiencing vomiting. In these cases, fluid replacement is absolutely essential.

Bottle-fed infants may benefit from formula that has been diluted (one-half formula and one-half water) to provide extra fluid. To ensure adequate intake of fluids for any infant, smaller feedings should be given more frequently. If the symptoms persist, oral hydration formulas may need to be added to the feeding schedule for both the bottle-fed and the breastfed infant (see table 11.2).

In formula-fed infants, brief use of a lactose-free formula (Isomil, Prosobee) may speed recovery from a diarrheal illness. Diarrheal illnesses may temporarily damage the intestinal enzyme that is required for digesting and absorbing lactose (see chapter 23). Feeding lactose-containing formula too soon may lead to poor absorption of lactose and more diarrhea.

Isomil DF, a soy-based formula with fiber, has been successful in treating some cases of acute diarrhea in infants. This formula should only be used for a short time (7 to 10 days), since long-term use can result in constipation.

For older children with diarrhea, liquids are essential to avoid dehydration. Small amounts given frequently should provide adequate hydration until symptoms subside. A toddler may be receptive to infant hydration formulas. Apple juice, ginger ale, and popsicles will probably be better received, but may worsen the diarrhea. These liquids provide calories and fluid but little else. Broths and bouillon provide added salt.

A popular therapy for diarrhea is the BRAT diet, in which intake is limited to bananas, rice cereal or rice, applesauce, and toast. The relative benefit of this diet over a soft diet (which can be tailored to a child's own particular food and drink preferences) remains to be proven.

Milk should be introduced slowly to ensure tolerance. As with infants, children may not absorb the lactose in the milk as efficiently as they did prior to their illness.

For children of all ages, you should seek medical advice if the diarrhea is more serious than usual, persists for more than 24 hours, or if there are signs of dehydration—namely, sunken eyes, no tears, dry mouth, or decreased urination.

Fever

An infant or child who is feverish will need more calories and more fluids, since a fever will cause the body's metabolic rate to rise. A child's caloric requirements increase 7 percent for every degree the fever rises above normal (98.6°F).

If an infant is not vomiting, feedings should be scheduled every two hours. Children should be offered cool liquids hourly. Water, fruit juice, ginger ale, popsicles, and sherbet should be well received. Slushy (partially frozen) juices may soothe the febrile child. As the temperature returns to normal, the diet can be modified, starting with canned fruits and cool pudding-type foods.

12

. . . .

Too Fat? Too Thin?

Many parents worry about their child's growth and weight gain during the course of development from earliest infancy through the end of adolescence. Depending upon the child's characteristics and the parents' attitudes, parents may be as concerned about excessive weight gain as they are about inadequate weight gain. Further complicating these issues are the child's eating patterns and the parents' approach to food.

Parents are not the only people who worry about weight and weight gain. Although many people assume that our society's emphasis on lean-

> **MYTH** A child in the 95th percentile for weight is too fat. **FACT** Weight and height must be considered together to determine whether a child is overweight. If that child is also at the 95th percentile for height, then the weight is fine.

ness affects only adolescents, a surprisingly large proportion of young children develop concerns about their body image. One recent study found 45 percent of boys and girls in grades three through six wanted to be thinner and 37 percent actively tried to lose weight. Many of these children also reported that they were influenced by the desires of their parents and friends to be thinner. Clearly in a culture that is obsessively concerned with weight, parents should have an accurate understanding of both normal growth patterns for children and their own child's actual growth patterns,

. . . .

Joseph Woolston ▪ Ed Strenkowski

and many parents will need to confront their own ideas and prejudices about body image in order to help their children develop realistic views.

Weight Curves

Both parents and children must remember that normal bodies come in a variety of sizes and shapes. In addition, there is considerable variation in patterns of growth and weight gain. Because of these natural and normal variations, parents should discuss their questions and concerns with their child's pediatrician or their family physician.

Some parents worry that their infant is too thin and frantically attempt to have him eat more, whereas others are concerned that their baby is overweight and may overly restrict his intake. They may imagine that their infant's body shape will become more and more pronounced as he becomes a child and an adolescent. They should be reassured that there is very little relationship between body shape before age 2 and body shape later in life.

Although it is virtually impossible to determine a child's nutritional status by just looking at her, the physician can rapidly assess the child's growth by plotting the child's height and weight on a standardized growth chart (see chapter 1 and growth charts appendix). The physician will note and explain the meaning of several important and related facts. First, the child's weight and height are compared to the range of weights and heights of other American children of the same age and sex. Second, one should not focus on weight alone, but rather on weight in relation to height. Typically, these growth curves are divided according to percentile groups. If a child's height and weight fall between the 5th percentile and the 95th percentile, growth is usually perfectly normal.

In assessing a child's weight, major changes

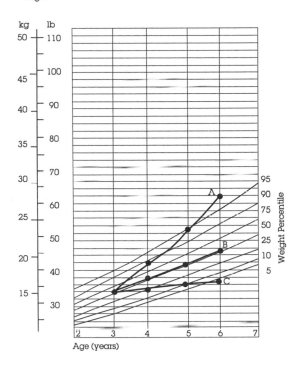

FIGURE 12.1
Changes in weight percentiles in three boys.

over time are more important than a single measurement. If, over a period of time, a child has shifted more than two percentile groups, then further evaluation may be indicated. Consider the weight curves of the three boys shown in fig. 12.1. At three years of age, all were approximately at the 50th percentile for height and continued to grow at a normal rate until six years of age. As shown in fig. 12.1, Boy A is clearly gaining weight too rapidly, and he needs a nutritional evaluation for obesity (see chapter 18). The weight curve of Boy C is also worrisome because it is falling. Such a decline in weight often indicates an underlying gastrointestinal or other medical problem. In this situation weight percentiles may fall even before growth in height is affected. By contrast, Boy B in

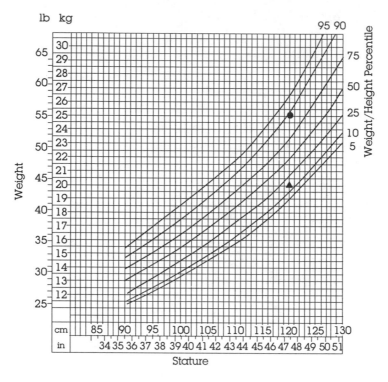

FIGURE 12.2
Variability in weight for height for two girls.

fig. 12.1 seems to have maintained a weight gain that is appropriate for his growth in stature.

At any given height, normal, healthy children show a wide variation in weight. To determine whether a child's weight is appropriate for the child's height, another standardized growth chart is used. This chart plots weight against height, essentially comparing weights for specific heights independent of the child's age. The normal variability in weight for height is illustrated by the two girls plotted in fig. 12.2. Although both are the same height (48 inches), one weighs approximately 60 pounds and the other 45 pounds, yet both fall within the normal range of variability.

Body Mass Index

Another commonly used method to evaluate weight in relation to height is to calculate the Body Mass Index (BMI), or Quetelet Index, which is the child's weight in kilograms divided by the square of the child's height in meters.

1. Divide weight in pounds by 2.2 = weight in kilograms
2. Divide height in inches by 39.4 = height in meters
3. Multiply height in meters by itself = height in meters squared
4. Divide the weight in kilograms (step #1) by the height in meters squared (step #3) = BMI

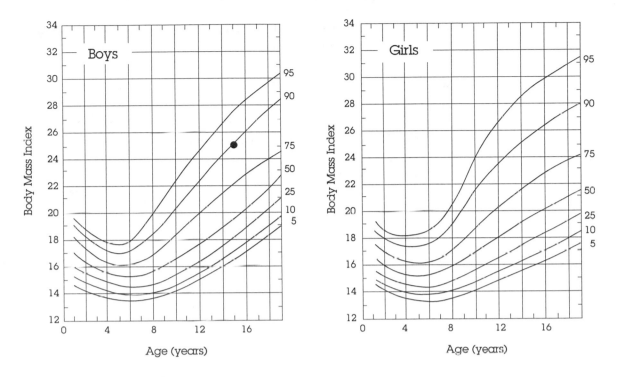

FIGURE 12.3
Body mass index percentiles for boys and girls showing the BMI for a 15-year-old boy.

In adults, a BMI above 27 defines obesity and is associated with greater medical risks. No such correlations have yet been determined for children, but standardized percentile curves for the BMI similar to the growth charts have been formulated for children and adolescents. For example, as shown in fig. 12.3, a 15-year-old boy who weighs 64 kilograms and who is 1.6 meters tall has a BMI of 25, a value that is at the 90th percentile for boys of his age. According to the recommendations of the National Institutes of Health Consensus Development Conference on Obesity, a BMI above the 85th percentile defines obesity in adults, but others have found a cutoff at the 95th percentile to be appropriate for a more conservative definition of obesity in children. Although a high BMI usually indicates obesity, there may be some exceptions. For example, body builders can have an elevated BMI that is attributable to increased muscle mass rather than to an increased amount of fat.

Other Assessments

Since a good deal of the body's fat is deposited under the skin, measurements of skin-fold thickness with special measuring calipers can also be used to assess obesity. Because the results can be influenced by differences in skin elasticity, compression times, and the skill of the examiner, these measurements are somewhat problematic as a means of assessing obesity. Skin-fold measurements are most useful in large population studies, but they can also be used to assess an individual's loss of body fat over time.

Two techniques for more directly measuring the percent of body fat are underwater weighing and estimating lean body mass by deuterium isotope methods. These methods are often impractical and difficult to use in children, but they have been employed in scientific studies.

The accumulation of fat around the abdomen or hips has important health implications for the obese child. This problem can be detected by simple visual observation, but the ratio between the size of the waist and hips will provide a framework for determining the severity of the problem, as discussed in detail in chapter 18.

13
· · · · · · · ·

Energizing the Young Athlete

Participating in athletics and physical activity offers a refreshing alternative to the typical American's sedentary lifestyle, and children who are interested in sports should be encouraged to be as active as their schedule will allow. Children have different dietary needs from adults, and special attention should be given to the nutritional requirements of the active child. In addition to training and talent, the foods athletes use to fuel their bodies can make the difference between sitting on the bench or being on the starting team.

The optimal sports diet for children builds on the basics of proper nutrition set forth by the

> **MYTH** Eating spinach makes strong muscles.
> **FACT** Spinach contains many vitamins, minerals, and fiber, but it does not promote muscle strength. Muscles are developed through regular exercise combined with a balanced diet.

Food Guide Pyramid (see chapter 4). This chapter will discuss the general dietary guidelines for athletic performance and the nutritional requirements of exercise as well as review various special considerations and controversial practices of young athletes.

General Guidelines for Athletic Performance

Whether the child is a competitive athlete or an exercise buff, developing a personalized training plan is fundamental for optimal physical performance. Do young athletes require different types of food? Actually, an ideal diet for a young athlete

· ·

Barry Goldberg ▪ Lisa Tartamella

includes the same types of food required for any other child and is described by the Food Guide Pyramid (see chapter 4). The pyramid advocates eating a wide variety of foods to ensure that the diet includes all the nutrients that active children need for growth and physical activity. The pyramid includes a range of servings for each of the food groups, but how much does an active child need on a daily basis?

CARBOHYDRATES Carbohydrates are one of the best sources of energy because they are used to fuel muscles during exercise. They are considered the foundation of an athlete's diet. The amount of carbohydrate used during exercise depends on the intensity level and duration of the activity. Brief, intense exercise, like lifting weights or running the 100-meter dash, uses glucose from the muscle's glycogen stores. Endurance sports, like cycling or running, first use glycogen for energy and then turn to the body's fat stores.

Young athletes should aim to obtain between 50 and 55 percent of their total calories from carbohydrates. Simple arithmetic can help determine the amount of carbohydrates needed each day. For example, a school-age athlete who requires around 2,500 calories a day should try to obtain at least 1,250 calories (50 percent) from carbohydrates. Since each gram of carbohydrate provides 4 calories, this individual should eat about 313 grams of carbohydrate per day (1,250 ÷ 4 calories/gram = 313 grams). Listed below is the carbohydrate content of various foods.

Food	Carbohydrate (in g)
1 slice bread	12
1 bagel	31
1 cup pasta	40
1 cup rice	59
1 medium baked potato	51
1 large waffle	26
½ cup corn	21
½ cup carrots	17
1 cup apple juice	29
1 cup grape juice	38
1 cup Rice Krispies	25
1 tsp sugar	4
1 tbsp jelly	14
⅔ cup raisins	79

It is especially important to eat carbohydrates as soon as possible after training because the glycogen in muscles needs to be replaced at that time. Juices are an excellent choice right after practice or competition since they are loaded with carbohydrates, vitamins, and minerals. A high-carbohydrate meal should follow two to three hours later to make sure that muscles are ready for the next training session. The above list provides a sampling of high-carbohydrate foods.

Since carbohydrates are the best form of fuel for physical activity, athletes often try to increase their stores of glycogen just prior to a game or event using a popular technique called carbohydrate loading. Carbohydrate loading is most effective for endurance events lasting longer than 90 minutes. Although athletes should try to eat a high-carbohydrate diet daily, carbohydrate loading involves a special diet designed to maximize the young athlete's carbohydrate consumption while reducing the amount of time the athlete spends in training on the day before competition. Rest is especially important, since this helps to load muscles with extra glycogen prior to endurance events. To prevent dehydration when carbohydrate loading, it is also important to drink extra water and juices.

PROTEIN Protein is another important part of the young athlete's diet, but will an extra steak or protein supplements lead to quicker quadriceps and bigger biceps? Although muscle is mostly made up of protein, excessive amounts of protein in the diet can hamper performance rather than enhance it, and eating extra protein does not make muscles larger or stronger. The extra protein in the diet is either burned up for energy or stored as fat. Too much protein without adequate water can also lead to dehydration, a condition that is detrimental to athletic performance.

Do young athletes need more protein than other children? Protein needs differ during different stages of a child's life cycle. Most healthy children need roughly 0.5 grams of protein per pound of body weight per day. Young athletes may benefit from slightly more protein since training may increase their needs. A general daily goal should be between 0.6 and 0.9 grams per pound of body weight. This may sound like a lot, but it really is not. The protein content of a few foods is listed below.

Food	Protein (in g)
1 cup low-fat or skim milk	8
3 oz chicken, lean meat, fish	21
(3 oz is about the size of a deck of cards)	
½ cup cooked dried beans or peas	7
1 large egg	7
1 oz cheddar cheese	8
2 tbsp peanut butter	9

Are supplements necessary? Plenty of protein and essential amino acids are available from foods, so protein supplements are unnecessary and can even be harmful if misused. Supplements are also expensive; the same types of amino acids present in supplements can be found in a glass of milk or a serving of meat and do not cost nearly as much.

FAT From our concern with heart disease and high cholesterol, fat has gotten a bad reputation. Indeed, the typical American diet includes much more fat than the body usually needs. When used in moderation, however, fat plays an important part in athletic performance and is essential for a growing child. Although carbohydrates are the primary fuel source for working muscles, fat is also used for energy when the exercise is performed for at least 30 minutes at a low intensity. Growing children need adequate dietary fat for normal growth as well as for endurance events. In addition, for children who are competing in sports with weight classes (like wrestling), restricting dietary fat can be dangerous because this fat provides an important source of energy.

VITAMINS AND MINERALS True or false?

- Megadoses of vitamins give an athlete extra energy.
- Taking extra iron will help an athlete run faster.

If you answered "true" to either of the above questions, it's time to talk about the real truth behind vitamin and mineral supplements.

Vitamins do not supply the body with energy because they do not contain any calories. Vitamins are necessary, however, for they help the body convert food into energy. Vitamins are like the spark plugs in a car—not the gas. Growing children need vitamins on a daily basis, but taking supplements and extra dosages will not make young athletes stronger or faster. Vitamin-rich foods can be found throughout the Food Guide Pyramid, and a balanced diet will supply sufficient amounts.

Minerals also play important roles in body functioning. Calcium is important for bone development. Calcium deficiencies are often linked to a higher incidence of stress fractures in athletes.

Athletes, like all children, should strive to include at least three servings of calcium-rich foods each day. Good choices include low-fat dairy foods like low-fat cheese, milk, yogurt, pudding, and custard. Iron deficiency can lead to poor stamina. Good sources of iron are meat, fish, and poultry. For those who do not eat meat, iron can be obtained from legumes and iron-fortified foods. Adolescent females may be at risk for iron deficiency, and in some cases supplements may be appropriate (see chapter 31).

All of the vitamins and minerals that a growing athlete needs should come from food. Active athletes generally require more calories and fluids than less active children, but a well-balanced diet will provide the additional vitamins and minerals naturally. Taking a vitamin and mineral supplement is not necessary and may provide a false sense of security. Supplements cannot compensate for poor dietary habits. Children with dietary restrictions should be sure that all their vitamin and mineral requirements are met by their permitted foods. Improved athletic performance comes from hard work, training, and talent; there is no evidence that extra vitamins or minerals will help at all.

Caloric Requirements

In addition to supporting growth, a young athlete's caloric needs should consider the energy requirements of the activity. Energy needs can be estimated by evaluating the athlete's growth rate, age, and activity patterns. It is crucial to provide adequate calories so that protein is spared for building muscle rather than being used to supply energy.

Energy expenditure during exercise is sport-specific. Consideration should be given to the athlete's training schedule, level of competition, time

TABLE 13.1
Energy Expenditure for Different Sports and Activities

Activity	Energy expenditure*	
	Per minute	Per hour
Basketball	6.9	414
Cycling 9.4 mph	5.0	300
5.5 mph	3.2	192
Football	6.6	396
Gymnastics	3.3	198
Running 9 min/mile	9.7	582
8 min/mile	10.8	648
7 min/mile	12.2	732
Tennis	5.5	330

*For a 110-lb (50-kg) adult.

spent training, and intensity of the training program. Since sport-specific caloric expenditures do not exist for children, adult values are often used as a guide. These assist in estimating the approximate amount of energy used per kilogram of body weight. Since children may be less efficient in their body movements than adults, however, these values are often on the low side. Examples of the amount of extra calories needed according to the type of exercise are shown in table 13.1.

The best way to determine whether the athlete is consuming adequate calories is to monitor growth patterns and changes in weight. Although growth rates vary among individual children, weight and height should remain proportional. Excessive weight loss is a danger signal (see chapter 12); another tell-tale sign of inadequate energy intake is a decline in physical performance. Before making any dietary changes, consult a pediatrician or registered dietitian for assistance in evaluating the athlete's daily intake and the need for changes.

Many parents and coaches believe that achieving a specific weight will give an athlete a competitive edge. Defining the "ideal" weight can often be misleading and impractical, however, since each child is unique. The appropriate body weight is a highly individual matter; it is a weight at which the athlete has a positive body image with ample energy to practice and compete.

Identifying athletes that could benefit from a program of weight loss or weight gain takes a skilled eye and is best left to the professional expertise of a pediatrician or registered dietitian. Much too often, children delve into the quick-fix promises of diet pills, fads, and supplements—all of which can be detrimental to a growing and developing body. Moreover, this continuous focus on food and weight loss or gain may foster abnormal eating behaviors. Children should establish sound nutritional habits that will serve them on the practice field as well as in adulthood.

Trying to drop a couple of pounds just before a competition to fit into a certain weight category is a poor choice for any athlete. Drastically reducing an athlete's intake can lead to a decline in stamina and performance, as well as poor growth. It is particularly risky to try to lose weight quickly with pills or powders. Rapid weight loss is usually associated with the loss of fluids and muscle tissue and may lead to dehydration, depleted muscle glycogen stores, needless fatigue, and poor performance. Most young athletes, particularly boys, are still growing in height and gaining weight. Trying to remain within a weight category by limiting food intake over long periods of time can adversely affect normal growth and development.

Obsessive concern with weight loss should be monitored carefully, especially in young female athletes. Extreme eating behaviors can lead to the development of eating disorders like anorexia or bulimia, which may require the assistance of a professional (see chapter 17).

Underweight athletes may not always have adequate energy to perform at their best; others may have a problem maintaining their weight. Gaining weight should be easy: eat more calories than the body burns. But this may not always be so simple for the young athlete, since adequate calories must also be consumed for growth and for continued athletic activity as well. When trying to gain weight, it is important to continue to exercise so that the additional calories contribute to gaining muscle mass rather than excessive amounts of fat. Weight goals should be realistic and should be designed by a pediatrician or registered dietitian. A slow weight gain, ½ to 1 pound per week, will help to ensure that lean body mass is being gained rather than extra body fat.

Competitive athletes may need to consume between 3,000 and 5,000 calories each day! The extra calories necessary for weight gain should come from foods that are high in carbohydrates rather than in fat. Below are some healthy techniques for gaining weight:

- Eat larger portions at mealtimes or eat smaller amounts more often.
- Eat high-carbohydrate snacks between meals.
- Eat plenty of both complex and simple carbohydrates; some favorites include pancakes with syrup, cereal with low-fat milk, lowfat yogurt, juice.
- Eat nutrient-dense foods (such as dried beans, lasagna, beef stew)

It may be easier to drink, rather than eat, the extra calories. One idea is to substitute high-calorie drinks for low-calorie ones by drinking juice instead of diet soda, for example. Commercially prepared supplements designed for weight gain may work well to add extra pounds, but they are often expensive. Instead, delicious homemade, high-calorie milk shakes can be concocted using instant breakfast, low-fat milk, and a banana. Raw eggs should be avoided. They may have worked for Rocky, but they pose too high a risk of salmonella. Fitting these snacks into busy days filled with competitive activities is considered later in this chapter.

Fluids and Electrolytes

The importance of water is well established. Approximately 60 percent of our weight is water, and an average adult will require 2.5 quarts each day to replace water that has been lost from the skin, lungs, and kidneys. Children require proportionately less water, but a physically active child requires a greater amount of water because water helps regulate body temperature during activity. In addition, ambient conditions (temperature, humidity, wind, and sun) can make it even more difficult to maintain appropriate body temperature and may make it necessary to consume extra amounts of fluid. In prolonged, high-intensity exercise, salt is also lost through sweat. For the competitive athlete, the replacement of both water and salt needs to be considered or diminished performance and heat-related problems may result.

Thermoregulation

During exercise, the body must rid itself of the extra heat produced by muscle activity. The body eliminates extra heat by increasing blood flow to the skin, by losing heat through ventilation, and by sweating. The environment in which the exercise is occurring can make it more difficult for the body to reduce its heat. The temperature zone between 25 and 27 °C (77 and 80 °F) and a relative humidity between 50 and 60 percent are considered neutral. As temperature and humidity rise, the body will respond with increased blood flow to the skin

and then with increased sweating to allow for the dissipation of heat by evaporation. Acclimatization occurs with repetitive exposure to exercise in hot or humid conditions. Acclimatization results in an increased sweating rate, an increase in the sensitivity of the sweating response to changes in core temperature, an increase in blood volume, and a decrease in the electrolyte content of sweat. Adults will become acclimated to heat or humidity in 3 to 4 days, but children may require 1 week.

Children do not respond to heat as well as older adolescents and adults. They have a lower sweating rate, deficient evaporative capacity, a lower cardiac output at a given work level, and diminished blood flow to the skin. At temperature extremes children are most susceptible to heat-related illness. Chronic diseases such as obesity, congenital heart disease, and cystic fibrosis magnify this risk. Children with anorexia nervosa or bulimia may not recognize their need for extra fluids, either because of their eating disorder or because the thirst center in their brain is not functioning properly. As exercise progresses, body fluids and salts are lost through sweating and breathing. Unless these fluids and salts are replaced, the body will enter a state of dehydration. Sweat rates can be as much as 4 to 6 cups per hour, but most athletes generally consume about 2 cups of fluid per hour. Thirst alone is an inadequate stimulus for children, and if left to drink on their own, only two-thirds of their lost fluid will be replaced. After repeated days of exercise, these cumulative losses may leave the child dangerously dehydrated. Another potential danger is the practice of losing weight through dehydration in order to qualify for a lower weight class in such sports as wrestling.

Dehydration can adversely affect performance and health. The heart rate rises by approximately 8 beats per minute for every 2.2 pounds of fluid that is lost. The increased heart rate reduces endurance and hinders strength and mental alertness. The blood flow throughout the body is also diminished by fluid loss, and core body temperature will rise by 0.6°F (0.3°C). A heat-related illness may be the result. Heat-related illnesses can include muscle cramps, headaches, fainting, giddiness, poor coordination, pallor or flushed skin, nausea, vomiting, chills, or exhaustion. The most serious condition, heat stroke, is a true medical emergency that can result in death. Body temperature rises, sweating usually stops, and the child may be disoriented, become comatose, or have a seizure. Immediate medical attention must be sought, and the child must be placed immediately in a cool environment. Body temperature can also be lowered by sponging with cool water.

Coaches and athletes must stay aware of temperature and humidity and modify the intensity of their training appropriately. When the temperature is greater than 80°F (27°C) and the humidity is greater than 70 percent, the following precautions are essential: wear light-colored cotton clothing to permit maximum skin ventilation, wear hats to decrease the absorption of radiant heat from the sun, institute rest periods in well-ventilated areas every 20 to 30 minutes, drink fluids during breaks, and reduce the intensity of the activities. Any child with an underlying medical problem should be closely monitored. When the temperature is above 90°F (32°C) and the humidity is greater than 70 percent, practices should be canceled or dramatically reduced.

Fluid Replacement

Fluid replacement during and after exercise is essential, although the amount needed depends on the athlete, the athletic activity, and the weather. Children and adolescents who are participating in sports cannot drink too much liquid. What their bodies do not need, they will eliminate through urination. Prior to practice or a game, an athlete should "overhydrate," particularly if it is a humid day, by taking 10 to 12 ounces of fluid 30 minutes prior to competition. If the activity lasts more than 90 minutes, 3 to 4 ounces of fluid should be consumed every 20 minutes, and if the activity lasts 3 hours or more, electrolytes and sugar must be replaced. Cool (55°F [13°C]) fluids will be more palatable. Flavoring the water will also help. In addition, fluids taken without solids will enhance stomach emptying and hasten absorption. After the activity, each pound of weight that was lost should be replaced with a pint of extra fluid.

Electrolytes, especially sodium and potassium, will be lost in sweat. These minerals are important regulators of fluid balance in the body (see chapter 33). They can be replaced by a normal diet as long as the activity is not prolonged beyond 3 hours or the temperature and humidity are not excessive. Most fluids for exercise replacement contain 50–110 milligrams of sodium and 25–85 milligrams of potassium per 8 ounces. Replacement solutions containing these minerals are shown in table 13.2. Salt pills with high concentrations of sodium should not be used. Fluids containing electrolytes (such as commercial sports drinks) should be used if a meal will not be consumed between prolonged endurance events.

Exercise is fueled by glucose (a simple carbohydrate), and there is good evidence that prolonged performance exercise can be improved through glucose supplementation during the exercise. Glucose in replacement fluids will act as a supplementary sugar source as long as the exercise does not exceed 75 percent of the child's maximum aerobic capacity. Several studies have shown that 120 to 400 grams of glucose supple-

TABLE 13.2

Carbohydrate, Sodium, and Potassium in Common Drinks (per 8-oz serving)

Product	Percent of carbohydrate	Carb. (g)	Type of carb.	Sodium (mg)	Potassium (mg)
Gatorade	6	14.4	Sucrose, glucose	110	25
Exceed	7.2	17.3	Glucose, polymer, fructose	50	45
Quickkick	4.7	11.3	Sucrose	116	23
10K	6.3	15	Sucrose, glucose, fructose	52	86
Orange juice	11.8	28	Sucrose, glucose, fructose	2.7	510
Coca-Cola	11.3		High-fructose corn syrup	9.2–28	Trace

Source: The Science of Gatorade, Beverage Comparison Chart.

mentation will improve endurance when the activity lasts longer than 90 or 120 minutes. Unfortunately, such high concentrations of glucose in a drink will limit fluid absorption due to the delayed emptying of the stomach. Nevertheless, for activities lasting beyond 90 to 120 minutes, carbohydrate replacement during the activity is of benefit and 4.7 to 7.2 percent (11 to 17 grams per quart) of carbohydrate is commonly found in sports drinks. Glucose polymers, found in some sport drinks, appear to be more effectively absorbed than pure fructose or glucose solutions.

Drinks containing caffeine actually increase urine production at the expense of hydration, which is not good for the young athlete. Increased fluid loss also occurs with high-protein diets because of the need to eliminate waste products. In hot or humid environments, high-protein diets should never be followed because they will promote dehydration and can result in a heat-related illness.

Meals before and after Competition

PRE-EVENT MEALS No magic bars or shakes will enable athletes to run faster or jump higher. The best energy booster is a well-balanced, high-carbohydrate diet that is observed throughout the training season. On the day of an event, it is a good idea to schedule a pre-event meal or snack to prevent hunger right before an event and to provide additional fuel for the muscles during exercise. Remember, this meal or snack is not intended to supply all of the energy needed for competition; this should come from the meals eaten the day and even the week before.

What are the best pre-event foods? There is no magical answer, but foods that are high in complex carbohydrates and low in fat are always good choices.

Larger meals take longer to digest than smaller snacks. To make sure that the athlete is not exercising on a full stomach, meals should be eaten 1 to 4 hours before practice or competition. Good choices 1 to 2 hours before an event include fruit or vegetable juice or a piece of fruit. Breads like bagels or English muffins, pasta, low-fat yogurt, or cereal with lowfat milk are smart ideas 3 to 4 hours before an event. Be sure to drink plenty of water.

Generally speaking, athletes should avoid eating sugary foods like candy or soda right before exercising. Eating or drinking a lot of sugar prior to physical activity makes some athletes feel dizzy or light-headed.

MEALS DURING EVENTS If the athlete is participating in all-day events, like swim and track meets, it is a smart idea to have energy-enhancing snacks on hand. Some ideas include fruits, bagels, pretzels, muffins, and, perhaps most important, plenty of fluids. Children should be encouraged to drink all day long. Making wise choices at the concession stand is also important. The high-fat and fried foods like hot dogs and French fries that are often popular at concession stands should be avoided, since they take longer to digest and do not provide the best form of energy for working muscles. Sports drinks are generally not necessary for young athletes, but they do provide carbohydrates for energy, as discussed above.

POST-EVENT MEALS After exercising, it is important to drink plenty of fluids, and it is also a good time to start thinking about fueling up muscles for the next workout and replacing electrolytes that have been lost. Since muscles are most efficient at storing glycogen 2 to 3 hours after exercising, a high-carbohydrate meal should follow about 2 hours after the event. Fruit juices are an excellent choice immediately after physical activity since they are easy to digest and are reasonable sources of vitamins and minerals. An 8-ounce serving of most juices contains about 30 grams of carbohydrate.

Ergogenic Aids

Ergogenic aids are practices or products that are believed to improve athletic performance. For example, a high-carbohydrate diet is a practice that has been successful in enhancing performance. Some products, like anabolic steroids, are illegal and can endanger the athlete's health. Nutritional ergogenic agents, such as powders, bars, and shakes, enjoy wide popularity, but few, if any,

have demonstrated efficacy in enhancing performance and many are expensive. The danger of nutritional ergogenic agents is that they may cause nutritional imbalances.

Preparations of amino acids have become available to athletes, often at a very high price. Arginine has most frequently been promoted for its ability to stimulate growth hormone, which may increase muscle mass. It has not, however, been demonstrated that oral arginine exerts a significant effect. Aspartic acid, branch chain amino acids, and glutamate have no proven beneficial effect on performance, although glycine, when given in dosages greater than 6 grams per day, can cause an increase in growth hormone. The benefits and risks of this increase have not been established. Lysine and ornithine have no proven ergogenic benefit, and tryptophan, though it can stimulate growth hormone, has been associated with significant toxicity and has been banned by the Food and Drug Administration. Ornithine alpha-2-ketoglutomate may be beneficial in protein synthesis and growth hormone secretion, but more research is required. Consuming certain fats has been postulated to improve performance in selected areas. Omega-3 fatty acids are long chains of polyunsaturated fatty acids that are thought to improve the delivery of oxygen to muscles and thus to enhance recovery after exercise. Medium-chain triglycerides, found in palm oil, coconuts, and milk, may act as an excellent energy source that will spare glycogen. These medium-chain triglycerides, however, are saturated fats, excessive amounts of which have been linked to heart disease and liver problems.

Athletes have frequently experimented with megadoses of vitamins to improve performance. The B vitamins have not demonstrably improved performance, even when taken in amounts beyond those normally recommended. Vitamin C works as an antioxidant, but it has not been shown to improve performance or regenerate muscle. Antioxidants are believed to reduce the damage by free radicals (toxic by-products) to muscle membranes, but this effect has yet to be proven. Excessive amounts of vitamin D have not been shown to have any benefit on athletic performance. Taking large amounts of vitamin C and the B vitamins is unlikely to be harmful because the body eliminates the unnecessary amounts in the urine. Excessive amounts of vitamins A, D, E, and K, on the other hand, can cause vitamin toxicity because they are stored in the fat cells of the body (see chapter 31).

Athletes have also tried megadoses of minerals. Calcium supplementation beyond established need has no proven ergogenic effect, although it can be of value for women or girls with low levels of estrogen whose bones are stressed from a heavy training regimen. Supplements of magnesium or phosphate have also not been shown to be of any benefit. Iron requirements appear to be greater in athletes than in the general population, but when body iron stores are normal, megadoses have no benefit and can be harmful. Excessive amounts of copper and zinc also have no established ergogenic role. Selenium may have a role as an antioxidant, and chromium has a possible role in increasing lean body mass and improving carbohydrate metabolism, though the effect of these minerals on athletic performance has not been proven.

Other dietary substances have received attention as ergogenic agents and are used by many athletes. Caffeine may improve the storage of glycogen and the metabolism of fat, but it is banned by the National Collegiate Athletic Association and the International Olympic Committee in levels greater than 12 to 15 milligrams per milliliter of urine (2 cups of coffee can result in a urine level of 3 to 6 milligrams per milliliter). Ferrulates— ferulic acid—are found in plants, function as antioxidants, and may stimulate growth hormone. No significant toxicity has been demonstrated, but neither have the studies of ferulic acid been adequate to demonstrate its efficacy. Gelatin has no demonstrated ergogenic effect. Ginseng may enhance performance, but studies are not as yet conclusive. Succinate and wheat-germ oil have no benefit on athletic performance, and pollen, though reported to be of some benefit by European studies, has not been shown to have any ergogenic effect in American studies. The benefits of brewer's yeast, carnitine, choline, kelp, lecithin, octacosanol, and royal jelly have also not been demonstrated.

Exercise places an increased burden on the body, particularly on the need for fluids and carbohydrates, and diet is an important component of athletic performance. None of the claims of so-called ergogenic nutritional aids have been substantiated, so eating nutritious meals and developing sound eating habits are the best way to optimize an athlete's performance. Coaches and trainers should encourage young athletes to achieve recommended nutritional goals. Appropriate weight gain and loss should be directed to enhancing performance levels and not pushed to extremes resulting in pathological conditions.

Resources

Clark, N. *Nancy Clark's Sports Nutrition Guidebook: Eating to Fuel Your Active Lifestyle.* Champaign, IL: Leisure Press, 1990.

Jennings, D. S., and S. N. Steen. *Sports Nutrition for the Child Athlete.* Chicago: American Dietetic Association, 1993.

Sports Nutrition. *A Guide for the Professional Working with Active People.* D. Bernardot, ed. Chicago: American Dietetic Association, 1993.

Steen, S. N. *Nutritional Assessment and Management of the School-Aged Child Athlete, Sports Nutrition for the 90s: The Health Professional's Handbook.* Gaithersburg, MD: Aspen Publishers, 1991.

14

. . . .

Acne and Diet: Is There a Connection?

Adolescence is a time of stress for both parent and child; the parent is learning to limit advice to significant issues, and the adolescent is striving for independence. This struggle can spill over into the physician's office when the family seeks treatment for teenage acne. Acne is, as parent and teenager both agree, an unwanted marker of the transition from childhood to adulthood. Acne may also become the focus of disputes over behavior modification, with the parent invariably looking to the physician to support the notion that the adolescent's "terrible eating habits" are at least making the acne worse, if not causing it.

MYTH Chocolate and fried foods cause acne.

FACT Research has not shown a connection between the consumption of chocolate or foods that are high in fat and the appearance of acne. Acne is primarily associated with hormonal changes in adolescence.

Generations of acne sufferers have been told to avoid foods that can purportedly cause acne: fatty foods, chocolate, candy, nuts, carbonated beverages, ice cream and other milk products, and even shellfish. At a time when our society is more food-conscious than ever before, when dietary factors are being implicated as the causes of such diverse illnesses as heart disease, diabetes, cancer of the bowel, and tooth decay, if teenagers change their eating habits and forgo some of their favorite foods, will it help them have clear skin?

. . . .

Ellen B. Milstone ▪ Leonard M. Milstone

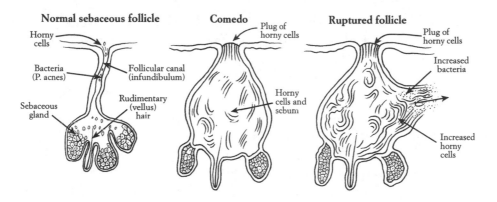

FIGURE 14.1
Development of comedo (whitehead or blackhead) to an inflamed pustule.

What Causes Acne?

Acne vulgaris results from many factors, including heredity, hormonal effects on hair follicles and oil glands, abnormal buildup of cells that line the hair follicle, excessive growth of bacteria that are normally found in the hair follicle, and probably other factors that are not yet fully understood. Acne is a disease of the pilosebaceous unit, a structure in which a hair follicle and an oil gland share a common opening to the skin surface (fig. 14.1). Acne occurs in virtually all adolescents and ranges in severity from an occasional "whitehead" or "blackhead" (comedo), to more inflamed pustules or severely inflamed cysts that leave scars after they resolve.

Pilosebaceous units occur on most areas of the body, but acne develops only in regions where the oil glands are the largest. The hormonal changes of adolescence cause those particular oil glands to enlarge and produce adult levels of the oily secretion known as sebum. Sebum production is a prerequisite for acne to occur, and increased sebum production and acne usually appear up to two years before other signs of puberty. The first stage in the development of acne is the accumulation of cells within the lining of the hair follicle

where it opens to the skin surface. This buildup of cells causes a plug that blocks the opening to the skin surface and slows the flow of sebum from the oil gland to the surface. Some bacteria, especially one named *Propionobacterium acnes,* are normally present in the pilosebaceous follicle, and the collection of sebum in the blocked hair follicle stimulates the growth of these bacteria. The bacteria produce minute amounts of substances that are very irritating to the skin and attract inflammatory cells to the pilosebaceous follicle.

When applied to the skin in a concentrated form, a number of naturally occurring oily substances contained in creams, lotions, hair care products, or coconut oil can aggravate acne by plugging the pilosebaceous follicle. Likewise, ingestion of certain industrial toxins (for example, tetrachlorodibenzodioxin, the toxic chemical in Agent Orange) can cause acne. Certain medical conditions (such as Cushing's disease) or medicines (such as cortisone) can make acne worse, and starvation diets lessen acne.

Acne and Food

Does the ingestion of normal foodstuffs by otherwise healthy individuals cause acne? Do omissions or additions to the diet aggravate or ameliorate acne? Many patients are absolutely convinced that certain foods cause their acne to flare up, and it would be unwise for the physician and parent to totally discount such observations. Yet, there are no well-documented studies linking diet to acne, although many anecdotal observations and poorly designed studies can be found in medical journals. Because the natural change in sebum production in early adolescence is closely associated with the onset of acne, many studies have examined the effect of diet on the rate of excretion and the fat composition of sebum. The results of those studies are conflicting, but most experts believe that although certain diets may alter the content and amount of sebum produced, none has been shown to have a direct effect on acne.

FATS Although applications of some fatty substances to the skin may aggravate acne, there is no convincing data that eating fatty foods does the same. This is because fats in the diet are digested and extensively metabolized by the body before being excreted to the skin surface by the sebaceous gland. There is no tendency toward increased blood levels of cholesterol or triglycerides in acne patients. Neither fat supplements nor restrictions alter the occurrence or severity of acne. In one study, however, low-fat diets sufficiently stringent to cause weight loss in obese patients also reduced the severity of their acne. In a double-blind study of patients who thought that chocolate worsened their acne, excessive intake of chocolate and fat in candy bars had no effect on their acne.

CARBOHYDRATES There is no evidence that individuals with acne have abnormal consumption or metabolism of carbohydrates. Attempts to treat acne by limiting sugar intake have been unsuc-

cessful. One study showed no difference in the amount of acne between patients on a restricted sugar diet and those allowed to eat unlimited amounts of sugar.

IODIDES Acne-like eruptions are seen in some patients given large doses of oral iodides as medication for other conditions. Although a controlled series in the 1930s did show worsening of existing acne from oral iodides, very large doses were administered that would never be consumed in a normal diet. Subsequent studies showed that supplements of iodized salt did not cause acne to flare up.

VITAMINS AND MINERALS It has been well established that insufficient intake of vitamins and minerals can cause skin disease, but recommended daily allowances established to maintain good health prevent those skin problems as well. Nonetheless, deficiency states can be caused by malabsorption or by an increased metabolic requirement in some people on otherwise adequate diets.

Several trace elements are necessary for normal development of the skin. Of these, zinc has been the one most carefully studied with regard to acne. Although some studies have suggested that dietary supplements of zinc improve pustular acne, other studies have shown no correlation. Furthermore, there is no indication that patients with acne are zinc-deficient.

Vitamin A deficiency causes early changes in hair follicles resembling the changes seen in acne, but there is no evidence that patients with acne are deficient in vitamin A. In very high doses (500,000 IU per day), vitamin A can be effective for acne, but severe toxic side effects to other organs preclude its use. These findings have led pharmaceutical companies to develop chemically altered forms of vitamin A that are effective in treating acne, are safe to use, and are available from your doctor. Since such treatments can still have adverse side effects, however, they must be carefully monitored by your doctor.

In summary, no well-documented evidence exists that diet aggravates acne or that dietary manipulation can improve acne significantly. This is important information because teenagers should not be made to feel that what they eat causes or worsens their acne. To date, no cure exists for acne, but no one needs to suffer with acne either. Eliminating acne can promote a teenager's self-esteem and reduce stress, and many good therapies that can control acne until it disappears are available from dermatologists or other qualified physicians.

Alcohol Use and Abuse in Adolescents

Alcohol is one of the most readily available and commonly abused drugs. Problems with drinking and alcohol abuse often begin early. A 1994 survey of high school students found that 92.2 percent had consumed alcohol at least once, and 66.4 percent admitted to drinking in the previous month. It is estimated that by the eighth grade, more than 300,000 children in the United States are binge drinkers, and this number doubles by tenth grade. Use and abuse of alcohol in teenagers is associated with failing grades, dropping out of school, serious accidents and injuries, violent crimes, and death. Alcohol is a factor in ap-

> **MYTH** You can't get drunk on beer.
>
> **FACT** Although beer contains less alcohol per ounce than wine or distilled liquor, a typical serving of each (12 ounces of beer, 5 ounces of wine, or 1½ ounces of distilled liquor) contains a comparable amount of alcohol.

proximately 40 percent of teenage drownings and more than 75 percent of fatal car accidents involving adolescents. Many teenage suicides are accompanied by the use of alcohol and other drugs, and at least 33 percent of serious crimes committed by adolescents are preceded by alcohol use.

Young people tend to drink less consistently than adults, but they drink more on any given occasion and are thus at greater risk for the behavioral and acute neurological impairments that accompany excessive alcohol intake. Moreover, if heavy drinking patterns are established at an early age, they may

· ·

Linda C. Mayes ▪ Teresa Fung ▪ Ed Strenkowski

TABLE 15.1

Relation Between Blood Alcohol Level and Neurological Impairments

Blood alcohol levels (g/100 ml)	Neurological effects
0.02	Feel warm and relaxed (usually the level reached after one drink in an adult)
0.05	Talkative; inhibitions, judgment, and restraint are reduced
0.08 (level of legal impairment in some states)*	Altered coordination, impaired judgment about capabilities (ability to drive, for example), slowed reaction time, impaired muscle coordination, numbness of arms and legs, tingling of hands
0.10 (level of legal intoxication in most states)*	Clumsiness, slurred speech, increasing impairment in muscle control and reaction time
0.15	Impaired balance and movement
0.2	Slurred speech, staggering, loss of balance, double vision
0.3	Lack of understanding of what is seen or heard; confusion, stupor
0.4	Loss of consciousness; clammy skin
0.45	Respiratory suppression, slowed respiration, coma
0.50	Lethal level

*Many states now have "zero tolerance" alcohol limits for underage drivers.

persist throughout adulthood. The acute physical consequences of too much alcohol, such as bleeding ulcers and an inflamed gastrointestinal tract (gastritis), occur in adolescents just as they do in adults.

Acute Effects of Alcohol

Excessive alcohol consumption causes some of the most severe and widespread adverse health consequences of any of the drugs of abuse. With chronic alcohol abuse, nearly every organ system suffers. Alcohol abuse in children and adolescents acutely alters judgment, learning, motivation, and peer relations. Alcohol produces euphoria and decreases appetite. However, alcohol is actually a depressant that sedates nerve cells, slows thinking and reaction times, and impairs decision-making capacities. Voluntary muscle control is impaired,

including those muscle systems involved in speaking (thus, the slurred speech of alcohol intoxication) as well as those reflexes required for quick action (while driving, for example). Despite impaired reaction times, the release of inhibitions by alcohol leads to faster and more reckless driving. Vomiting is one of the body's self-defense mechanisms to prevent one from drinking more alcohol. As neurological sedation progresses with continuing consumption, the drinker first loses consciousness and then the basic brain functions regulating respiration and body temperature are suppressed. If untreated at this stage, the individual lapses into a coma and may die.

The specific acute effects of alcohol on the brain depend on the blood alcohol level (BAL; grams/100 milliliters). The degree of neurological impairment provides a general guide to the degree of overconsumption. For persons not accustomed to alcohol, a low BAL may lead to a greater degree of functional impairment than for an individual who is used to drinking alcohol. Table 15.1 provides the correlation between BAL and neurological and psychological symptoms for a person unaccustomed to alcohol.

Binge drinking, with its attendant high BAL, is common among adolescents. Many experts believe that occasional bingeing episodes may be more harmful to the brain and nervous system than regular but small to moderate amounts of drinking that do not result in intoxication.

Additional effects of excessive alcohol consumption include mildly elevated blood pressure, a modest decline in body temperature, dilatation of peripheral blood vessels (leading to the flushing and sense of warmth that accompany alcohol ingestion), and increased salivary and stomach secretions. Alcohol increases urine production by the kidneys by suppressing a hormone that controls the amount of urine produced. Therefore, though alcohol is a liquid, it actually has a dehydrating effect, since it increases urination. This helps explain the dry mouth that accompanies a hangover. Alcohol also interferes with the regulation of blood-sugar levels, and with increasing BAL, blood-sugar levels may decrease to dangerously low levels, producing hypoglycemia. Thus, the risk of severe intoxication involves the combination of dehydration, hypoglycemia, loss of consciousness, and lowered body temperature.

Long-Term Effects of Alcohol Abuse

With long-term alcohol abuse, virtually every organ system is affected. Among the most severely affected are the central and peripheral nervous systems and the gastrointestinal and cardiovascular systems. Damage to the brain and spinal cord is manifest as memory loss and confabulation (making up stories), degeneration of the nerves that control eye movements, and a loss of balance control. Additionally, with chronic alcohol abuse, alcohol-associated dementia results, and for some alcoholics, there is a decrease in overall brain size, probably because of alcohol-associated brain cell death. The severe liver disease associated with alcohol abuse also contributes to neurological problems including impaired sleep-wake regulation, mood swings, impulsive behavior, and ultimately confusion, disorientation, and coma. Alcohol-induced degeneration of the nerves to the trunk and the extremities causes the severe burning pains in the hands and feet that are often reported by alcoholics.

The gastrointestinal system, and in particular liver function, represents another area of serious organ damage. Because alcohol alters the metabolism of fat, excessive fat is deposited in the liver leading to an enlarged liver. Alcohol also causes chronic inflammation of the liver, leading to abnormal liver function and to scarring and death of areas of the liver, a condition known as cirrhosis. With abstinence, the fat deposits are reversible but cirrhosis is not. With the reduction of liver size caused by scarring and death, the usual patterns of blood flow through the liver are blocked; this leads to increased pressure in the abdominal venous system. Such pressure leads to the accumulation of fluid in the abdomen (ascites) and the development of varicose veins around the esophagus, which may rupture and bleed. Esophageal inflammation causes scarring and narrowing, further compromising the alcoholic's already lowered nutritional state. The third digestive organ to be severely compromised is the pancreas. Chronic inflammation from alcohol ingestion results in loss of function and, ultimately, diabetes and pancreatitis. The absorption of protein and essential vitamins declines as a result of the poor functioning of the liver and the pancreas. Even before the later stage complications of alcoholism set in, heavy alcohol consumers may be deficient in the vitamins thiamine and folate because of decreased appetite and poor nutrition, and these deficiencies can cause some of the neurological problems associated with alcohol. In alcohol treatment centers, many patients are given thiamine, folate, and a multivitamin to replenish the vitamins that have been lost. Chronic alcohol abuse also increases the risk of cancer of the mouth, esophagus, rectum, and lung.

Hypertension, cardiac arrhythmias (irregular heartbeat), increased deposits of fat in the coronary arteries, and a damaged heart muscle represent the cardiovascular complications of alcoholism. Although these problems are most clearly evident after years of alcohol abuse, even early alcohol abuse has direct cardiovascular effects. The direct toxic effects of alcohol, as well as concomitant poor nutrition, also lead to gradual loss of skeletal muscle and of muscle mass in the arms and legs. Deteriorating strength limits the capacity to exercise, which further limits cardiovascular conditioning. An additional cardiovascular stress comes from the anemia of alcoholism, which is caused by nutritional deficiencies and the blood loss from bleeding ulcers and esophageal varices. Anemia places a greater workload on an already stressed and compromised heart.

The severest aspects of alcohol abuse do not occur in adolescents, but it is important to realize that the process of reaching these end-stage complications begins in the earliest years of alcohol abuse. Even adolescents are at risk for the poor nutrition associated with alcohol use and for diminished cardiovascular condition. Alcohol abuse that begins during adolescence also has a number of indirect but potentially serious long-term consequences: the choice of peer group or of an in-creasingly solitary lifestyle, poor performance in school, and negative self-image. Some adolescents may use alcohol as a method of self-medicating psychological and psychiatric conditions like depression that warrant professional evaluation and treatment.

Alcohol Consumption and Nutrition

Alcohol provides 7 calories per gram but no nutrients other than calories. Because alcohol does not require any digestion, it is readily absorbed. As much as 20 percent of the ingested alcohol is absorbed immediately in the stomach. The rate of absorption also depends on amount, concentration of alcohol in the beverage, and the type of beverage. Carbonation (such as that in champagne or cocktails made with soft drinks) increases the rate of absorption, but the presence of food in the stomach delays it. The only organ that metabolizes alcohol is the liver.

If alcohol is consumed in addition to a normal diet, an adolescent may gain weight. Even with a gain in weight, however, an adolescent can still become malnourished due to vitamin B deficiencies. Adolescents who drink but do not eat will probably lose weight. The calories from the alcohol consumed throughout the day will cause a decrease in hunger and a loss of appetite. This pattern can also lead to protein, mineral, and vitamin deficiencies. For growing children and adolescents, the combined effects of decreased food intake and impaired nutrition may seriously compromise growth. Weekend binging —heavy drinking on Friday and Saturday night— may not produce the same nutritional concerns as daily drinking, but this pattern is certainly just as life-threatening, especially in regard to driving and the risks of loss of consciousness and death that accompany extreme intoxication.

Alcohol Addiction

Most adolescents who experiment with alcohol do not become addicted. Many who try alcohol stop soon after their initial exposure because they do not like it. Others may use it for several months or even years but eventually stop or reduce their use dramatically. Unfortunately, some teenagers do become seriously addicted over a period of months or years. Initial alcohol use for most adolescents is social—they drink with friends on weekends and find that alcohol helps them feel more a part of the group and alleviates, at least temporarily, social anxieties and stresses. Adolescents also cite the novelty of the experience, the sense of a rite of passage, the need (and attendant anxiety) to prove their sexual maturity, the recreational properties, and relief of boredom or depression as other reasons to use alcohol. If their use increases, adolescents may enter a phase of actual abuse in which they maintain their own supplies of alcohol and even drink by themselves outside of the social group. At this level of use, the adolescent begins to develop a tolerance for alcohol and thus requires more alcohol to achieve the same psychological effect.

Once individuals progress to nearly daily use, they may be considered addicted, and it has been suggested that adolescents progress to addiction more rapidly than adults. Adolescents who drink alcohol at this level may experience frequent blackouts (can't remember what they did when they were under the influence of alcohol) and are more likely to drink by themselves. Gradually their peer group shifts to involve only others who drink daily, and they grow increasingly isolated and become focused only on obtaining sufficient alcohol to support their addiction. At this stage, most individuals will deny that their alcohol use

is a problem. Their relationships with family and friends as well as their performance at school or work begin to deteriorate, and the adolescent may have his or her first encounter with the law for driving under the influence or for drunk and disorderly conduct.

Once an adolescent is physiologically addicted, trying to reduce use is a very difficult process. Because such withdrawal symptoms as severe craving, tremors and nervousness, nausea, hyperactivity, increased startle response, elevated heart rate and blood pressure, hallucinations, sleeplessness, and nightmares may occur, most adolescents cannot stop alcohol use at this level without outside intervention.

Four models are used to explain the varying risks of addiction to alcohol and other drugs—biological, psychological, social, and disease models. The biological model suggests that persons who become addicted to alcohol or other drugs have a biologically based susceptibility. For example, studies of identical twins have shown that if one twin is alcoholic, the other twin has at least a 50 percent chance of also becoming addicted, whereas for nonidentical twins the shared risk decreases to approximately 25 percent. Among adopted children, males whose biological fathers were alcoholics have a risk for alcoholism that is four times greater than that for adopted males whose fathers were not alcoholics. Not all individuals with an alcoholic parent progress to alcoholism, of course; factors other than biological susceptibility are also causative.

The psychological model of alcohol abuse suggests that certain personality traits and types as well as other psychological conditions, such as depression, predispose one to alcoholism. Alcohol use may temporarily relieve certain emotional states such as chronic or acute anxiety. According to this model, alcohol use is a form of self-medication and is secondary to the underlying psychological condition. Little evidence exists to support the so-called addictive personality, but among those addicted to alcohol, there is a high incidence of long-term depression, difficulties in school and work, and repeated traumas, some of which appear to predate the addiction.

The social model takes into account the environmental and experiential influences that contribute to alcohol use. Living in a family or associating with a peer group that frequently uses alcohol may contribute to a familiarity with alcohol as a way of reducing stress or of identifying with families and friends. Experiential factors associated with alcohol abuse include poverty, repeated personal losses, family chaos and discord, school or job failure. Clearly, these factors intensify the level of disorganization and stress in the individual's life, and with the accumulation of these factors, the incidence of alcohol addiction increases, but this model does not explain individual variation in the rates of addiction among adolescents growing up in these environmental and experiential conditions.

The disease model treats alcoholism as a pathological state with expected signs and symptoms, a predictable course if left untreated, and varying outcomes with different treatments. The disease model allows for an interplay between biologic, psychologic, and social factors and views addiction as a loss of control over the use of alcohol, despite the known adverse consequences. Alcoholism is characterized as a diagnosable disease or condition with a specific and multifaceted treatment plan. Additionally, the disease model underscores the chronic nature of the condition by emphasizing that individuals who have once been addicted can never return to social drinking.

Recovery Diet

To aid the recovering alcoholic in combatting the addiction, the recovery diet should stress well-balanced meals and snacks—if necessary—throughout the day. Hunger may be confused with a feeling associated with needing a drink, so the goal is to prevent feelings of extreme hunger. If the recovering adolescent is overweight, meals and snacks of lower caloric content should be planned. If the individual is underweight, extra snacks of good nutritional quality should be included to aid in regaining the lost weight (see chapters 17 and 18).

Adequate protein and complex carbohydrates are important for someone recovering from alcohol abuse or trying to decrease alcohol intake. This diet is similar to that used to treat hypoglycemia. In hypoglycemia (low blood sugar) if the blood sugar drops low enough, one may feel weak, experience shakiness, and even sweat. Prolonged periods of not eating caused by drinking can lead to low blood sugar and the same symptoms. The dietary treatment for hypoglycemia is designed to keep the blood sugar at a constant normal level and to avoid the symptoms that accompany a sudden decrease in blood sugar.

A daily multivitamin is also beneficial and will help restore vitamins and minerals that may have been depleted due to alcohol use and poor diet.

Alcohol abuse in adolescents differs in important ways from that of adults. Adolescents are still in the process of developing physically and psychologically; they have not developed adult coping skills or judgment, and they are struggling with the intense developmental pressures of emerging sexuality and impending emancipation and independence from parents and home. Alcohol use interferes with all the physical and psychological tasks of adolescence.

16

. . . .

Diet Tips to Keep That Winning Smile

Dietary factors are known to affect oral health in three major ways: (1) a balanced diet provides the essential nutrients needed for the growth and development of healthy gums and teeth, which in turn provide resistance to oral disease; (2) fluoride, a trace mineral, is known to protect tooth surfaces from destruction and demineralization; and (3) various foods play a role in the promotion or prevention of dental caries (cavities or tooth decay).

MYTH A baby falls asleep better with a bottle of juice or milk.

FACT An infant should *not* be put to bed with a bottle containing juice or milk. Liquid from the bottle can pool on the baby's teeth and cause severe tooth decay.

Good Nutrition in the Development of Teeth

A nutritionally adequate diet is an essential ingredient for the growth and development of healthy teeth, gums, and jaws. Children need essential minerals, including calcium, phosphorus, and appropriate levels of fluoride, as well as protein and vitamins for well-formed, decay-resistant teeth, and healthy oral tissues (see chapter 31). Because teeth start to develop during the sixth week of

. . . .

Donald Kohn ■ Ellen Liskov

pregnancy and begin to calcify as early as the third month, expectant mothers should make sure their diets contain sufficient nutrients throughout their pregnancy.

Fluoride and Dental Health

A balanced diet provides all the nutrients most children and adults need for good oral health, with the possible exception of fluoride. Fluoride is a naturally occurring mineral that plays a crucial role in developing and maintaining healthy, decay-resistant teeth.

When developing teeth are exposed to *systemic* fluoride that is swallowed and absorbed into the body and deposited in the calcifying tissue via the bloodstream, they become harder and more resistant to the acid attack of bacteria that starts the tooth decay process. When erupted teeth are exposed to *topical* fluoride that is applied to the surface of the teeth through the use of fluoridated toothpaste, mouthwash, or fluoride treatments, the decay resistance of their outer enamel layers is enhanced. A combination of systemic and topical applications of fluoride appears to provide optimal decay prevention.

Many natural springs and wells have sufficient fluoride to provide this important protection, and a fluoridated water supply is certainly the easiest and most effective way to enjoy the systemic benefits of this important mineral. In areas where the community water supply does not contain enough fluoride (about one part fluoride per million parts water), the level of fluoride can be adjusted. If fluoridated water is not available in your community, a pediatric dentist or pediatrician should be consulted to prescribe a supplement to provide the appropriate amount of fluoride.

Even children who drink fluoridated water will benefit from the topical effects of fluoride-containing toothpaste and mouthwash, as well as from regular, periodic topical fluoride treatments provided by dentists. All of these products are designed for topical use and should not be swallowed. Too much fluoride can cause problems. If very young children swallow excess amounts of fluoride (such as in pleasantly flavored children's toothpaste) over a prolonged period of time, white flecks called fluorosis may develop on their permanent teeth. This is one reason why pediatric dentists recommend that no more than a tiny, pea-sized drop of fluoride toothpaste be used by young children, and that the use of fluoridated mouthwash be avoided by children under the age of 6. Dental care products that have been tested for safety and effectiveness carry the Seal of Acceptance of the American Dental Association.

The Impact of Diet on Cavities

For decades, sugar has been the main focus of dietary advice concerning a child's risk of getting cavities. Many health campaigns have discouraged the consumption of foods with a high sugar content because they promote dental caries. In recent years, however, this has been an area of considerable controversy and debate.

Strong scientific evidence supports the involvement of sugar, a form of carbohydrate, in the development of cavities. Dental caries develop when bacteria, especially *Streptococcus mutans,* attach to the surface of the tooth and form a sticky coating called dental plaque. These bacteria metabolize carbohydrate from food, producing acid in the process. An acidic environment in the mouth demineralizes the surface of the teeth, making them less resistant to the bacteria and therefore more susceptible to destruction. When a food containing carbohydrate is eaten, the resulting acid attack on the teeth may last for twenty minutes or more. The more frequently carbohydrates are eaten throughout the day, the greater the opportunity for acid demineralization. Keeping teeth clean by brushing, flossing, and regular visits to the dentist so that plaque does not accumulate will minimize the effect of diet in the development of cavities. In addition, fluoride provided by the water supply, applied topically, or taken in supplements will help reduce the tooth's susceptibility to the bacterial attack that causes dental caries.

All types of sugar—sucrose, fructose, glucose, and lactose, for example—may contribute to cavity formation, given poor dental hygiene or inadequate exposure to fluoride (for more on carbohydrates, see chapter 29). Sucrose, the type of sugar obtained primarily from both white and brown sugar, is also present in many fruits and vegetables, particularly bananas, beets, potatoes, sweet potatoes, and melons. Natural sweeteners such as honey, corn syrup, and molasses have often been considered good alternatives to refined sugar. Not only do these sweeteners contain naturally occurring sucrose, fructose, and glucose, but they may actually be more harmful than refined sugars, for they are stickier and are not as easily removed from the tooth surface by saliva!

New evidence has also suggested that dietary fat can reduce the incidence of dental caries. Foods such as nuts and cheddar cheese which naturally contain fat can help neutralize the acids that demineralize the surface of the teeth and may thus help protect against caries.

As far as diet is concerned, the principles are balance and moderation. Here are a few simple tips:

- According to the dietary guidelines and the Food Guide Pyramid, fats and sweets should be eaten in moderation but not eliminated. Added sugars (refined sugar, honey, corn or maple syrup) should comprise no more than 10 percent of a child's daily calories.

- Sugars appear to have the most negative effects on the teeth when they are eaten frequently throughout the day. If a child wants a sugary treat between meals, reinforce tooth brushing afterwards. Appropriate healthier snacks could include fresh fruit slices and yogurt, celery sticks stuffed with peanut butter (natural, without added sugar), and low-fat milk, low-fat cheese and crackers with juice, or half a sandwich with some fruit. Sugars are less damaging to teeth when eaten as part of a meal where there is the buffering action of fats and where more saliva is produced to wash away the residual sugar on the tooth surface. So, consider serving desserts as part of a meal to reduce their cavity-causing potential.

- Limit a child's intake of the sticky foods that are least likely to be cleared from the surface of the teeth such as honey, caramel, gumdrops, nougat, or toffee. Even foods such as raisins or dried fruits may be troublesome, particularly if eaten between meals. Again, reinforce the importance of good brushing and flossing habits.

- Sweet treats that prolong the exposure of sugars to the surface of the teeth should also be limited. This includes sugar-containing chewing gum, mints, lollipops, and similar long-lasting candies.

- Although fruits, milk, and grains do provide naturally occurring sugars, they contain much more nutritive value than does refined sugar. Therefore, foods such as fruits and fruit juices, milk, yogurt, pudding, crackers, and pretzels are still more sensible snack choices than soda, candy, fruit leather, or baked items.

So, food choices traditionally considered safe

or healthy for children's teeth may actually have some negative effects, while other foods provide surprising protection against cavities. All foods, including sucrose, fructose, lactose, and all other types of sugars, can fit into a child's everyday diet. It would not be appropriate to try to completely eliminate any of these types of sugar because in wholesome foods, sugars provide an important source of calories, calcium, vitamin D, vitamin A, and other nutrients that are essential for growth, development, and good health. Nor would it be wise to give children only nuts, cheese, and other high-fat foods for meals and snacks. A diet too high in fat may precipitate different health problems (see chapter 30).

Helping Children Stay Cavity-Free for Life

Every child should be given the opportunity to grow up with a healthy, attractive smile. Children who are given the benefit of early dental care can develop healthy habits that continue into adulthood. A healthy smile gives a growing child the ability to eat and speak comfortably and contributes to a positive self-image. Those who avoid problems with their primary (baby) teeth are more likely to have healthy and attractive permanent (adult) teeth as well. Children with dental problems often experience needless pain and infection, which can interfere with their overall health and well-being as well as with eating, speaking, and concentrating. The following are a few tips to keep children free of dental problems.

1. Avoid putting a baby to bed with a bottle or allowing babies with teeth to nurse themselves to sleep. Babies should be held during bottle feedings and should never be left unattended with a "propped up" bottle. Try to discontinue bottle use by the child's first birthday. If a child must have a bottle for comfort after the age of 1, only plain water should be in the bottle.

2. The key to good dental hygiene is daily cleaning. Begin by gently wiping an infant's mouth and gums with a clean, damp gauze pad or washcloth after feedings. As teeth grow into the mouth, they should be brushed by an adult at least once a day with a soft, nylon-bristle toothbrush. Most children do not develop the dexterity to brush their own teeth effectively until the age of 5½ to 6 years. A pediatric dentist can help with the selection and use of products for home dental care and may recommend sealants to coat cavity-prone pits and grooves on teeth.

3. Cavity-free children begin preventive care as babies! Pediatric dentists recommend that the first preventive visit take place around the first birthday, shortly after the first teeth begin to erupt. At this visit, the dentist will make sure the baby's teeth and jaws are developing properly and on schedule; discuss teething, feeding recommendations, mouth cleaning, oral injury prevention, and pacifier use; and check that the baby is receiving the proper amount of fluoride. Regular preventive visits should take place every six months, or more often if recommended by the pediatric dentist.

Baby Bottle Tooth Decay

Baby bottle tooth decay (BBTD), a preventable condition, is caused by prolonged exposure of the teeth to carbohydrates such as sucrose, fructose, or lactose, which allows the *Streptococcus mutans* bacteria in plaque to produce acids and demineralize the teeth. These carbohydrates are present in cow's or breast milk, fruit juice, for-

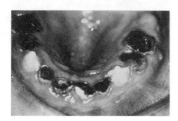

FIGURE 16.1
Baby bottle tooth decay.

mula, or any sweetened liquid. As soon as the first teeth erupt in a baby's mouth, decay can begin to develop. BBTD often appears initially as chalky white spots or lines on the upper front teeth; as decay progresses these areas turn brown.

The most common cause of BBTD is allowing a child to sleep or nap with a bottle, which leaves the teeth exposed to carbohydrate-containing liquids for a long period of time. Saliva plays an important role in preventing BBTD, but during sleep the production of saliva diminishes. Frequent feedings, not being weaned off a bottle by the age of 1, and the use of pacifiers dipped in a sweet liquid or honey are other important risk factors. The upper front teeth are most commonly affected, since they are among the first teeth to erupt and are heavily exposed to any liquid that remains in the mouth. Over time, other teeth may be affected as decay spreads to areas where the teeth are more sheltered by the tongue from exposure to liquids.

To prevent this condition:

- Establish and keep to regular feeding schedules as much as possible.
- Discourage night feedings for bottle-fed babies; water is a safe alternative for children who need a bottle for comfort.
- Do not allow breastfed babies to nurse for unlimited amounts of time, especially at night.
- Make it a goal to wean the child from a bottle by the age of 1.
- Refrain from using pacifiers dipped or coated with sweet solutions.
- Wipe the teeth and mouth with a clean cloth or gauze before bedtime daily.

PART THREE

Beyond the Basics:
Special Challenges in Nutrition

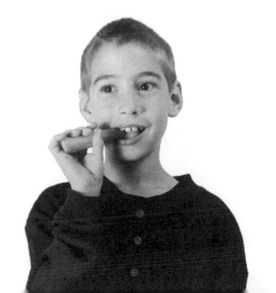

17

Eating Disorders

Most children go through at least a brief episode of giving their parents a hard time about food and eating. Food refusal, eating only a very narrow selection of foods, sneaking food, eating at the "wrong" time, and exhibiting rituals around food are among the more common complaints parents report about their children's eating habits. What sets eating disorders apart from more minor eating-related concerns is the fact that they represent enduring patterns of behaviors that are associated with serious health problems and marked psychological disturbance. Although eating disorders are most often associated with girls, they do occur in boys as well. In the first section of this chapter, we describe three major eating disorders: anorexia nervosa, bulimia nervosa, and binge eating disorder. In the second section we describe ways to reestablish healthy eating patterns in children or adolescents suffering from each disorder.

Anorexia nervosa, bulimia nervosa, and binge eating disorder share at least two of these three core features: (1) body-image disturbance; (2) extreme efforts to control one's body weight; and (3) loss of control over eating. Although the precise distinction of the three eating disorders described below may be helpful for

> **MYTH** A child with an eating disorder is very skinny.
>
> **FACT** Although individuals with anorexia are usually very underweight, those with bulimia or binge eating disorder are often of normal weight or are even overweight.

Ruth H. Striegel-Moore ▪ Ed Strenkowski

planning treatment, it is important to note that in many cases, the symptoms in the same person may change over time from one disorder to another. For example, it is estimated that up to 50 percent of girls with anorexia nervosa eventually meet diagnostic criteria for bulimia nervosa. Moreover, many of the treatment suggestions provided later in this chapter apply to all three disorders.

Anorexia Nervosa

The key symptoms of anorexia nervosa are a failure to maintain a minimal body weight, morbid fear of weight gain, body-image disturbance, and, in females, failure to menstruate (amenorrhea). Anorexia nervosa is a rare disorder which occurs in less than 0.5 percent of girls or women. The disorder is likely to occur during two critical age periods: around puberty, and around 18 years of age. There are two subtypes of anorexia nervosa: restricting type and binge eating/purging type. Restricting anorexics become emaciated by severely restricting their food intake, and they do not engage in bingeing or purging behavior. Binge eating/purging type refers to those who engage in binge eating and/or purging.

Most people think of dramatic weight loss as the key symptom of anorexia nervosa, yet among children who have not yet reached their mature height and weight, failure to gain an adequate amount of weight (rather than weight loss) may be the key symptom. In either case, emaciation is the consequence of the child's refusal to maintain a minimal body weight. In our thinness-preoccupied society, many parents may not notice right away that their child is not putting on enough weight, or that the child is losing too much weight. Dieting to lose weight is common among adolescent girls, and in many instances a teenager's attempts to lose a few pounds do not result in

a serious health problem. Moreover, parents may welcome a child's efforts to maintain weight or to lose weight as a sign of maturity. However, a precipitous drop in weight, or a marked slowing of weight gain (measured against the expected growth curve), is cause for concern.

Fear of gaining weight is the motivational core from which the other symptoms of anorexia nervosa develop. It is often the first symptom to emerge, particularly in young girls and in girls who are already thin. Again, because of our society's emphasis on thinness and widely shared negative views about being overweight, this symptom may be difficult to identify. Persistent expression of concern about fear of fatness should be taken seriously, however. It is often helpful to explore with children what it means to them to be preoccupied with this fear and to ask what makes them feel bad about the possibility of gaining weight. Many young people fail to appreciate that the growth spurt of puberty is associated with a normal increase in body fat, especially in girls, and that this increase in fatness does not continue to the point of causing obesity.

Children with anorexia nervosa almost always have misperceptions in the ways in which they view or think about their bodies. They feel fat even when clearly underweight, or perceive parts of the body, such as cheeks or thighs, as grotesquely fat, even though these parts are normal. Many affected children believe that losing weight is the most important goal in life. Typically, anorexic children experience profound shame about the body, which often results in avoidance of social situations, such as refusing to participate in a sport that requires wearing clothes that reveal parts of the body, like gym shorts or bathing suits. Not all children report the same symptoms, and in many instances these symptoms may not be readily acknowledged if the child suspects that admission of these symptoms will confirm a parent's or health professional's concern about an eating problem. Many adolescents feel awkward or embarrassed about their bodies. Parents can help them feel more comfortable by acknowledging that the physical changes of puberty can be difficult, by maintaining a respectful attitude toward their children's appearance, and by not teasing them or criticizing them for the way their bodies look. Parents can also help them view their bodies in positive ways that are not tied to physical appearance by encouraging the development of skills in a particular sport or activity.

Failure to menstruate, or amenorrhea, is another important symptom of anorexia nervosa. Absence of three consecutive menstrual cycles, or failure of girls to start menstruating by age 16 or within three years of starting pubertal development, should be evaluated by the pediatrician. Growing medical literature attests to the considerable negative long-term consequences of such menstrual abnormalities, including an increased risk of osteoporosis. Therefore, even in the absence of other symptoms of anorexia nervosa, menstrual dysfunction requires medical evaluation and treatment.

Even though the diagnostic criteria for anorexia nervosa do not specify particular weight loss behaviors as core symptoms of this disorder, severely restrictive dieting is a major part of the picture. In the restricting form of anorexia nervosa, the child eliminates almost all food from her diet and manages to subsist on very small amounts of often very limited types of food (only carrots, or only fruit). Many of the food rituals associated with anorexia nervosa (hoarding food, excessive preoccupation with food in the form of constant cooking or baking and offering others food, extensive collecting of recipes) are a direct result of the physiological and psychological side effects of starvation. In addition to restricting food intake, many anorexic individuals engage in excessive and often ritualized exercise, such as running up and down stairs a predetermined number of times or doing hundreds of jumping jacks. As with dieting to lose weight, the anorexic child's exercise behavior may not be readily seen as pathological. American culture values fitness and admires individuals who can "go for the burn" and perform astonishing athletic feats. However, when exercise is done to the point of exhaustion, or when it is continued despite illness or injury, or when the person becomes highly irritable when unable to exercise, chances are that exercise is no longer a healthy activity. In children with diagnosed anorexia nervosa, it is important to impose limits on the amount of exercise they may do. For example, a child on a high school track team should not be permitted to train or compete if his or her weight is dangerously low.

In many cases, as starvation continues, abstaining from food becomes increasingly difficult, and many children with anorexia nervosa eventually engage in episodic binge eating. In essence, the only major difference between anorexia nervosa with binge eating and bulimia nervosa is the fact that for a diagnosis of anorexia nervosa, the child has to be below minimum weight for his or her height and age. (Problems associated with binge eating are described under bulimia nervosa.) Starvation contributes to serious psychological as well as physical disturbances, including severe depression, anxiety, irritability, and in many cases changes in cognitive functioning. In an advanced state of emaciation, anorexic patients' ability to make informed decisions about treatment is even impaired. This poses a particular challenge in those instances where the anorexic child refuses treatment. Anorexia nervosa is a serious, life-threatening illness, and early detection is important so that the child can be treated and the risk of complications due to prolonged illness may be reduced.

Bulimia Nervosa

The core features of bulimia nervosa are recurrent episodes of binge eating, followed by inappropriate compensatory behavior like vomiting or excessive exercising. Bulimia nervosa, which typically begins during mid- to late adolescence, occurs in approximately 2 percent of adolescents and adults. Two types of bulimia nervosa have been recognized: purging bulimia nervosa and non-purging bulimia nervosa. Persons with the former disorder regularly engage in purging by means of vomiting or use laxatives, diuretics, or other medications for weight control purposes.

Binge eating episodes are characterized by consuming a large amount of food in a limited time period to the point of physical discomfort due to stomach distention, accompanied by a sense of loss of control. The person feels unable to stop eating or unable to prevent such episodes from happening. Although many individuals experience occasional episodes of overeating, such as during a holiday meal, binge eating encompasses incidents in addition to those where good food and good company let us forget our limits.

Compensation for binge eating may take many forms. Although vomiting is commonly thought to be the main bulimic symptom aside from binge eating, many bulimics compensate for their binges by means of prolonged starvation, or by use of laxatives, diuretics, and, in some cases, drugs like amphetamines or cocaine. Often compulsive exercise is an additional form of compensatory behavior. These various "weight control strategies" worsen the problem by leaving the individual completely famished, thus setting her up for the next binge. For some, vomiting takes on added signifi-cance by representing a means for releasing tension. Once purging becomes a firmly established habit, binge eating becomes very difficult to control.

Individuals who suffer from bulimia nervosa invariably say that weight or body shape is extremely important to their sense of self. They believe that their worth as a person is directly related to their body size: the thinner they are, the better they feel about themselves. It is often difficult to determine where to draw the line between normal concerns about physical attractiveness and unhealthy preoccupation. When weight becomes the single most important domain of aspiration and achievement, the individual needs help to regain perspective.

In many cases, the eating patterns of children with bulimia nervosa are characterized either by complete chaos, in that eating follows no regular meal pattern, or by restraint (for example, not eating breakfast or lunch), followed by excessive eating. Bulimia nervosa is associated with a disturbance in appetite and satiety: individuals with this disorder often can no longer tell whether they are hungry, and in most cases they can no longer tell when they are "full." Moreover, many bulimic individuals feel that normal eating will result in significant weight gain, even though scientific evidence suggests that a majority of bulimics do not gain weight when they adopt a healthy, regular eating pattern.

Like anorexia nervosa, bulimia nervosa is often associated with significant depression and anxiety. In addition, children with bulimia nervosa experience other problems with impulse control. In many cases, the disturbed eating pattern represents a coping effort to manage such aversive emotional states as anger, sadness, or frustration. Afflicted individuals fear that without binge eating or purging, they will be unable to maintain control over other aspects of their lives. Bulimia nervosa is a serious disorder, for purging behaviors in the form of vomiting, laxative abuse, or drug abuse represent a serious health risk, and it is important for sufferers to seek medical and psychological treatment.

Binge Eating Disorder

It was not until the early 1990s that binge eating was defined as an eating disorder. As with bulimia nervosa, binge eating disorder is characterized by recurrent episodes of binge eating, but unlike bulimia nervosa, the episodes are not followed by the regular use of inappropriate compensatory behaviors. Not surprisingly, individuals who binge eat but do not compensate for their eating binges are often overweight or obese. The age when children or adults develop binge eating disorders appears to be less clearly limited to a particular developmental stage than is the case for anorexia nervosa or bulimia nervosa. Initial studies of this disorder show that in some cases it may begin in early childhood. Approximately 2 percent of adolescents and adults suffer from binge eating disorder.

In many cases individuals who suffer from this disorder eat relatively large amounts of food even when not binge eating. In contrast to children with anorexia nervosa or bulimia nervosa, children with binge eating disorder need help to learn to eat less. Parents can help their children learn to eat appropriate amounts by permitting children to choose from among a variety of healthful food and by permitting an occasional treat of sweets, snack foods, or fast food. Food selection should be neither extremely restrictive nor overly permissive in order to help children regulate their own food intake. Parents can also help their children establish healthy eating patterns by ensuring regular mealtimes and by modeling healthy eating

behavior. Parents should emphasize the importance of eating in response to hunger (which also means not pushing a child to eat when the child is not hungry) and eating only until comfortably full (which includes allowing the child to stop when he or she feels full rather than when the plate is empty).

General Nutritional Interventions in the Treatment of Eating Disorders

The treatment of eating disorders is a complex process. Psychotherapy, medical monitoring, and nutrition counseling are all part of the therapy. This discussion focuses on the nutritional aspects of treatment. Parents are involved in the process when needed, but the nutrition counseling is conducted primarily with the child. The individual with an eating disorder needs to establish a relationship with a dietitian based on support and trust. There needs to be an honest exchange of ideas as to goals and expectations. This includes what the child or adolescent is able or willing to do at the outset of recovery in terms of eating. It may be easy to outline a meal plan on paper, but getting someone with a long history of disordered eating to adhere to the plan may be quite challenging. The dietitian can also provide factual nutrition advice while weeding out fads, fallacies, and unsound nutrition information. The child needs to be able to trust the advice given by the dietitian, while the dietitian needs to be committed to what may become a long-term intervention.

For the three eating disorders, several general interventions are critical. The child needs help in establishing a reasonable weight goal. In anorexia nervosa, this weight goal will be significantly above the weight the child may feel comfortable with, and, invariably, the child needs to gain weight during the initial treatment phase. In bulimia nervosa, the child's current weight may already be in a healthy weight range, so weight maintenance may be all that is needed. In binge eating disorders, many clients are overweight and may benefit from moderate weight loss.

Regardless of the specific type of eating disorders, these children and teenagers need to learn the pattern of eating three meals and one or two snacks a day. In anorexic children, the pattern of undereating needs to be changed; in bulimic individuals, the frequent pattern of eating too little during regular mealtimes needs attention. In binge eating disorder, the habit of eating large regular (nonbinge) meals must be adjusted. Some binge eaters, who exhibit a pattern of eating continuously throughout the day ("grazing"), need to establish regular eating patterns at established mealtimes.

For each of these disorders, it is useful to have the child keep a food diary to track progress made in treatment and to identify problematic times (many binge eaters overeat in the evening) or problematic events such as whenever the child becomes upset, sad, frustrated, and so on.

Nutritional Treatment of Anorexia Nervosa

There are two stages of nutrition intervention with the anorexia client—recovery and maintenance. The first phase of treatment is to recover to the goal weight (based on pediatric growth charts). In conjunction with the psychotherapist, the dietitian will establish a goal weight that the client needs to achieve and maintain. The dietitian will determine the appropriate calorie and protein needs based on the Recommended Dietary Allowances (RDA) established by the National Research Council. Individual needs during the recovery period of eating include consuming extra calories to pro-

mote weight gain. Slow and gradual weight gain is encouraged, with a goal of a 2-pound increase per week. Any extraordinary calorie expenditures, such as exercise, need to be considered and compensated for. If exercise and expended calories increase, the number of consumed calories should also increase. If this is not followed, the child may stop gaining or even begin to lose weight. All exercise programs should be discussed between the child and the psychotherapist. Exercise should be helpful and healthy and not used to "burn off" calories consumed. Once the goal weight is achieved, the daily caloric requirements can be adjusted to the level that will account for exercise and maintain the child's appropriate weight.

Accurate weighing at appropriate time intervals is an important part of both recovery and maintenance stages. Body weight measurements may vary based on factors such as the time of last meal or the amount of clothing worn. Body weight should therefore be measured at the same time each day wearing as little clothing as possible, ideally first thing in the morning after urinating. This method is a good way to monitor the gradual weight increases as well as monitoring maintenance weight.

After calorie needs are established for recovery or maintenance, a daily meal pattern is formulated. The total number of calories should be spread throughout the day into meals and snacks. It may be difficult for recovering children to eat more food than they are used to eating. Distributing the calories over frequent feedings, such as three meals and two snacks, allows for smaller meal sizes. The content and pattern of meals and snacks should be discussed and agreed upon by the child and dietitian. The feedings should be realistic and changeable while fitting into the child's daily lifestyle. Counting exact number of calories is not necessary and may reinforce previous disordered eating behavior. Emphasis should be placed on numbers of servings and types of foods. For example, breakfast could consist of juice, a bagel, and peanut butter. The child should be instructed that a breakfast of juice, cold cereal, and skim milk is of similar caloric content and may be exchanged for the other breakfast. Considerations for lunch include whether the child eats at school and, if so, what foods are available there. A combination of school food and food from home can provide greater variety, which is an important part of following a diet. When the same foods are eaten repeatedly, boredom or frustration may increase, and the child may not follow the diet. Most dinners are constructed around the family's typical pattern. Children should be encouraged to interchange snacks for variety, and the snacks should be easy to prepare, like fruits or yogurt.

To help with the adjustment of taking in more calories, it may be helpful for the child to try small amounts of calorie-dense foods or snacks. For instance, adding cereal and/or honey to low-fat yogurt increases calories without increasing the volume of food appreciably. Similar adjustments in calories can be made by adding condiments such as margarine, jelly, cream cheese, and mayonnaise to toast, bagels, and sandwiches.

Many individuals with eating disorders have aversions to some foods, especially those high in sugar or fat. They may want to plan a diet that omits sweets and includes only fat-free foods. It is possible to do this, but these restrictions will require an increase in the volume of food that has to be eaten. For example, one has to drink 14 ounces of skim milk to get the same amount of calories as one gets from 8 ounces of whole milk. These are areas that the child and dietitian need to discuss in order to develop a practical diet. In addition to daily meal plans, children would probably benefit from an age- and sex-specific daily vitamin and mineral supplement. In many instances a supplement can help restore nutrients that have been depleted during the starvation phase of anorexia nervosa.

Nutritional Treatment of Bulimia Nervosa

Bulimics are usually in a healthy weight range, as opposed to binge eaters, who are typically overweight or obese. The recovering bulimic child usually needs nutrition education about appropriate serving sizes and calorie intake to maintain weight. After patterns of bingeing or fasting, many bulimics or binge eaters fear that they will gain weight, even when they eat normal amounts. The dietitian must be able to convince the child that it is possible to eat and maintain one's weight without having to binge or fast.

Goal weights, calorie requirements, and exercise patterns need to be established, as previously discussed with anorexia nervosa. Calories should be calculated to maintain the goal weight while accounting for exercise. These issues need to be discussed and a realistic meal pattern for the child established by the dietitian. The meal pattern needs to fit the lifestyle of the child and family and take into consideration previous bingeing patterns. For example, if evening was a time of heavy bingeing, the recovery diet should not include an evening snack of previously binged foods. The goal of the diet should be at least three meals per day, each of approximately equal amounts so as not to induce any feeling of overeating (bingeing) at any particular time. With the bulimic child, snacks may be more helpful at times the child previously did not binge, such as midmorning or midafternoon.

Bulimic or binge-eating children may also benefit from guidance concerning their eating habits. Meals or snacks should be eaten at the table, rather than while reading or watching television. Activities while eating (such as reading) may encourage the child to linger with the activity and therefore overeat. An oven timer may be helpful to quantify the length of the mealtime. When the timer goes off, the child is reminded of the time and can go on to the next activity or task. These issues need to be discussed with the psychotherapist as they are one part of the recovery process.

It may be difficult to reintroduce foods that were once binge foods, such as ice cream or sweets. If the child wants to try these foods, it is best to try them at a previously nonbinge time and in a nonbinge setting. For example, if ice cream was an evening binge food, the child can try to eat a small amount of ice cream at school. In this setting the fear of purging may decrease as well. Again, these are behavior issues that should be discussed with the psychotherapist.

The recovering bulimic may benefit from keeping a food diary. Diet and exercise patterns and adjustments can be noted. Any time that a fear of bingeing occurs, the child should jot it down. Diet and snack patterns can then be changed to prevent the return to bingeing. The diary can be used to record positive changes, thus providing positive reinforcement and support on a path to a healthy weight and healthy eating.

Nutritional Treatment of Binge Eating Disorder

Treatment for the child with binge eating disorder is similar to treatment of the bulimic child in that it focuses on relearning how to eat in response to hunger, until one feels full, and in appropriate contexts. However, since many binge eaters are overweight, calorie needs should provide for weight loss as necessary. Because many binge eaters have chaotic eating patterns, it is helpful to introduce a regular eating schedule. By spacing meals at established intervals throughout the day, the child eventually will experience hunger prior to meals, because the body is being retrained to anticipate food at a certain time of day.

Binge eaters also benefit from instruction regarding the appropriate meal size. Often these children simply do not know how much constitutes a healthy meal. They need to understand that, initially, because of their past pattern of overeating, they may not feel full after a regular meal. The dietitian works with the child to help promote needed behavioral changes. For example, the dietitian can suggest alternative activities (letter writing, playing a game, bicycle riding) that take the child's mind off food.

Resources

American Anorexia/Bulimia Association, Inc. (AABA), 133 Cedar Lane, Teaneck, NJ 07666. (201) 836-1800.

Anorexia Nervosa and Associated Disorders, Inc. (ANAD), P.O. Box 271, Highland Park, IL 60035. (312) 831-3438.

Levenkron, S. *The Best Little Girl in the World.* New York: Warner Books, 1979.

O'Neill, C. B. *Starving for Attention.* New York: Continuum, 1982.

Childhood Obesity

Obesity is becoming the most common and serious nutritional disorder in children in the Western Hemisphere. It is estimated that 10–25 percent of children in North America are substantially overweight, and the prevalence of this disorder is on the rise (see chapter 12 for the definition of obesity). Most important, an obese child has a much higher likelihood than a nonobese child of becoming an obese adolescent and adult. Furthermore, studies have shown that adults who were overweight during adolescence had a twofold greater risk for coronary heart disease than those who were not overweight. Prevention and treatment of obesity should start at a young age in order to avoid adult obesity and the health problems associated with it.

> **MYTH** A "miracle diet" can make the pounds melt away.
>
> **FACT** Obesity is a multifaceted disease. Successful weight reduction requires long-term lifestyle changes, including changes in food selection, exercise, and attitude. There is no quick fix to this complicated disease.

What Causes Obesity

Childhood obesity is a complex disease that results from an imbalance of energy intake and expenditure. Children gain weight when the amount of food energy (calories) that is eaten exceeds the amount of energy that is used by the body for activity and growth. The excess energy is stored as fat. Becoming overweight is usually a gradual

Sonia Caprio ▪ Nancy A. Held

process, and overeating is not always so obvious. For example, if a child only eats 50–100 calories (equivalent to five to ten potato chips) more each day than the child uses up in energy, then the child will gain about 5–10 pounds of fat per year. Thus many parents are confused and surprised that their children are overweight even when they don't appear to be overeating. How do parents know that their child has a problem? The growth chart (see chapters 1 and 12) shows the range of optimum weight for height by age. Children who are gaining weight faster than they are growing in height are eating more than their bodies need.

Both genetic and environmental factors have been implicated as causes of obesity, yet the basic mechanisms underlying the development of childhood obesity are not entirely clear. The transmission of human obesity within families is well known. If parents are obese, there is a good chance that their children will be as well. Genetic factors influence when a person feels full, where fat is stored in the body, and the rate that the body burns energy. Yet a family tendency toward obesity is not necessarily a genetic predisposition, as family members share not only common genes, but also diet, cultural background, and many other aspects of lifestyle. However, studies of identical twins who were reared apart established more firmly the importance of genetic factors. Despite different diets and environmental factors, the adult weights and body shapes of these twins remained remarkably similar. However, these findings do not mean that fatness or obesity is determined at conception and that environment has no effect. Genetic factors can be altered by an individual's diet and exercise. Nevertheless, the individual who is prone to obesity must continuously struggle against these genetic factors in order to maintain a healthy body weight. It is often hard for the child to accept that his or her body build has a strong genetic component. This is often most difficult if one parent is thin and the other is overweight, and the child physically takes after the heavy parent.

The continuing rise in obesity among children suggests that environmental factors affect the genetic predisposition toward obesity (see chapter 12). Watching television appears to be a strong predictor of obesity. The more time a child spends in watching television, the less time he or she spends doing something more active. In addition, some television commercials promote eating and influence children's snack preferences, as the foods advertised are often calorically dense (high in sugar and/or fat). A child between 6 and 11 years old may watch an average of twenty-four hours of television a week. Watching more than twelve hours a week has been shown in some studies to affect school performance negatively.

Other psychosocial and environmental factors also influence the development of obesity. Emotional overeating—when a child disregards hunger and satiety cues and eats in response to emotions (sadness, anger, stress, boredom, and the like)—can contribute to weight gain. How parents relate to their children also affects youngsters' ways of dealing with food. A child who has never had limits set may never have learned when to stop watching television—or when to stop eating. Parents need to explain that eating half a bag of cookies or watching five hours of television a day is not acceptable. When a child is indulged, he or she learns unhealthy habits. Yet when one or both parents are distant and a child is not nurtured and supported, the child may seek out food as comfort in order to feel better. In this case a child may well be trying to fill a void.

Three potentially critical periods have been identified in childhood for the development of later obesity and its associated metabolic and cardiovascular complications. The periods are pregnancy and early infancy, the time from 5 to 7 years of age, and adolescence. The body mass index (BMI) increases during the first year of life, decreases thereafter, and increases again at approximately 5 years of age. Children who gain weight or whose BMI increases earlier than age 5 seem to have a greater risk of obesity. The mechanisms responsible for the increased risk associated with obesity at these ages are not clear. The increased incidence of obesity during these critical periods should serve to focus preventive measures on these developmental stages.

Another factor associated with obesity in children is a high fat intake. Not only is fat more calorically dense than carbohydrate and protein, it is also easily absorbed and stored in fat tissue.

Diagnostic Criteria

There are a number of ways in which excess body fat can be measured. Both direct and indirect measures have been used to describe this state, with somewhat arbitrary cut-offs defining overweight and obese on the upper end of a continuum (see chapter 12).

However, a major recent advance in our understanding of the medical consequences of obesity relates to the importance of the distribution of fat in the body. Obese adults can be broadly divided into two main categories: individuals in which the greater amount of fat is stored in the hips and legs (lower-body obesity) and those in which the greater proportion of fat is stored in the abdomen (upper-body obesity). People with upper-body obesity are more likely to develop diabetes, hypertension, and coronary artery disease than those with lower-body obesity. Indeed, it is the fat that is deposited inside the abdomen, around the liver and other abdominal organs, that really appears

to be the culprit. This is called visceral abdominal fat.

The simplest way to determine fat distribution is to measure the waist-to-hip circumference ratio. This is determined by measuring the waist at its most narrow point and dividing it by the measurement of the widest area of the buttocks. The ratio is useful because it distinguishes upper-body obesity from lower-body obesity and is also easy to measure. Individuals with a high ratio (waist larger than hips) tend to have increased amounts of visceral fat. However, this measure in children does not indicate the extent of visceral fat. Additionally, the ratio does not directly distinguish visceral from subcutaneous fat deposits. Visceral (intra-abdominal) fat can be directly measured using magnetic resonance imaging (MRI). As MRI poses no known health risks, repeated studies can be done. These techniques are currently being used in several studies examining the causes of medical complications in childhood obesity.

Medical Complications of Childhood Obesity

Many organ systems are adversely affected by childhood obesity. Elevated blood pressure (hypertension) is a common cardiovascular complication present in children with moderate to severe forms of obesity. Other risk factors for cardiovascular disease are increased levels of lipids such as triglycerides and decreased levels of high-density lipoproteins commonly known as the "good cholesterol" (see chapters 20 and 30). Of particular interest is the fact that these alterations are correlated with the excess accumulation of visceral intra-abdominal fat.

In morbid or severe forms of obesity the respiratory system is often severely affected. These children get short of breath easily and are at risk for potentially catastrophic episodes of sleep apnea (momentary cessation of breathing while asleep). Increased daytime sleepiness, snoring, and bed-wetting are also seen in very obese children. Several orthopedic conditions that occur in children with this condition may be attributable to the extra weight placed on the joints. Given the serious health consequences of childhood obesity there is a need to prevent and treat this disorder at the earliest stage. Preventive measures should be taken for children who are at increased risk by virtue of family history.

Metabolic Complications

Excess body fat in children is associated with alterations in the metabolism of glucose. Although the reasons are not yet understood, obesity almost invariably causes the body to be less responsive to insulin than normal. To keep blood glucose levels normal, the pancreas secretes much more insulin, so insulin levels in the blood rise (hyperinsulinemia). The oversecretion of insulin and hyperinsulinemia cause further problems. Obese children often have increased insulin levels together with a decreased action of insulin on target tissues. Eventually, overwork of the pancreas can lead to the development of diabetes in adults. However, diabetes secondary to obesity is not as common in children as it is in obese adults. Hyperinsulinemia is proportional to the degree of fatness and maintains obesity by promoting the deposition of fat and decreasing the breakdown of fat from fat cells. The disturbances seen in the cholesterol and lipoprotein levels of obese children (high triglycerides and low high-density lipoprotein) are also related to hyperinsulinemia. Hyperinsulinemia also may be a cause of high blood pressure because it favors retention of salt in the body (see chapter 33) and contributes to hardening of the arteries in obese adults. Obese adults are thus at increased risk for heart attacks, strokes, and circulation problems in the legs.

Psychological Issues

Obesity during childhood can result in problems with social and psychological adjustment. Overweight children may be laughed at or teased or be isolated from peers. Obesity often leads to a negative body image and low self-esteem, and it can make adolescence more difficult than it is for teenagers of normal weight. Children who are obese may be stereotyped as lazy or lacking self-discipline and they may be blamed for the weight, when, in fact, many factors contribute to the development of obesity. Simply putting a child on a diet is not sufficient or effective in producing weight loss. Psychological issues need to be addressed, depending on the extent of problems. Often family therapy is necessary in addition to nutrition, exercise, and behavioral counseling.

Secondary Forms of Obesity

Parents often seek a physiologic cause of the obesity. However, rare genetic disorders or endocrine causes account for less than 1 percent of childhood obesity. The rare genetic forms are often associated with other physical features, such as almond-shaped eyes, V-shaped mouth, high, arched palate, and/or mild to moderate mental retardation. Hormone abnormalities like underactive thyroid (hypothyroidism) and overactive adrenals (Cushing's syndrome)—often thought of as causative factors for obesity—are rarely the reason for obesity. Prolonged use or high doses of cortisone-like drugs also cause obesity. A common feature of most of the secondary forms of obesity is that the children are short or not growing at a steady rate. Normal growth in height in an obese child makes one of the secondary causes of obesity very unlikely.

Treatment

Obesity during childhood often stems from a number of causes and develops over a number of years. Consequently, treatment is not quick nor is it limited to one approach. Many parents of overweight children seek professional help and expect a medical prescription: a doctor fixes the problem with medicine. Unfortunately, no such pill currently exists, so treatment is directed at changes in lifestyle that need to be individualized for the child. On the one hand, a child who is mildly overweight and fairly sedentary may simply require encouragement to increase activity and to eat appropriate types of food. In this example, the parents may or may not need help with implementing the changes (setting rules about watching less television and getting more exercise, for example). On the other hand, an extremely obese teenager who eats a poor diet, participates in minimal physical activity, and has a strong family history of obesity will need more in-depth intervention. This treatment would include education and behavioral strategies in appropriate eating and exercise, as well as individual and family counseling to address psychoemotional problems that commonly occur in tandem with this disease.

In general, there are three prerequisites to treating obesity in children: family involvement; a balanced, lower-calorie intake; and increased physical activity. Family involvement is essential. Research has shown that programs for weight loss that included one or more parents and the child had more success than those that included only the child. This is not surprising, since parents are responsible for food provided in the home and supervision of the child's activity. If a home is stocked with potato chips, cakes, and cookies, the child will eat these calorically dense foods. Parents and other family members set examples of both eating and exercise behaviors for children. If parents eat poorly and are sedentary, these are the behaviors that the child will copy. It is useful for families to have rules about eating, just as there are rules about bedtime, homework, and so on. These should not be punitive but should provide a child with clear expectations of behavior and the knowledge that meals and snacks will be provided on a regular schedule. For example, children would be expected to sit at the table with the family and would not be permitted to eat in front of the television.

Children whose parents attempt to control the child's intake with food bribes and rewards are less able to respond to their own internal hunger and fullness cues. Studies have shown that children who do not adjust their energy intake — to eat smaller amounts of food if it is calorically more dense — have greater fat stores. Children who are taught to focus on external controls, such as amount remaining on the plate and time of day, also are less able to adjust their own energy intake. Parents should have control over what kind of food is brought into the house, but even when trying to lose weight, the child should determine how much he or she will eat. If parents disagree with each other on appropriate nutrition and are not consistent in their philosophy, an overweight child will be less successful in achieving and maintaining a lower body weight (see chapter 9).

Parents need to recognize the need to change and to provide a healthier model for their children. Children cannot be expected to make changes on their own.

Specific goals of treatment will vary with each child, depending on the various causes of obesity.

As a child develops, growth in height is normally accompanied by weight gain. For a young child or preteen who is obese yet still growing, small amounts of weight loss or weight maintenance is appropriate. For obese adolescents who have completed their growth, slow weight loss of 1 to 2 pounds per week is appropriate.

There is no one method or diet that works for everybody. Structured, overly restrictive diets for weight loss are generally inappropriate for children. These diets arbitrarily impose a caloric limit which may not meet the child's growth needs and are usually viewed as unpleasant, short-term solutions to a weight problem—something to abandon once the weight is lost. Other approaches to help with food selection are grouping foods according to caloric density, with emphasis on the lower-calorie foods, or the Food Guide Pyramid (see chapter 4). A registered dietitian should teach the family and child how to make appropriate food choices. Parents and children need to learn how to choose balanced meals, including foods from different food groups. Children need to learn to respond to internal cues (feelings of hunger and fullness) and stop eating when full, even if food is still on the table or on the plate.

Other behavior and habit modification techniques include self-monitoring (keeping food intake and exercise records), role playing, contracting, and goal setting. Eating slowly, minimizing distractions during eating, and using a small plate can also help the child. Parents may need to be trained by a dietitian to support habit changes. Positive reinforcement and praise are very effective in helping children and teens make difficult adjustments to new ways of eating and thinking about food. Negative reinforcement or no reinforcement is not effective. For example, a response such as "You only ate one cookie, that's great," is appropriate, whereas "Why did you have to eat a cookie and spoil your diet?" is not.

Younger children, in particular, may worry that they won't get enough food. They should be reassured that they are eating enough. If their intake is not restricted, they may ignore feelings of satiety and eat more than they need. If young children know that they will get what they need, they can better respond to internal cues.

Generally very low-calorie diets (less than 800 calories a day) are not appropriate for children. However, some medical centers are using a very low-calorie, protein-sparing modified fast to promote weight loss in both children and adolescents. Protein is increased to preserve lean body mass while fat is lost with the reduction in overall calories. Concerns about these diets include impact on height growth and ability to adhere to a nutritionally balanced low calorie intake after the diet is completed.

Exercise

Exercise is a necessary component in the treatment of obesity. Physical activity is important for many reasons, primarily because children have fun and enjoy exercise. Improved fitness also enhances self-esteem. Exercise increases caloric expenditure, which leads to weight loss if food intake does not increase.

General lifestyle exercise—playing outside with friends or family, riding bicycles, playing soccer, basketball, and the like—is an important part of everyday health. Parents should not only encourage their children to be active, but also make exercise a priority for the entire family. Exercising together can improve family relationships. Lifestyle activity promotes caloric expenditure, but doesn't improve fitness to a great extent because these activities are usually of low intensity.

Fitness is defined by aerobic capacity, body composition, and muscular strength and endurance. To improve fitness levels, more intense exercise must be done. This can be accomplished with a structured program of aerobic exercise (running, walking, bicycling, swimming) a prescribed number of times per week and of set duration and intensity. It is important that a child or teenager begin a program that is of appropriate intensity, as it is easy to become discouraged with a program that is too difficult. Exercise intensity is actually a predictor of whether people adhere to their exercise program.

Just as the causes of childhood obesity are com-plex, long-term successful solutions are also complex. Family dynamics, eating patterns, and exercise should all be evaluated when developing a plan of action. The child's pediatrician, as well as a registered dietitian, should play an integral role in evaluating and monitoring progress.

Resources

Mellin, Laurel. *Shapedown* series (workbooks and guides for overweight children, teens, and their parents). Balboa Publishing, Library Place, San Anselmo, CA 94960, 415-453-8886.

The Weight-Control Information Network, 1 Win Way, Bethesda, MD 20892-3665, 1-800-WIN-8098, WINNIDDK@aol.com.

19
· · · · · · · ·

Food Allergies

The many kinds of adverse reactions to foods have led to confusion and controversy over food allergy. Food allergy has been blamed for a wide variety of symptoms, including hyperactivity and learning disabilities, chronic fatigue syndrome, behavior disorders, asthma, and anaphylaxis, though in most instances there is no scientific evidence for such an association. Much of the popular press that discusses food allergy relates to anecdotal experiences which do not stand up to rigorous examination.

MYTH "My teenager must be allergic to milk; it gives her diarrhea."

FACT Although gastrointestinal symptoms are common in infants with milk allergy, in older children, diarrhea after drinking milk is more commonly due to lactose intolerance, which is a digestive problem.

The broad term used to describe these reactions is *adverse reactions to foods.* These may be classified as allergy if they are mediated by the immune system. In a food allergy, repeated ingestion of the particular food causes the development of an allergy antibody (IgE). Nonimmunologic reactions to food are those that do not involve the immune system, including symptoms associated with bacterial, viral, parasitic, or chemical contaminants, psychological aversion, and deficiency of digestive enzymes.

· ·

Frank Gruskay ▪ Kathy French

Non-Immune and Immune Reactions to Food

Nonimmune reactions
Enzyme deficiencies such as lactose intolerance
Food poisoning, toxins, microorganisms
Pharmacologic food reaction, such as stimulative effect from coffee or "Chinese restaurant syndrome" (reaction to MSG)
Scombroid reaction—fish containing high levels of histamine

Immune reactions
Hypersensitivity
   Systemic—anaphylaxis, hives
   Local—colic, diarrhea, vomiting
Atopic dermatitis (eczema)
Milk-induced pulmonary disease (Heiner's syndrome)
Celiac sprue

Incidence

Although the incidence of adverse reactions to foods may be large, allergic reactions have been estimated to occur in only 0.5–7 percent of children, with the frequency decreasing with age. The incidence is higher in children with hereditary disposition for allergy.

Research has shown that in only 39 percent of children whose parents were convinced of the presence of food allergy was food allergy proven by double-blind placebo-controlled challenge. In this kind of study neither the investigator nor the patient knew if the patient received the suspected food or a placebo. This study confirmed that food allergy does exist, but that it is less common than generally believed. Although any food may cause allergic reactions, 95 percent of food allergies are caused by seven foods: milk, soy, fish, wheat, egg, peanuts, and tree nuts. Reactions to more than one food are unusual. The eating habits of the individual may determine which foods are more allergenic. Hence, milk allergy is most common in small children, soy allergy is more prevalent in Japan, and fish allergy is more common in Scandinavian countries. Long-term studies have shown that children tend to lose their sensitivity to milk and soy between the ages of 2 and 5. However, tree nut, peanut, and shellfish allergies are usually persistent throughout life and may cause severe symptoms and even anaphylactic death.

Mechanism and Sensitization

There is evidence that in the normal individual, minute amounts of undigested or partially digested food proteins (allergens) are absorbed by the cells (enterocytes) which line the intestine (see chapter 2). These allergens are transported into the intestinal wall, where a local immune response produces specific antibodies that inactivate the allergen. This antibody (secretory IgA) inhibits penetration of large amounts of protein into the bloodstream and prevents the development of allergy antibodies. When the natural immune defense mechanism is disrupted, excessive allergen may enter the blood and lead to sensitization and disease. In the young child, it is easier for allergens to penetrate the intestinal wall because of immature local defense mechanisms and low or no production of secretory IgA. Local damage to the intestinal wall by small allergic reactions may allow large quantities of unaltered protein to gain access into the circulation and thereby lead to generalized allergic symptoms. As the child grows older and intestinal and immune functions mature, food allergy becomes less prevalent.

Prevention of Food Allergy

Over the past thirty years many studies have documented a marked decrease in food allergy in children of allergic families who were put on a prevention regimen. While the incidence of allergic disease (atopic dermatitis, asthma, hay fever, hives) in the child with no history of allergy in parents, siblings, grandparents, aunts, or uncles is about 10 percent, it climbs to 30–40 percent if one side of the family has a history of allergy, and to 60–70 percent if both parents' families have an allergy. Children from high-risk families who were treated with the prevention regimen had up to a 50 percent decrease in the chance of developing allergic diseases.

Prevention measures are as follows. Most formulas are based on cow's milk and soy milk, which contain "foreign" (nonhuman) protein, and thus must be excluded from the infant's diet. Mothers are encouraged to breastfeed their infants because breast milk has only human protein and contains large quantities of secretory IgA, which helps the infant's intestine exclude allergens from entering the blood. The mother cannot consume milk products during lactation, as cow's milk protein has been found in breast milk when the mother ingests milk products. If the mother chooses to bottle-feed, "nonallergic" formula (Nutramigen and Alimentum, for example) is recommended. Other baby foods are intro-duced after 4–6 months of age, with the exception of highly potent sensitizers such as eggs, citrus fruits, tomato, tree nuts, peanuts, and fish, which should not be introduced until 18–24 months. Breastfeeding mothers should avoid these sensitizers as much as possible, as well. Because the intestine matures and its permeability to allergens decreases to near adult levels after 12 months of age, cow's milk and soy are not allowed until that time. In addition, pets, dust mites, and cigarette smoke should be excluded from the infant's environment to help prevent respiratory symptoms in allergy-prone children.

Common Symptoms

Allergic reactions to foods may produce symptoms that vary, depending on the age of the child, the amount of food ingested, and other medical problems. Symptoms may be related to the gastrointestinal tract alone or to the body as a whole. Gastrointestinal symptoms are common in infants due to milk allergy, which can cause abdominal cramps (colic), vomiting, and/or diarrhea. Generalized reactions include hives and swelling of the face, lips, throat, eyes, and extremities; atopic eczema; asthma; nasal allergy (rhinitis); or systemic anaphylaxis (difficulty in breathing, hypotension, shock). These symptoms typically occur within two to four hours after the food allergen is eaten, but the most severe reactions occur within minutes. Delayed reactions occurring several hours or days later have been reported, but these have rarely been verified in placebo-controlled challenge tests.

Diagnosis

Diagnosis requires a thorough review of the patient's history to verify that the food in question causes an allergic reaction to the exclusion of other causes. Symptoms of hives, itching, and swelling are due to the release of histamine and other substances when an allergen combines with its specific allergic antibody (IgE) on cells that produce histamine. The presence of the specific IgE may be demonstrated by skin tests with reliable food allergens. Negative skin test results indicate that the child is not allergic to that food. While positive skin test results indicate that the child is sensitive to that food, only about one-third of those children actually have allergic symptoms.

Radio-allergosorbent test (RAST) is a blood test that measures specific allergic IgE antibodies. Like the skin tests, RAST testing shows that only the higher degree of hypersensitivity is correlated with clinical symptoms on food challenge. RAST has no practical advantage over the skin test except when the skin is unsuitable for skin tests, as in generalized dermatitis. RAST is more difficult to perform and more costly, and its results are somewhat less reliable than skin testing.

Food diaries, food elimination, and food challenge tests (individual foods are given to a child in a controlled setting to observe any adverse response) are all useful in the detective work sometimes necessary to make a proper diagnosis.

Clinical and laboratory tests such as provocative testing, subcutaneous and sublingual titration, in vitro cytotoxic food tests, and the pulse index have been used by some clinicians for several years. These have been shown in several studies to be unreliable and may occasionally lead to anaphylaxis.

Living with Food Allergies

The mainstay of allergy management for any allergic disease is identification and avoidance of the offending substance. Children on diets of multiple food elimination must be careful to receive a balanced and nourishing diet with supplements of calcium, iron, and vitamins, if appropriate. Careful reading of food labels and alertness for foods that commonly contain the offending substance is important. After age 3 or so, a child may develop immune tolerance. The offending food may be cautiously reintroduced into the diet in the physician's presence where a severe allergic response can be treated (but not in the cases of tree nuts, peanuts, or shellfish as they can cause rapid shock, coma, and death).

There is no evidence at present to support oral desensitization or injection immunotherapy in the treatment of most food allergies. However, a small preliminary study on the use of injection immunotherapy for peanut allergy has shown positive protective results, and this provides a future line of clinical investigation for the treatment of this potentially fatal disease. Clinical studies with the use of the drug cromolyn sodium to prevent food allergies have been inconclusive.

For people susceptible to anaphylaxis, it is highly recommended that they carry an epinephrine kit (bee-sting kit) and wear a medical emergency information bracelet at all times. Fatal anaphylaxis is more common with bee stings, but it also can occur with food allergies. Of seven patients who were reported to have died after anaphylaxis, four had ingested peanuts, and the other three had eaten pecans, crab, and fish, respectively. In all cases there was a lack of prompt adequate treatment (early use of epinephrine) in hopes that the symptoms would get better.

Cow's Milk Allergy

Cow's milk allergy is thought to occur in the range of 0.5 percent to 3 percent of children; as age increases the incidence decreases. This condition occurs when the immature gastrointestinal tract and immune system react to the antigens found in cow's milk. Milk allergy should not be confused with lactose intolerance, which in general does not appear until ages 3–5 and is the result of an inability to digest lactose, the sugar in milk (see chapter 23).

Formula-fed infants who display symptoms of abdominal discomfort, diarrhea, and vomiting may be allergic to cow's milk. Eliminating all sources of cow's milk protein from the diet is the standard method of treatment. A breastfeeding mother should avoid all milk and milk products in her diet, as cow's milk protein can be transmitted through breast milk. A formula-fed infant may be changed to a soy formula. However, a casein hydrolysate formula in which the protein is already predigested, such as Nutramigen or Alimentum, may be substituted because up to 50 percent of infants with cow's milk allergy will become sensitized to soy protein as well. As table food is introduced into the toddler's diet, all milk and milk products must be avoided. All commercial foods which contain the ingredients listed below must also be avoided.

Milk Products

Butter	Ice cream
Buttermilk	Margarine
Calcium caseinate	Milk chocolate
Casein	Milk solids
Cheese	Powdered milk
Condensed milk	Sherbet
Cottage cheese	Sodium caseinate
Cow's and goat's milk	Whey
Cream	Yogurt
Evaporated milk	

Milk and milk products are the primary source of calcium in the diets of children, and exclusion of these foods can lead to calcium deficiency. Infants will obtain adequate calcium via breast milk or formula. The daily calcium needs of the growing child (which range from 800 milligrams for children to 1,200 milligrams for teenagers) may be difficult to meet without the aid of a calcium supplement, however (see chapter 31). The calcium content of milk and other foods that contribute calcium to the diet are listed below.

Calcium	(mg) in selected foods
Milk (8 oz)	300
Calcium-fortified orange juice (8 oz)	300
Lactaid milk (8 oz)	300
Cereal (Total) (1 oz)	250
American cheese (1 oz)	174
Nutramigen (8 oz)	150
Spinach (½ cup)	84
Soy milk (8 oz)	10

Milk and milk products are also important sources of protein, vitamins, and minerals other than calcium. Careful planning is required to meet protein requirements, in particular, if a milk substitute is not used. The child needs a wide variety of foods to receive adequate vitamins and minerals, including one or two servings per day of a protein-rich source such as eggs, meat, poultry, fish, or legumes.

As studies suggest that 33–66 percent of children outgrow a cow's milk allergy after 2 to 3 years of age, periodic trials of small amounts of milk are recommended to reintroduce this important nutrient source.

Wheat and Gluten Allergies

Wheat is the most allergenic of the grain family; for this reason it is added to the infant's diet after rice and oats. A child with an intolerance to wheat products will need to eliminate all forms of wheat, not only "whole" wheat products.

Wheat Products

Bran	Pasta (durum and
Farina	semolina)
Graham crackers	Soy sauce
Graham flour	Wheat bread
Malt	Wheat flour
Malt syrup	White bread
	Whole-grain bread

Gluten intolerance is also known as celiac spruc or gluten-sensitive enteropathy. Gluten is a protein found in wheat, rye, oats, and barley. The protein damages the small intestine of susceptible individuals and interferes with the absorption of all nutrients. The condition may be discovered when an infant is first introduced to cereal, but often is not diagnosed until adolescence or adulthood.

Symptoms include abdominal pain, diarrhea, and weight loss. Infants may be excessively irritable and fail to thrive. Foods to be avoided include most baked products, cereals, and pasta (see list).

Foods Containing Gluten

Barley	Rye seeds, rye flour
Bran	Salad dressings
Cola drinks	Soups: barley, cream,
Graham flour	noodle
Kasha	Soy sauce
Malt	Wheat and wheat
Millet	products (see list
Mustard (prepared)	above)
Oats, oatmeal, oat	Worcestershire sauce
flour	Vinegar (distilled white)
Root beer	

Products that include flour as a thickener, such as soups and sauces, must also be avoided.

This disorder interferes with the absorption of all nutrients until a diagnosis is made and gluten is eliminated from the diet; therefore, nutrient deficiencies may occur, and vitamin and mineral supplementation may be required. In addition, the absence of breads and cereals from the child's diet removes excellent sources of B vitamins, iron and fiber. Because the diet excludes many basic foods, families are encouraged to contact the American Celiac Society for recipes and wheat-free product information. Careful meal planning with wheat-free, gluten-free products should avoid further nutritional deficiencies.

Egg Allergy

As a general rule, whole eggs should not be introduced into the infant's diet until the age of 12 months. Although most infants tolerate the egg yolk, the protein in the egg white is a powerful allergen. Any child who is sensitive to eggs must avoid many commercially prepared foods. These include most cakes and cookies, waffles, pancakes, and French toast. In addition to eggs and egg products, albumin, globulin, ovamucin, and vitellin should be avoided. Although eggs are an excellent source of protein, eliminating them from the diet does not compromise a child nutritionally, as meats and dairy products, which are common in a child's diet, are good sources of protein. Note that egg substitutes eliminate cholesterol but not egg protein, which is the cause of the egg allergy. They should therefore be avoided on an egg-free diet.

Citrus Allergy

Citrus fruits and juices should not be introduced until a child has reached the age of 12 months. As with any potentially allergenic food, citrus fruits should be introduced in small amounts over the course of several days with careful monitoring for symptoms like skin rashes. If a citrus allergy is suspected, citrus fruits as well as strawberries and tomatoes should be avoided. Although citrus fruits are an important source of vitamin C, this nutrient can be readily obtained from other sources, including broccoli, potatoes, spinach, and cabbage. Also, many fruit drinks that do not contain citrus juice are fortified with vitamin C.

Corn Allergy

An allergy to corn may be diagnosed in infancy, as corn oil is a component of some baby formulas. As it is considered a fairly common allergenic food, it should be introduced carefully into the infant's diet. Should a corn allergy be suspected, the foods listed below should be eliminated.

Corn Products

Alcohol	Dextrin
Caramel color	Dextrose
Corn: fresh, canned, or frozen	Fructose
	Lactic acid
Cornmeal, corn muffins, corn bread	Maltodextrins
	Mannitol
Corn oil	Mixed vegetables that
Cornstarch	contain corn
Corn syrup	Sorbitol

A corn-free diet will require careful label reading for hidden sources of corn but should not nutritionally compromise a child.

Soy Allergy

An allergy to soy may be discovered in infancy with the introduction of a soy-based formula. Unfortunately, up to 50 percent of babies with a cow's milk allergy are also allergic to soy. Casein hydrolysate formulas, such as Nutramigen or Alimentum, may be used for these infants. For the older child with a soy allergy, labels must be read carefully, as the use of soy products is widespread in commercially prepared foods. Should a soy allergy be suspected, all soy-containing foods, including tofu, miso, and tempeh, should be eliminated from the diet. In addition, nonspecific ingredients such as emulsifiers, flavoring stabilizers, lecithin, shortening, or vegetable oil on a food nutrition label may indicate that soy was used in processing.

Peanut Allergy

Peanuts are part of the legume family, not the nut family: many individuals who are sensitive to peanuts can tolerate other nuts. However, as the reaction to peanuts can be severe, the introduction of other tree nuts should be well monitored. In addition, any commercial product whose label lists nonspecific ingredients like chopped nuts or nut topping should be avoided, as peanuts may be present. Although an allergy to peanuts may require careful label reading, a child on a peanut-free diet should not be nutritionally compromised.

Resources

American Celiac Society, 45 Gifford Avenue, Jersey City, NJ 07324. (201) 432-2986.

Food Allergy Network, 10400 Eaton Place, Fairfax, VA 22030-5674. (702) 691-3179.

Gluten Intolerance Group, P.O. Box 23053, Seattle, WA 98102-3053. (206) 325-6980.

Hagman, B. *The Gluten-Free Gourmet: Living Well without Wheat.* New York: Henry Holt, 1990.

Kidder, B. *The Milk-Free Kitchen: Living Well without Dairy Products.* New York: Henry Holt, 1990.

Learning to Live with Food Allergies. Available from Food Allergy Network.

Novick, W. L. *You Can Do Something about Your Allergies.* New York: Macmillan, 1994.

Nutrition Guide to Food Allergies. Available from Food Allergy Network.

Off to School with Food Allergies. Available from Food Allergy Network.

20
· · · · · · · ·

High Blood Cholesterol

Cholesterol and triglycerides are fats, also called lipids, which are carried in the bloodstream. Individuals in whom these values are abnormally high have hypercholesterolemia, or hyperlipidemia, respectively. This is an inherited disorder, although occasionally hyperlipidemia may be due to some secondary causes like certain illnesses, medications, or dietary habits. Both dietary and medical treatment can help to correct elevated lipid levels.

> **MYTH** Cholesterol in food is the major factor which raises blood cholesterol.
> **FACT** While dietary cholesterol has some effect on blood cholesterol, saturated fat has the greatest impact on blood cholesterol.

Why Be Concerned?

The most frequent cause of death among adults in the United States is atherosclerosis (thickening of the arteries due to accumulation of lipids in the artery walls). Such thickening leads to coronary heart disease, stroke, and circulation problems in the legs. Many research studies have identified high blood cholesterol levels and diets high in cholesterol and saturated fat as important factors in coronary heart disease development. One well-known project is the Framingham, Massachusetts, study, which has followed town residents since 1948. This study has made it possible to follow the natural history of heart problems over many years in those with normal cholesterol levels as

· ·

Ruth Whittemore ■ Lisa Devine

well as those with high cholesterol levels. This and other projects have documented high cholesterol levels and high-fat diets in a large percentage of those who had evidence of coronary heart disease. The higher cholesterol levels were associated with higher mortality rates among middle-aged men.

It is also known that the process of cholesterol deposition in major arteries begins in childhood. Children, even at the age of 3, can develop fatty streaks in the walls of the aorta and inner lining of the main blood vessels. Studies on soldiers during World War II and the Korean War showed that 70 percent of the soldiers killed in battle (average age 23) were found to have the beginning of atherosclerosis in the lining of the aorta and large blood vessels. Even more advanced hardening of the arteries was seen in soldiers killed in the Vietnam War. Therefore, preventive measures should start in young children to slow down this process, particularly if there is evidence of high lipid levels or if there is a family history of heart attacks before the age of 50.

What Are Cholesterol, Triglycerides, and Lipoproteins?

Cholesterol and fats in the diet and in the bloodstream are discussed in detail in chapter 30. Briefly, cholesterol is carried in the blood in association with blood proteins in three main types of particles called lipoproteins: low-density lipoprotein (LDL), very low-density lipoprotein (VLDL), and high-density lipoprotein (HDL). On the one hand, the presence of a high level of LDL (greater than 130 milligrams/deciliter) seems to be the greatest culprit in the early development of hardening of the arteries. On the other hand, HDL appears to be the "good" lipoprotein, and higher levels are associated with lower risk of heart disease (see fig. 20.1).

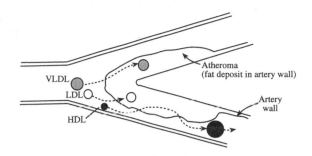

FIGURE 20.1
Lipoproteins and fat deposits in arteries. LDL and VLDL increase the risk of atherosclerosis because they add lipids to fat deposits in artery walls, whereas HDL removes lipids from fat deposits and lowers the risk of atherosclerosis.

Large amounts of saturated fats and cholesterol in the diet are associated with higher levels of LDL in the blood. However, some children and adults with hyperlipidemia have genetic defects that reduce the rate at which LDL is removed from the bloodstream. These individuals have high LDL levels even when they are eating an average amount of fat and cholesterol.

Pediatricians should often check cholesterol levels in healthy children if there is a family history of atherosclerosis in adults younger than 50 years of age. If it appears that there is a family trend to hyperlipidemia, it is recommended that the immediate family be screened to identify any members who may not know that they have a problem. This includes all children over the age of 2 years and both parents. This lipid profile should include at least total cholesterol, HDL, LDL, and triglyceride levels. Acceptable, borderline, and abnormal lipid levels are given in table 20.1.

Pediatricians should also screen for hyperlipidemia in children who are taking medications (such as contraceptives, retinoic acid derivatives,

TABLE 20.1
Blood Levels of Lipid Profiles in Children (milligrams/deciliter)

	Total cholesterol	HDL	LDL	Triglycerides
Acceptable	<170	>35	<110	<130
Borderline	170–199	30–35	110–129	130–150
Abnormal	>200	<30	>130	>150

Note: HDL is the only fraction where higher is better.

or steroids) or have conditions that elevate blood cholesterol levels such as those listed below.

Diabetes mellitus   Lupus
Hyperinsulinism   Nephrotic syndrome
Hypothyroidism   Obesity
Liver disease or
    obstruction

Conversely, a high cholesterol level may be the first sign of one of these other medical problems. Moreover, effective treatment of some of these disorders (like diabetes and hypothyroidism) may lower cholesterol levels as well.

Common Types of Hyperlipidemia

The disorders of lipoprotein metabolism fall into several main categories that have distinctive characteristics and genetic patterns of inheritance.

Familial hypercholesterolemia occurs in about 1 in 500 people and is most commonly associated with a family history. The primary problem is not only the elevation of the total blood cholesterol level but also an increase in LDL. A child with this condition usually has a cholesterol level of 250 milligrams per deciliter or more with an LDL cholesterol level above 200. This disorder is inherited as an autosomal dominant gene, meaning that a child of an affected parent has a 50 percent

chance of having the disorder, even though the other parent does not carry the genetic trait.

Most children are identified by screening blood tests because there are usually no clinical manifestations. Rarely, cholesterol deposits cause swellings on tendons, yellow deposits between the fingers, similar deposits on the eyelids of some adults, or a whitening around the cornea of the eye. Rarely, a child may have small yellowish deposits in the skin and have a very high cholesterol level which may require intensive work-up and treatment.

Familial combined hyperlipidemia. This type of hyperlipidemia is the most frequent and occurs in about 0.5 percent of all children (1 in 200). A slight elevation of cholesterol may be all that is seen in the child at first. An increase in the triglyceride level is often not seen until later in the teens or early adult life, when the cholesterol level also increases. In families with this type, one normal blood cholesterol and lipids test result may not be significant. Repeat studies should be done at least every 5–10 years to ascertain possible triglyceride involvement. Treatment should be the same as with children who have hypercholesterolemia until hypertriglyceridemia is diagnosed, at which time further modifications of diet or medications are often needed to lower triglycerides. These families are prone to early coronary heart disease, especially if the LDL is high and the HDL is lower than normal (30 grams per deciliter).

Hypertriglyceridemia. A rare family has pure hypertriglyceridemia (2–3 in every 1,000 adults), often not manifested until early adulthood. The level in these individuals is usually between 200 and 500 milligrams/deciliter, while normal is 50–150. Reduction in fat intake and weight loss usually can control this. Individuals with a low HDL are more vulnerable to develop coronary heart disease than those who have a normal HDL. Children in early stages of diabetes can sometimes have the same lipid picture as seen in these families. Some changes in diet are usually recommended for the child. Special medication is rarely needed in childhood, but may be recommended in adolescence to control cholesterol as well as triglyceride levels.

There are less frequent hyperlipidemias which should be treated by a clinic that specializes in lipid disorders. A condition of excessively high cholesterol inherited from both parents occurs in one child in a million. These children usually have clinical symptoms early in life and should be treated at a specialty clinic center at as early an age as possible. Experimental procedures such as plasma pheresis or partial liver transplant may be recommended. Some of these children (often infants) have benefited from a liver transplant.

Diet Therapy

When the type of the hypercholesterolemia or hyperlipidemia has been identified and other causes of hypercholesterolemia have been excluded, the first line of treatment is diet modification, although it need not be overwhelming. The younger the child, the easier it is for him or her to become accustomed to the recommended diet. This may start as nothing more than a healthy, balanced diet, as has been discussed in many other chapters in this book. Medication is not considered until the response to diet is determined.

Parental concerns include the reaction and response of their child. Most young children accept the new plans, sometimes as an adventure, but a great deal depends on the circumstances and how well the family is counseled. Older children, especially teenagers, may feel overwhelmed when they learn they have the same problem as a near member of the family who has had a heart attack or even died suddenly. Some children rebel, some become depressed, others may try to deny the problem. Counseling allows the children to talk out feelings with someone with whom they feel comfortable. Social workers, psychiatrists, and the dietitian, as well an understanding physician (such as the pediatrician), may well serve this purpose. It is important for the clinic to identify how the child is dealing with the situation and address concerns. Another potential source of frustration for the adolescent and young teenager is peer pressure from friends, especially concerning dietary restrictions.

THE STEP-ONE AND STEP-TWO DIETS Diet management for hypercholesterolemia is achieved in two steps, the Step-One and Step-Two diets, which are designed to reduce dietary intakes of saturated fat and cholesterol progressively. In 1991, the National Cholesterol Education Program (NCEP) issued recommendations for implementing the Step-One and Step-Two diets in the management of hypercholesterolemia in children. These recommendations were derived from a first-time consensus among pediatric specialists, lipid researchers, and nutrition experts regarding the role of diet in children and their risk for cardiovascular disease. The goals of diet therapy are to

TABLE 20.2

Recommended Intake in Step-One and Step-Two Diets

	Step-One diet	*Step-Two diet*
Total fat	Average no more than 30% of total calories	Same
Saturated fatty acids	Less than 10% of total calories	Less than 7% of total calories
Polyunsaturated fatty acids	Up to 10% of total calories	Same
Monounsaturated fatty acids	Remaining total fat calories	Same
Cholesterol	Less than 300 mg/day	Less than 200 mg/day
Carbohydrates	About 55% of total calories	Same
Protein	About 15–20% of total calories	Same
Calories	Sufficient to promote normal growth and development and to reach or maintain desirable body weight	Same

reduce blood cholesterol levels while maintaining a nutritionally adequate diet and promoting normal growth.

The Step-One diet is indicated in children with total cholesterol levels greater than or equal to 170 milligrams per deciliter or an LDL cholesterol level that is greater than or equal to 110 milligrams per deciliter. As shown in table 20.2, the Step-One diet consists of a total fat intake of no more than 30 percent of total calories, saturated fat intake of less than 10 percent of total calories, cholesterol intake of less than 300 milligrams per day, and calorie intake sufficient to promote normal growth and maintain desirable body weight. It should be noted that the Step-One diet is identical to the NCEP recommendations for the general U.S. population in promoting good health and preventing cardiovascular disease. It is compatible with the Dietary Guidelines for Americans, as well as the American Heart Association guidelines. In other words, all Americans over the age of 2 years are urged to adapt an eating pattern as described in the Step-One diet. The diet becomes therapeutic when implemented in a medi-

cal setting with specific counseling and support of a treatment team.

If the goals for reducing blood cholesterol are not reached after three to six months on the Step-One diet, the child should begin the Step-Two diet (table 20.2). This calls for further reduction in intake of saturated fat to less than 7 percent of total calories and cholesterol intake to less than 200 milligrams per day. The Step-Two diet is more difficult to adhere to and requires careful planning. It should be followed for six months to one year before medication is considered. Fortunately, such therapy is necessary in only a very small percentage of children.

When the Step-One diet is recommended for a child, many questions may go through a parent's mind: Does my child have to eat diet foods? Will he or she have to stop eating school lunch? Can he or she still eat pizza? Will he or she get enough vitamins and calcium? Often the Step-One diet can best be achieved by changing several food choices in the child's diet. Buying low-fat or nonfat dairy products and lean meats and opting for fruits over high-fat snack chips and desserts may be enough to bring a cholesterol level down. Parents and children can use the guidelines in table 20.3 to make wise decisions about food selection. In a therapeutic setting, a dietitian evaluates the child's diet through a detailed nutrition history and uses the information to set goals for dietary changes where necessary. Educating the family about snack foods is an additional focus. The parent who shops for the family has an important role and should read food nutrition labels carefully. When all the foods available in the home are healthful, parents won't have to worry about what the kids are eating when they are not there to supervise.

Meat, Poultry, and Fish

Meat, poultry, and fish are good sources of protein, iron, and vitamin B_{12}. Meat and poultry (with skin) are also significant sources of saturated fat, total fat, and cholesterol. Lean beef, pork, poultry, and fish all have similar cholesterol contents, averaging 66 to 76 milligrams per 3-ounce serving. Beef, pork, and lamb should be lean cuts, such as those that come from the round or loin, and should be well trimmed before cooking. Ground beef should be at least 85 percent lean (90 percent for Step-Two) and should be blotted on paper towels after cooking. Lean meat can be eaten every day within allowed portion size, as will be discussed below. Once skin is removed from poultry, it is generally low in fat and saturated fat. Ground turkey and chicken are fine alternatives to ground beef if they contain only white meat, as saturated fat content rises considerably in ground poultry which contains skin and other parts. Labels should be checked carefully when buying these products. There are several brands of low-fat and fat-free processed meats and poultry available for hot dogs, bologna, pastrami, and

so forth. Generally, good choices are those with 3 grams or less total fat per ounce. Liver and other organ meats are very high in cholesterol and should be permitted no more than once a month.

Seafood in general is low in saturated fat. Although shrimp, crayfish, and squid are low in saturated fat, they should be consumed in limited quantities, as they are high in cholesterol.

Dairy Products

Although dairy products provide calcium, phosphorus, and protein, like meats they may contribute substantial amounts of saturated fat and cholesterol if consumed as whole-milk products, full-fat yogurt, regular cheeses, and fat-loaded frozen treats. When shopping in the dairy aisle, choose 1 percent or skim milk, low-fat yogurt, and low-fat cottage cheese. Look for low-fat cheeses containing no more than 6 grams of fat per ounce and frozen desserts with less than 5 grams of fat per half-cup serving. Any product stating that it is "low-fat" means it contains 3 grams or less of fat per serving. Therefore, "low-fat" on a label should signal a green light (see chapter 36 on reading food labels).

Eggs

Eggs are a good source of protein and iron; however, they are high in cholesterol. A large egg contains approximately 215 milligrams of cholesterol, which is more than two-thirds the daily allotment in the Step-One diet. Thus, it is advisable to limit consumption to no more than four eggs per week. For the Step-Two diet, no more than two whole eggs should be consumed per week. A fine alternative for eggs are egg substitutes, which contain mostly egg whites (the egg white is the high-protein, cholesterol-free part of the egg). Espe-

TABLE 20.3
Foods to Choose and Decrease for the Step-One and Step-Two Diets

	Choose	*Decrease*
Meat, poultry, and fish	Beef, pork, lamb—lean cuts, well trimmed before cooking	Beef, pork, lamb—fatty cuts, spare-ribs, organ meats, sausage, hot dogs, bacon
	Poultry without skin	Poultry with skin, fried chicken
	Fish, shellfish (broiled, baked, grilled, poached)	Fried fish, fried shellfish
	Processed meat prepared from lean meat (e.g., turkey, ham, tuna, hot dogs)	Regular luncheon meat (e.g., bologna, salami, sausage, hot dogs)
Egg	Egg whites (two whites equal one whole egg in recipes), choles-terol-free egg substitute	Egg yolks (if more than 4 per week on Step-One or if more than 2 per week on Step-Two); includes eggs used in cooking
Dairy products	Milk—skim or 1 percent fat (fluid, powdered, evaporated), buttermilk	Whole milk (fluid, evaporated, condensed), 2 percent milk, imitation milk, milk shakes
	Yogurt—nonfat or low-fat yogurt or yogurt beverages	Whole milk yogurt, whole milk yogurt beverages
	Cheese—low-fat natural or processed cheese (part-skim mozzarella, ricotta) with no more than 6 g fat per oz on Step-One, or 2 g fat per oz on Step-Two	Regular cheeses (American, blue, Brie, cheddar, Colby, Edam, Monterey Jack, whole-milk mozzarella, Parmesan, Swiss), cream cheese, Neufchatel cheese
	Cottage cheese—low-fat, nonfat, or dry curd (up to 2 percent fat)	Cottage cheese (4 percent fat)
	Frozen dairy desserts—ice milk, frozen yogurt (low-fat or nonfat)	Ice cream
Fats and oils	Unsaturated oils—safflower, sun-flower, corn, soybean, cottonseed, canola, olive, peanut oils	Coconut oil, palm kernel oil, palm oil
	Margarine made from unsaturated oils listed above, light or diet margarine	Butter, lard, shortening, bacon fat
	Salad dressings made with unsatu-rated oils listed above, low-fat or oil-free	Dressings made with egg yolk, cheese, sour cream, whole milk
	Seeds and nuts—peanut butter, other nut butters	Coconut
	Cocoa powder	Chocolate

TABLE 20.3
Continued

	Choose	*Decrease*
Breads and cereals	Breads—whole-grain bread, hamburger and hot dog buns, corn tortillas	Bread in which eggs are a major ingredient, croissants
	Cereals—oat, wheat, corn, multigrain	Granola made with coconut
	Pasta	Egg noodles and pasta containing egg yolks
	Rice	
	Dry beans and peas	
	Crackers, low-fat—animal, graham, saltines	High-fat crackers
	Homemade baked goods using unsaturated oil, skim or 1 percent milk, and egg substitutes—quick breads, biscuits, corn bread and muffins, pancakes, waffles	Commercial baked pastries, muffins, biscuits
Vegetables and fruits	Vegetables—fresh, frozen, or canned	Vegetables prepared with butter, cheese, or cream sauce
	Fruit—fresh, frozen, canned, or dried	Fruit served with cream
	Fruit juice—fresh, frozen, or canned	
Sweets and modified fat desserts	Beverages—fruit-flavored drinks, lemonade, fruit punch	
	Sweets—sugar, syrup, honey, jam, preserves, candy made without fat (candy corn, hard candy), fruit-flavored gelatin	Candy made with chocolate, coconut oil, palm kernel oil, palm oil
	Frozen desserts—sherbet, sorbet, fruit ice, popsicles	Ice cream and frozen desserts made with ice cream
	Cookies, cake, pie, puddings prepared with egg whites, egg substitutes, skim milk or 1 percent milk, and unsaturated oil or margarine (for example, gingersnaps, fig bar cookies, angel food cake)	Commercially baked pies, cakes, doughnuts, high-fat cookies, cream pies

Source: National Cholesterol Education Program, *NCEP Report on Blood Cholesterol Levels in Children and Adolescents,* September 1991.

cially for the Step-Two diet, egg substitutes may replace eggs, totally or partially, in baked goods and egg dishes.

Breads, Cereals, and Grains

Breads, cereal, and grains should account for the majority of calories in one's diet (for children and adults), and this is usually easy to achieve. Most breads, cereals, and grains are low in fat and cholesterol-free—in their purest form. For instance, rice, oats, and whole-wheat bread are low in fat and have no cholesterol, but change these into pork fried rice, oatmeal cookies, and French toast, and the fat and cholesterol content has increased considerably. Choose whole-grain cereals at breakfast and snack times, and include pasta, rice, potatoes, and legumes frequently at mealtimes as part of the main entrée. For adolescents who need to cut down on portions of meat, try offering mixed dishes like pasta with meat sauce, chicken and vegetables over linguini, stir-fried beef over rice, and chili.

Fruits and Vegetables

Servings of fruits and vegetables—excellent sources of several vitamins, especially vitamins A and C, minerals, and fiber—should be increased to meet the goals of the Food Guide Pyramid (see chapter 4): two to four servings of fruits, and three to five servings of vegetables per day. Fruits and vegetables can replace higher-fat foods as well as improve fiber content in the child's diet.

Fats

In the Step-One and Step-Two diets, the aim is to consume a small amount of fats and oils, but enough to allow normal growth. In addition, the diet promotes unsaturated fat over saturated fat. Saturated fat is found in animal products and tropical oils, namely, palm kernel, coconut, and palm oils. Saturated fat is also found in products containing hydrogenated oils (see chapter 30). The Step-One and Step-Two diets allow for some saturated fat, which is primarily derived from the recommended lean meats and low-fat dairy products already mentioned. The diet strictly limits saturated fat, which is in many bakery goods, candies, cookies, processed meats, and fast food. Unsaturated fat is found in vegetable oils like canola, corn, cottonseed, olive, soybean, safflower, sunflower, and peanut oils. These oils should be used in cooking, while lard and shortening should not be. Tub margarine (which contains less saturated fat) should be used in place of butter, and the polyunsaturated to saturated oil ratio on the label should be at least two to one. Look on food labels for no saturated fat, preferably, but no more than 4 grams of saturated fat per serving in entrées and side dishes and 2 grams of saturated fat per serving in desserts and snack foods. When reading the food label, compare the label serving size to how much the child normally eats. If the child eats two servings, twice as much fat will be consumed.

Meal Planning

A child on the Step-One or Step-Two diet need not eat special "diet" food. For example, a child may have pizza as long as a few adjustments are made. Homemade pizza is best because parents can control the amount and type of ingredients used (for example, low-fat cheeses, vegetables, or low-fat meat). Restaurant or take-out pizza can be allowed from time to time if it doesn't have meat toppings and extra cheese. Eating out at fast-food restaurants should be limited to about once a week. Strict adherence to the diet can be relaxed

TABLE 20.4

Step-One Diet Nutrient Recommendations in Servings per Day for Children of Different Ages

	All children			Boys	Girls	Boys	Girls
	2–3	4–6	7–10	11–14	11–14	15–18	15–18
Meat, poultry, and fish (oz per day)	2	5	6	6	6	6	6
Eggs (per week)	3	3	3	3	3	3	3
Dairy products	3	3	4	4	4	4	4
Fats and oils	4	5	5	7	5	10	5
Breads and cereals	5	6	7	9	8	12	8
Vegetables	3	3	3	4	3	4	3
Fruits	2	3	3	3	3	5	3
Sweets and modified-fat desserts	1	2	2	4	3	4	3

Source: National Cholesterol Education Program, *NCEP Report on Blood Cholesterol Levels in Children and Adolescents,* September 1991.

for a birthday party or other special occasion as long as most meals eaten in a given week are low in saturated fat and cholesterol.

School lunch menus vary tremendously from school to school (see chapter 30). Some schools have adopted healthful menus and encourage students to choose nutritious foods in the lunch line through health awareness programs. In contrast, some schools have contracts with fast-food chains, thereby giving students the choice of burgers and fries, fried chicken and biscuits, or pizza on a daily basis. Parents are strongly encouraged to become familiar with their child's school lunch menu and learn, with the child, ways to incorporate favorite meals into the recommended diet. For example, it may be acceptable to choose the school lunch three times a week and bring a lunch from home twice a week. Menus of hot dogs with tater tots and grilled cheese with fries can be skipped, whereas spaghetti with meat sauce, turkey sandwich with carrot sticks, and cheese pizza with salad can be chosen.

Table 20.4 translates Step-One dietary recommendations into servings per day for different ages. For most children, appetite should guide food consumption. However, parents must be in charge of providing the appropriate balance of foods and giving the child the opportunity to choose from among healthy foods (a "win-win" situation). The recommended servings per day also set the stage for a nutritionally adequate diet that is safe and consistent with normal growth and development. The Step-One and Step-Two diets meet the Recommended Dietary Allowances (RDAs) for all nutrients and provide adequate calories for growth when properly followed. Some reports of stunted growth have surfaced, but these were the result of inadequate consumption of calories by young children who followed these diets improperly. Table 20.5 shows sample menus for school-age children, including a typical diet for comparison. Calorie levels are similar in each, but fat content decreases from greater than 35 percent to less than 30 percent in the Step-Two diet. Cholesterol content also decreases significantly. Some may find it surprising that the Step-One and Step-

TABLE 20.5
Sample Menus for Children Ages 8–11 with School Lunch

Typical	Step-One	Step-Two
Breakfast		
Orange juice, ½ cup	Orange juice	Orange juice, ½ cup
Toaster waffles, 2	Toaster waffles, 2	Toaster waffles, 2
Soft margarine, 2 tsp	Syrup, 2 tbsp	Syrup, 2 tbsp
Syrup, 2 tbsp	1 percent milk, 1 cup	Skim milk, 1 cup
Whole milk, 1 cup		
School lunch		
Grilled cheese sandwich	Grilled cheese sandwich	Lean ham, 2 oz, and reduced-fat American cheese, 1 oz, sandwich on white bread with lettuce, tomato, pickles and light mayonnaise (2 tsp)
Italian green beans, ½ cup	Italian green beans, ½ cup	Italian green beans, ½ cup
Canned pears, ½ cup	Canned pears, ½ cup	Banana, 1
Whole milk, 1 cup	1 percent milk, 1 cup	Skim milk, 1 cup
Snack		
Barbecue-flavor potato chips, 2 oz	Graham cracker squares, 6	Graham cracker squares, 6
Soda, regular, 1½ cups	Peanut butter, 1 tbsp	Peanut butter, 1 tbsp
	Apple, sliced, 1	Apple, sliced, 1
	Soda, regular, 1½ cups	Soda, regular, 1½ cups
Dinner		
Spaghetti and meatballs, 1 cup	Spaghetti and meatballs (lean beef), 1 cup	Spaghetti and meatballs (extra lean beef), 1 cup
Tossed salad, 1 cup	Tossed salad, 1 cup	Tossed salad, 1 cup
Vinaigrette dressing, 1 tbsp	Vinaigrette dressing, 1 tbsp	Vinaigrette dressing, 1 tbsp
Dinner roll, 1	Dinner roll, 1	Dinner roll, 1
Butter, 1 tsp	Soft margarine, 1 tsp	Soft margarine, 1 tsp
Applesauce, ½ cup	Applesauce, ½ cup	Applesauce, ½ cup
2 percent milk, 1 cup	1 percent milk, 1 cup	Skim milk, 1 cup
Snack		
Vanilla ice cream, ½ cup	Low-fat vanilla ice cream, ½ cup	Frozen yogurt, ½ cup

Two menus include snacks, soda, and cookies. The diet isn't meant to be boring or overly restrictive, and it certainly need not be.

Parents are role models and must have a positive attitude about food selections, especially for children who may not understand why they need to change what they eat. Ideally, the entire family should eat the same healthful diet, but if this is not realistic, the following tips may make things easier.

- Focus on what foods the child can eat rather than what he or she cannot.
- Involve the child in food shopping and preparation.
- Keep favorite healthy snacks on hand.
- Include foods the child should eat as part of the daily meal pattern for the entire family.
- Remember to think of the child as a child, not a sick patient.
- Accept that there will be times when children make poor food choices. React calmly, and encourage them to do better next time.
- Praise healthy food choices, especially in difficult situations.

Medical Follow-Up

Follow-up appointments are important especially in the early stages after diagnosis. It is usually advisable for the child to be seen by the doctor, as well as the dietitian, every six weeks to three months at first and to make dietary changes according to how the blood lipid levels are responding. The child may need several months to adjust to the change in eating habits. Parents should discuss with the physician any difficulties with following the diet. If the blood lipid results show improvement, diet therapy alone may be all that is necessary. It should be stressed that these dietary changes are lifelong. With good response, return visits may be decreased to every six months and later to once per year, usually after the first year.

Medications

If medication is necessary, it is chosen based on the specific lipid disorder, the age and maturity of the child, and the child's capability of taking the medication. Medication may not be necessary until the child is around 10 years old, although many times it is necessary to start earlier. Some medications used for children, their action, dosage, administration, and possible concerns are discussed here.

Cholestyramine (known as Questran commercially) is a bile acid sequestrant that congeals bile acid (important for the absorption of fat in the intestinal tract). When cholestyramine is given, fat from ingested food is solidified and passes out in the stool rather than being absorbed into the bloodstream. Therefore, some of the lipids in the diet do not get absorbed into the circulation. This medication is a coarse powder which, when placed in water or juice, becomes slightly gelatinous but is still granular in texture. A preparation with added orange flavor has been more acceptable to some children. Children take this in a glass of water or juice about one half hour before a meal. The child may be somewhat constipated and complain of stomachache the first few days. An increase in the fiber content of the child's diet (such as fresh or dried fruits) is most helpful at this time, and the child must drink plenty of water. If a child who starts taking cholestyramine is also taking vitamins, the cholestyramine should be taken at least 4 hours away from the vitamin supplement. If this timing is inconvenient, the child can be given liquid vitamins. After four to six months, Questran may lower the cholesterol level by 15–20 percent, as well as decrease the LDL level.

Colestipol HCl acts in the same way as cholestyramine with the same results and concerns.

Niacin is another medication of choice if diet and cholestyramine do not produce adequate results. Niacin not only lowers cholesterol, LDL, triglycerides, and VLDL; it also appears to increase HDL. The action of niacin in lowering lipids and lipoproteins is not well understood, and it is used only with caution in older children under very close scrutiny. In adults, it has been quite satisfactory in the majority of cases. However, there are potential problems with this medication. Flushing, or a sensation of heat with redness and possible rash, is a problem which an individual may feel for a short time after taking the tablet, but this becomes more tolerable over time. This sensation is due to the fact that niacin causes small blood vessels in the skin to dilate. Giving an aspirin tablet a short time before the niacin reduces the discomfort from the flushing. Niacin should be taken with or after the meal, not on an empty stomach, and alcohol should never be consumed while an individual is on this medication. Niacin should be started with a low dose and gradually increased with care. Liver function must be closely watched during the gradual increase of this medicine, and should be compared with the premedication liver function tests. Niacin should not be used if there is any question of liver or gallbladder problems or any evidence of peptic ulcer.

Gemfibrozil (Lopid) primarily reduces the production of triglycerides and VLDL by decreasing the hepatic extraction of free fatty acids, the precursors of triglycerides. This is used in adults to lower high triglycerides, but rarely in children. Complications from this medication can include liver or kidney dysfunction and gallstones.

HMG-Co-A reductase inhibitor medications (Mevacor and others) are newer medications that markedly reduce total and LDL cholesterol and increase HDL. They have not been recommended for children as yet, although trials are under way concerning their use in children.

In all instances, a modified diet is to be maintained throughout life, often with continued use of cholestyramine or other medication, if indicated.

Conclusions

Despite the reduction in the coronary heart disease mortality rate over the past two decades, the condition remains the number one cause of death in the United States. Clinical and epidemiological studies demonstrate that elevated blood cholesterol contributes to the atherosclerotic process. Preventing or slowing down the development of cardiovascular disease early in life, especially for those children at high risk, can extend the years of healthy living for many Americans.

This can be accomplished with dietary modifications that are nutritionally sound, easy to adopt, and far from dull. One hopes that the typical American diet will continue to become more healthful, with our children as beneficiaries.

Resources

National Cholesterol Education Program. *Report of the Expert Panel on Detection, Evaluation, and Treatment of High Blood Cholesterol in Adults.* Bethesda, MD, U.S. Department of Health and Human Services, Public Health Service, National Institutes of Health, National Heart, Lung, and Blood Institute. January 1989, NIH Pub. No. 89-292.

National Cholesterol Education Program. *Report of the Expert Panel on Blood Cholesterol Levels in Children and Adolescents.* Bethesda, MD, U.S. Department of Health and Human Services, Public Health Service, National Institutes of Health, National Heart, Lung, and Blood Institute. September 1991, NIH Pub. No. 92-2732.

21

......

Diabetes

Diabetes mellitus (derived from the Greek words for sweet urine) is one of the most common chronic childhood illnesses, affecting 1 in 500–600 children under 18 years of age in the United States. Diabetes in childhood presents parents, children, and physicians and other clinicians with special challenges. On the one hand, diabetes is a very difficult condition to treat, involving daily insulin injections and multiple finger pricks to test blood glucose levels. On the other hand, the more effectively diabetes is regulated during childhood, the fewer health problems the child with diabetes will have when he or she reaches adulthood. Moreover, careful attention to diet and good nutritional principles is one of the cornerstones of therapy for diabetes.

> **MYTH** Eating sweets will cause diabetes in children.
> **FACT** Diet has no impact on the development of diabetes in children. Diabetes in children is caused by genetic, immunologic, and environmental factors.

What Is Diabetes?

The basic problem in individuals who have diabetes is that their bodies are not making enough insulin. Insulin is the hormone produced by the pancreas that regulates the body's production and use of glucose. Glucose is the form of sugar that circulates in blood (see chapter 29) and provides the main source of energy for the brain and other tissues. The body regulates the blood glucose concentration normally at a level between 70 and 140

....

William V. Tamborlane • Nancy A. Held

milligrams/deciliter. When the person is not eating, blood insulin levels fall and this allows the body to produce glucose from stores in the liver to keep blood glucose levels from falling too low. Conversely, after eating, insulin is secreted by the pancreas to allow the tissues of the body to take up the extra glucose from the meal, which keeps blood glucose levels from going too high. Insulin also has important effects on other nutrients, helping to build protein and muscle and to increase body stores of fat.

There are two main types of diabetes. Type I, or insulin-dependent diabetes mellitus (IDDM) is the type of diabetes that afflicts most children with diabetes; it was once called juvenile diabetes. The other is Type II, or non-insulin-dependent diabetes (NIDDM), which is seen most often in adults. The characteristic that distinguishes the two types of diabetes is not age (either type can occur at any age), but rather the degree of insulin deficiency. People with IDDM have severe deficiency of insulin and require insulin injections in order to survive. Individuals with NIDDM, in contrast, make some insulin, but their bodies don't respond as well to insulin as they should. This is called insulin resistance. Individuals with NIDDM can be treated, at least initially, with pills that lower blood-sugar levels instead of insulin shots, because the medication helps increase the body's secretion of and response to insulin. Parents often ask whether children who have been treated with insulin injections will be able to switch to pills once they become adults. This is not possible because the pills work only if the pancreas is able to make some insulin. Because the vast majority of children with diabetes have Type I, or IDDM, this chapter concerns IDDM unless otherwise noted.

When the pancreas cannot make enough insulin, the level of glucose (sugar) in the blood rises because too much glucose is being produced and not enough is being utilized. Values in untreated diabetic people can exceed 1,000 milligrams/deciliter, whereas the normal range is 70–140. The body tries to get rid of the extra sugar by excreting it in the urine. Each sugar molecule acts like a little sponge, drawing water with it and causing excessive urination. This may be most obvious at night, when the child gets up several times or when bed-wetting recurs in a previously trained child. The extra urination leads to increased thirst and drinking; in girls, sugar in the urine may contribute to the development of vaginal yeast infections. Children will begin breaking down muscle rather than building it up, and weight loss despite adequate food intake is another warning sign of diabetes.

Many children are diagnosed by the early warning signs of increased drinking, urination, and weight loss at a stage where they are still making some insulin. If diabetes is not recognized, insulin levels continue to fall and more severe problems develop. The child begins breaking down excessive amounts of fat, and levels of ketones (by-products of fat metabolism) increase in the blood. Ketones cause abdominal pain, vomiting, acidosis (too much acid in the blood), and dehydration. The term for this is diabetic ketoacidosis, and, if unrecognized, it can lead to coma and death. Persons with diabetic ketoacidosis require hospitalization, often in an intensive care unit. This is the most severe stage of uncontrolled diabetes.

What Causes Diabetes?

Although the precise cause of diabetes has evaded researchers so far, knowledge about the underlying disease process has progressed a great deal

TABLE 21.1

TABLE 21.1

Approximate Risks of a Child Developing
Insulin-Dependent Diabetes Mellitus (IDDM)

General population	0.2–0.3%
Parent or sibling with IDDM	3–5%
Identical twin with IDDM	30–40%
Tests positive for antibodies against the pancreas	25–50%
Tests positive for antibodies against the pancreas and has reduced insulin secretion	80–90%

since the mid-1980s. Three major areas of interest are the roles of genetic, environmental, and immunologic factors.

Several lines of evidence indicate the importance of genetic influences in the development of diabetes. Specific gene patterns are commonly associated with IDDM, but many unaffected individuals also have the same gene patterns. IDDM runs in families; if a parent or child has IDDM, the risk that an unaffected child will get diabetes increases from 1 in 500 (0.2–0.3 percent) to 3–5 in 100 (3–5 percent). If an identical twin gets diabetes, the chance of the other twin getting it goes up to 30–40 percent (table 21.1). However, if IDDM were purely a genetic problem, one would expect the risk for an unaffected identical twin to get diabetes to be 100 percent. Therefore, it appears that individuals inherit a tendency toward diabetes, but other factors are needed for its full expression.

Individuals with a genetic tendency to diabetes may have to come in contact with the right environmental factors in order to develop the disease. Feeding infants with cow's milk has been suggested as one factor, but this remains extremely controversial. Many viruses have also been implicated as causes of diabetes. In these cases, the virus itself does not infect the pancreas. Instead, certain proteins on the surface of the virus (called antigens) are similar to proteins on the surface of beta cells, the insulin-producing cells of the pancreas. In the process of killing the virus, the body's immune system becomes sensitized against its own beta cells and starts attacking the pancreas.

A condition like IDDM that is caused by the immune system is called an autoimmune disease. With IDDM, the immune attack leads to a gradual loss of insulin-producing cells over a period of months or even years. During this "prediabetic" phase, the immune system's antibodies that attack the pancreas can be detected by blood tests. The tests are not perfect predictors of who will get IDDM, because in some individuals the immune process may stop on its own and diabetes may never develop.

Treatment of Diabetes

Insulin, diet, and exercise are the three cornerstones of treatment of IDDM. The overall goals of treatment are to balance these factors in order to minimize symptoms of high or low blood-sugar levels and to promote normal growth and development. Any chronic illness like IDDM can have adverse psychological effects that clinicians try to minimize by providing an education program that stresses independence and self-management skills. Why bother? That's the question that most of our teenagers with diabetes ask when we ask them to do the things that are needed to take care of their diabetes. The simple answer is that they'll be healthier when they grow up, that good diabetes control can delay or prevent the long-term complications of diabetes. High blood glucose levels over many years cause damage to the eyes, kidneys and nervous system that can result in blindness, kidney failure, pain and numbness. The 1994 results of a landmark ten-year study (Diabetes Control and Complications Trial or DCCT) have shown that many of these complications can be avoided or delayed by lowering glucose to levels as close to normal as possible.

Insulin Therapy

Insulin is a protein hormone that is composed of two chains of amino acids of very specific structure. It must be given by injections and not as a pill because, like any other protein, it would be broken down to its individual amino acids and deactivated during the digestive process. Stabilizing agents are added to the basic insulin molecule to produce three types of insulin, based on their time-course of action: fast (regular), intermediate (NPH and Lente), and long-acting (Ultra-Lente) insulins.

An aim of insulin therapy is to maintain blood insulin levels that are as close as possible to those seen in children without diabetes. Practical considerations regarding how many insulin injections children are willing to take each day may limit what can be done toward this goal. As an acceptable compromise, most newly diagnosed children receive two daily insulin injections: one before breakfast and one before dinner. Both injections consist of a mixture of fast- and intermediate-acting insulins. In the morning, the fast-acting insulin is supposed to reproduce the normal surge of insulin with breakfast, and the intermediate insulin takes care of lunch. In the evening, the fast-acting insulin covers supper, and the intermediate insulin fulfills the overnight insulin requirement.

Early in the course of IDDM in children, there may still be some insulin-secreting cells in the pancreas that begin to work better once insu-

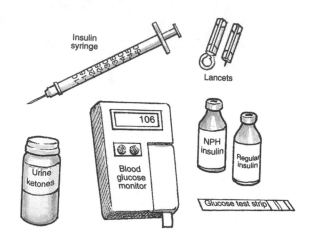

FIGURE 21.1
Equipment and supplies used in the management of diabetes.

lin therapy has been begun. Insulin doses often drop dramatically as the child goes through a partial remission of diabetes (called the "honeymoon" phase). This phase is usually short-lived because the immune system continues its attack on the pancreas. After the honeymoon phase, children with diabetes need steadily increasing doses of insulin to account for growth. A common misconception is that the need for ever larger insulin doses means that the child's diabetes is "getting worse." This is not true. More insulin is needed because weight and caloric intake increase with age in children and because the hormonal changes of puberty make the body less responsive to insulin.

One of the major advances in the ability to determine how much insulin is needed was the development of small, portable, accurate monitors that children and families can use at home to measure the child's blood glucose levels. People with diabetes should check their glucose levels two to four times a day to make sure that they're not getting too little or too much insulin. In order to do so, the child must prick his or her finger each time with a specially designed needle (lancet) to obtain a drop of blood. A great deal of support from parents, nurses, and doctors is required to encourage the child to do this every day.

If good control prevents complications, why doesn't everyone do it? Part of the reason is that treatment of diabetes with insulin injections is far from perfect. It is very easy to give too much insulin and cause blood glucose to fall to dangerously low levels, which is called hypoglycemia. When the blood glucose level falls too low, the brain is deprived of its main source of energy, which can cause loss of consciousness and seizures. In the Diabetes Control and Complications Trial, the individuals with the best control also had the most problems with severe hypoglycemia. To avoid these problems, people with diabetes may need to do more blood tests at home and take more frequent doses of insulin. That's why it is difficult for many people to manage their diabetes as well as they would like.

Team Management of Childhood Diabetes

Because coping with childhood diabetes can be so difficult, children and adolescents with IDDM should be routinely referred to a diabetes center that uses a multidisciplinary team that is knowledgeable and experienced in the management of children with diabetes. This team should ideally consist of a pediatric endocrinologist, a nurse educator, a dietitian, a social worker or a psychologist, and be able to refer the child to other specialists for eye, kidney, nerve, and other problems.

One of the concerns regarding changes in health care reimbursement in the United States is that some insurance carriers will not always allow referral of children with IDDM to the appropriate diabetes treatment center. Therefore, parents and other caregivers need to know what specialty services their insurance plans cover.

Exercise

Diabetic children are encouraged to participate in regular exercise and sports, which have positive effects on psychological as well as physical well-being. Children and parents should be advised that different types of exercise may have different effects on blood glucose levels. For example, sports that involve short bursts of intensive exercise like hockey may increase rather than decrease blood glucose levels. On the other hand, long-distance running and other prolonged activities are more likely to lower blood glucose levels. Aerobic endurance exercise is thus preferred to weight lifting and other activities that involve straining and increase blood pressure.

At some treatment centers, children are discouraged from exercising if they have high blood glucose levels (greater than 240 milligrams/deciliter). However, if such a prohibition were enforced in young people with diabetes, few teenagers would be allowed to exercise. Therefore, moderate exercise should be encouraged, unless the child is not feeling well.

Nutritional Management of Diabetes

Nutrition plays a key role in diabetes management. Dietary treatment has gone through many changes over the years. When insulin was first discovered, a low-carbohydrate, high-fat diet was recommended, then a moderate carbohydrate and fat diet. More recently, a high-carbohydrate, low-fat diet was suggested. The current guidelines emphasize that a low-saturated-fat diet is appropriate and that the carbohydrate content may be variable and should be individualized.

In addition to helping achieve optimal glucose levels and normal growth and development, nutritional management of diabetes in children is aimed at reducing the risk for other diseases, including obesity, high blood cholesterol, and high blood pressure. Underlying all of these is the establishment of sound eating patterns which include balanced, nutritious foods and consistent timing of food intake.

MEAL AND SNACK TIMING AND COMPOSITION
In managing diabetes, the aim is to match the insulin doses with food intake. To do so, food intake should be as consistent as possible with respect to timing, amount, and types of food eaten each day. For example, if a child typically eats a small breakfast and one day eats a much larger breakfast, the blood glucose level will be much higher after the big breakfast. Younger children, in particular, normally eat varying amounts each day, so this guideline can be difficult to maintain. Parents can encourage consistency by serving meals and snacks at predictable times.

Being aware of food composition and the child's current blood glucose level helps, also. For instance, if a child does not want a scheduled snack and the blood glucose level is high, then that snack can be reduced in size or omitted. In situations when a child is more active than usual, extra food often needs to be eaten. Insulin doses can also be varied according to the size of the meals. However, it is simpler and more predictable if meals include approximately the same amount of food each day.

Different types of food have different effects on blood glucose. Carbohydrate (simple, as in sugar, or complex, as in starch) raises the blood glucose quickly, whereas the impact of protein and fat on the blood glucose is slower and more long lasting. In other words, a dinner that consists of pasta, tomato sauce, bread, and diet soda will have a different blood glucose response than a meal of chicken, scalloped potatoes and margarine, broccoli, and 2 percent milk. The first meal is very high in carbohydrates, whereas the latter contains less carbohydrate and more protein and fat.

Children should eat each meal and snack about the same time each day. This practice helps to prevent low blood glucose levels if meals are skipped or delayed and high blood glucose levels if meals are eaten too close together. All children, with or without diabetes, benefit from eating on a predictable schedule, as this promotes sound eating behaviors. An effective routine permits a child to eat before getting too hungry, but allows enough time for him or her to get hungry enough to eat a good meal. A predictable meal or snack time provides a youngster (especially toddlers and preschoolers) with a feeling of security. Although it is important to adhere to a pattern, there are no set times or standard amounts a child should eat. The pattern is determined by each family's lifestyle or typical schedule.

Sometimes insulin doses or types of insulin are adjusted to meet the needs of a child's schedule. When children and teenagers use multiple injections of insulin or insulin pump therapy, food intake can be more flexible from day to day. For instance, if a child loves spaghetti and usually eats a large portion, the family can calculate how much extra carbohydrate will be eaten and how much extra insulin will be needed to cover it.

Children obtain a significant portion of their calories from snacks, and parents should make every effort to provide nutritious items. Snacks help to prevent low blood sugar, as well as to satisfy hunger. Foods from the bread group and fruit group are good choices, but may need to be combined with milk or other protein food, depending on the time of day or the amount of time between meals. Often 15 grams of carbohydrate (for example, a piece of toast or a piece of fruit) is sufficient for a morning snack, whereas more may be necessary for the afternoon snack. Because there is usually more time between lunch and dinner, children are often very hungry when they arrive home from school. However, it is important for them not to overeat in the afternoon, as it raises pre-dinner blood-sugar levels and decreases the chance that a good dinner will be eaten.

Although the ideal composition of the diabetic diet for children and teenagers is the subject of controversy, there are a few points that are clear. Whatever meal plan is chosen, it should be realistic and one that the child and family will be able to stick to. A meal plan that looks great on paper but is not followed is useless.

Many people think that children with diabetes should not eat candy or sweets. Children "cheating" on their diet is a common complaint among parents. The recommendation to restrict sugar in the diabetic diet was based on the assumption that simple sugar would elevate blood glucose levels too rapidly and create swings in blood glucose levels (see chapter 29). However, current research has determined that this is not necessarily true. Instead, there appears to be a wide range of overlapping blood glucose responses from starches and sugars. When equal amounts of simple and complex carbohydrate were compared, no significant differences were found in the blood glucose responses. These new findings suggest that the blood glucose increase is more dependent upon the total amount of carbohydrate eaten and not on the form (sugar versus starch). It may seem to those with IDDM that foods high in sugar raise their blood sugar excessively, but if a food is high in sugar, it is also high in carbohydrate. If it is higher in carbohydrate than a food usually eaten at that time and there is not sufficient insulin to cover

it, the blood glucose level will increase. Dietitians often recommend limiting juice consumption for children with diabetes because it apparently raises the blood glucose more than other carbohydrates. One reason is that people tend to drink juice in large quantities. A 12-ounce glass of juice has 45 grams of carbohydrate, compared with a 4-ounce glass that has 15 grams. Also, carbohydrate in liquid form is digested more quickly than solids and may cause blood sugar levels to increase more rapidly.

Although the current recommendations allow for more flexibility in the diet, foods with sugar should continue to be limited for a number of reasons. For anyone, too much sugar promotes dental caries. Also, foods high in sugar are often high in fat and not very nutritious. Sweet foods can be included in the diet of a child with diabetes in the context of an overall balanced and nutritious diet. The sugar must be counted in the total carbohydrate allowance for the particular meal or snack.

The recommendations regarding fiber for children with diabetes are the same as for those without diabetes. Often children have low fiber intakes and therefore eating fruits, vegetables, cereals, and grains should be encouraged.

For most people with Type I diabetes, a low-fat diet is appropriate, as hardening of the arteries is a common problem when children with Type I diabetes become adults. Specifically, less than 30 percent of calories should be from fat (less than 10 percent from saturated fat), with the remainder derived from protein and carbohydrate. These recommendations are the same as those from the National Cholesterol Education Program (NCEP) for children without diabetes and are discussed in depth in chapters 20 and 30. Fat should not be restricted in children under 2 years of age.

Protein should comprise about 10–20 percent of calories. High-protein foods include meat, fish, poultry, eggs, milk, peanut butter, and beans. Many people in developed countries eat more protein than they actually need, which increases the fat and saturated fat content of a diet. Protein tends to increase blood flow to the kidneys, which can cause problems in diabetic patients with kidney disease. There is some evidence that vegetable protein (peanut butter, beans) is not as damaging to the kidneys as animal proteins. Very restricted protein diets have been used in adults with kidney problems, but these diets are not recommended for children because they do not provide enough protein for growth.

SWEETENERS There are two kinds of sweeteners: caloric and noncaloric. Fructose, sorbitol, maltitol, and hydrogenated starch hydrolysate (HSH) provide calories. Other caloric sweeteners are fruit juice concentrates, honey, molasses, dextrose, corn syrup, and maltose. The latter group offers no advantage over sucrose (table sugar) in its effects on blood glucose levels or calories. Fructose produces somewhat less of a blood-sugar rise, but it may increase lipids. Fructose as an added sweetener is not recommended unless it is from natural sources such as fruits. Sorbitol and maltitol cause less of a blood glucose rise than sucrose, but they have gastrointestinal side effects (loose stools, bloating, flatulence) and contain about the same amount of calories as table sugar.

Noncaloric or nonnutritive sweeteners include aspartame, saccharin, and acesulfame K. The nonnutritive sweeteners are very useful for children and adults with diabetes because they reduce the carbohydrate content of foods and add sweetness to foods without making them high in carbohydrate. Saccharin (Sweet 'N Low) is primarily used as a tabletop sweetener, but it is also added to fountain carbonated drinks and some prepared foods. This sweetener was deemed safe after review of all scientific data available. Aspartame (NutraSweet) has been proven safe in children as well as adults and pregnant women. It is now used in beverages, juices, frozen desserts, mints, and teas. Acesulfame-K (Sweet One) is sold primarily as a tabletop sweetener.

Meal Planning Approaches

A number of methods can be used for meal planning. The aim of most methods is to encourage day-to-day consistency in the amount of food eaten at each meal. The exchange system has been traditionally used for teaching the diet principles in diabetes, although other methods may be more appropriate for certain children. The exchange system divides food into six groups, based on similar nutrient content. Foods on each list can be substituted or "exchanged" with other foods on the same list. The exchange lists are starch, fruit, milk, vegetables, meat and meat substitutes, and fat. For example, three-quarters of a cup of unsweetened cereal equals one slice of bread or half a small bagel. The exchange system promotes consistency in the diet, as well as teaching food composition by making individuals aware of how much carbohydrate, protein, fat, calories, sodium, and fiber is in various foods.

The exchange system can also be a basis to teach other meal planning approaches, for instance, carbohydrate exchange counting and gram counting (see table 21.2). Carbohydrate (from any source) affects the blood glucose level more rapidly than protein and fat, so it is most important to keep track of carbohydrate intake. A system of counting only carbohydrate exchanges simplifies planning and offers more flexibility than the exchange system that accounts for six food groups. The exchange groups of starch, fruit, and

TABLE 21.2
Daily Meal Plans According to Three Methods

Meal	Exchanges	Carbohydrate (choices)	(g)
Breakfast	Milk 1	4	57
	Fruit 1		
	Starch 2		
	Fat 1		
Snack	Fruit 1	2	30
	Starch 1		
Lunch	Milk ½	4½	71
	Vegetable 1		
	Fruit 1		
	Starch 3		
	Meat 2		
	Fat 2		
Snack	Starch 2	2	30
	Meat 1		
Dinner	Milk 1	5	77
	Vegetable 1		
	Fruit 1		
	Starch 3		
	Meat 3–4		
	Fat 2		
Bedtime snack	Milk ½	1½	21
	Starch 1		

Note: Based on 2,400-calorie daily meal plan.

milk all have approximately the same amount of carbohydrate per exchange (15 grams in starch and fruit, 12 grams in milk), and can be called one carbohydrate choice. Vegetables have 5 grams of carbohydrate per serving and can be eaten in any quantity without affecting the blood glucose level. An individual meal plan would list the number of carbohydrate choices for each meal or snack with guidelines for fat and protein. This approach is appropriate for anyone but is particularly suited to young and school-age children because of its simplicity and flexibility.

Another method is carbohydrate gram counting. This can be used with any insulin regime, but is particularly useful for intensive insulin management because it is more precise than the traditional exchange system or carbohydrate exchange counting. A meal plan consists of an allotment of grams of carbohydrate, and the amount of insulin needed for each gram of carbohydrate is calculated for each meal and snack. This information can be used to increase or decrease insulin doses before a meal when more or less carbohydrate than usual is eaten. This meal planning approach is appropriate for very motivated individuals. Many children and teenagers may find this method too burdensome, since label reading and more involved calculations are necessary.

In summary, the dietary recommendations for children with diabetes have changed dramatically. No longer are sweets and simple sugars prohibited out of hand. Instead, they are incorporated in limited amounts as is recommended for all children. The current approaches in meal planning for children with diabetes focus on consistency in the total amount of carbohydrate eaten at each meal rather than the type of carbohydrate.

Resources

American Diabetes Association, 1660 Duke Street, Alexandria, VA 22314. (800) 232-3472.

American Dietetic Association, 216 West Jackson Avenue, Chicago, IL 60606-6995. (800) 877-1600.

Juvenile Diabetes Foundation, 120 Wall Street, 19th floor, New York, NY 10005. (800) JDF-CURE (533-2873).

Travis, L. B. *An Instructional Aid on Insulin-dependent Diabetes Mellitus,* 9th ed. Austin, TX: Century Business Communications, 1995.

22

. . . .

Cystic Fibrosis

What Is Cystic Fibrosis and How Does It Affect Nutrition?

Cystic fibrosis (CF) is an inherited disease that affects the secreting glands (exocrine glands) of the body. These glands are located in the respiratory tract,

MYTH Drinking milk makes a child produce more mucus. **FACT** Research has not shown a connection between milk intake and the quantity of mucus produced.

these glands get plugged up they do not work efficiently or correctly. Consequently, the body processes that depend on them, such as digestion and breathing, suffer.

the digestive tract, the reproductive tract, and the skin. The exocrine glands produce watery secretions such as mucus, digestive juices, saliva, and sweat. These secretions are essential for normal bodily functions. In CF, instead of producing thin, watery secretions the exocrine glands in the respiratory and digestive tracts secrete thick, sticky mucus which often clogs up the glands. When

Digestion, a fairly complicated process (see chapter 2), requires the organs in the digestive tract (the stomach, pancreas, and small intestine) to work together so there is breakdown and absorption of nutrients as well as transport of waste through the digestive tract. Normally, when food enters the stomach it triggers the exocrine glands of the pancreas to make digestive enzymes — chemicals that the body uses to digest food. The pancreas secretes these enzymes into the small

. . . .

Lisa Devine ▪ Marie Egan ▪ Teresa Fung

intestine for the digestive process. In most children who have CF, the exocrine glands of the pancreas are defective, so that instead of producing thin, watery secretions filled with enzymes, they produce thick, sticky secretions. These thick secretions can clog the glands so that the digestive enzymes never reach the small intestine. Without these enzymes food cannot be properly digested and absorbed, a condition called malabsorption. Although individuals with malabsorption eat enough food, the food cannot be used by the body because many nutrients, especially fat and protein, are excreted in the stool. Malabsorption of protein and fat leads to poor growth, malnutrition, and deficiencies of fat-soluble vitamins. Poor growth in children with CF is not solely due to malabsorption, however. Children who have cystic fibrosis have increased energy demands (that is, they need more calories) because of mucus accumulation in the lungs. Thick mucus is difficult to clear and increases the energy required for breathing. Chronic lung infections are common with CF and require energy for continued repair of the lung. Both of these processes require a tremendous amount of extra calories. Ironically, even though children with CF need to eat more than the normal amount of food, they often have a blunted appetite because of their chronic illness.

If fat is not digested and absorbed, it exits the digestive tract in the stools. High fat content in the stools (known as steatorrhea) will result in bulky, greasy stools that have a very unpleasant odor. These stools can be difficult to pass and can lead to a condition known as rectal prolapse where the rectum protrudes out the anus. Fat malabsorption can also lead to excessive gas.

Fatty stools can lead to a number of vitamin deficiencies. Vitamins A, D, E, and K are absorbed only when accompanied by fats, so if there is sig-

nificant fat malabsorption, these vitamins will not be absorbed well. Vitamin deficiencies can lead to a number of problems, including anemia, skin rashes, vision disturbances, neurologic symptoms, bone abnormalities, and clotting problems.

Abdominal pain and discomfort can be a problem for many children with CF. This can be caused by muscle soreness from chronic coughing, partial blockage of the intestine, or from fat malabsorption. Intestinal blockage, which can be a repeated problem for individuals with CF, occurs when the abnormal thick, sticky secretions in the intestine are mixed with poorly digested food.

Children with CF are also at greater risk for developing diabetes mellitus. Why this happens is not entirely clear. However, it is believed that the scarring that results from blockage of the pancreatic ducts damages the insulin-producing cells of the pancreas and leads to diabetes. If this occurs, it can be treated with insulin therapy.

The liver can also be affected in children with CF. The liver has small passages that allow bile to drain into the digestive tract. In some individuals with CF these ducts become plugged with secretions. This can cause liver damage called cirrhosis.

Gastroesophageal reflux can occur in infants with CF and in individuals with significant lung disease who suffer from severe coughing episodes. It is the prolonged presence of stomach acid into the esophagus (see chapter 2). This can irritate the esophagus and result in heartburn that can be unrelenting and can make eating a painful experience. Gastrointestinal reflux can be treated with medications that decrease the acid production of the stomach.

Nutritional Intervention

NUTRITIOUS BALANCED DIET WITHOUT FAT RESTRICTIONS The increased nutrient demands of

CF plus the normally high nutrient needs for growth make it a special challenge for children with CF to obtain adequate calories and nutrients. In general, children with CF should eat a diet which contains a variety of foods from all food groups (breads and grains, meats, dairy products, fruits, vegetables) and should eat as much as they want to help ensure adequate intake of calories, protein, vitamins, and minerals. There are no specific foods that a child with CF should avoid, unless the child is lactose intolerant or has diabetes mellitus. In the case of CF-related diabetes mellitus, concentrated sweets and excessive carbohydrates are generally the only limitation (see chapter 21). Although foul-smelling stools due to fat malabsorption is one of the key symptoms of CF, dietary fat restriction is unnecessary if the child is receiving pancreatic enzyme replacements.

Nutritional management aims to achieve and maintain optimal nutritional status and to promote growth appropriate for the child's age. Children with CF should be encouraged to maintain a good level of outdoor physical activity, as this may enhance appetite and vitamin D synthesis through exposure to sunlight. The best way to determine nutritional adequacy is by monitoring growth.

A high-calorie, high-protein diet is essential to meet increased energy needs in children with CF. The disease imposes an extra 20–50 percent energy demand on top of the amount required for growth and physical activity. Energy needs are further increased during acute illness and infections or in children with advanced pulmonary disease. Complications of CF such as excessive coughing, cough-induced vomiting, and gastrointestinal discomfort can interfere with appetite and increase the risk of malnutrition. In some children, emphasis on food intake and weight gain may heighten stress and anxiety at mealtimes.

ENZYME SUPPLEMENTS In 85 percent of individuals with CF, the pancreatic enzymes cannot reach the small intestine because the ducts are blocked by thick mucus. Without these enzymes, much of the fat, protein, and carbohydrate is malabsorbed. To help prevent malabsorption due to enzyme deficiency, many CF patients take pancreatic enzyme supplements. In order to be effective, enzyme supplements should be taken at the beginning of each meal and snack. Most enzyme supplements come in capsule form and the amount needed varies, depending on the individual's age and weight, the size of snack or meal, and how much the pancreas is affected by CF. Therefore, the dosage of enzyme supplements is determined by the physician. The goals of enzyme therapy are to minimize malabsorption, prevent intestinal discomfort, and promote normal growth and development. For infants and children who are unable to swallow capsules, the capsules can be opened and the beads mixed into soft foods such as applesauce, baby foods, mashed banana, fruit yogurt, and mashed potato. Beads should not be mixed into foods with a high pH such as milk, custard, and ice cream which will destroy their enteric coating and their potency. The beads should not be chewed or crushed for the same reason. Adjustments in enzyme dosage and sometimes additional medication may be necessary from time to time to prevent malabsorption and to maintain a normal stool pattern.

HIGH-CALORIE, HIGH-PROTEIN DIET To achieve a high calorie intake, the child should be encouraged to increase consumption of all regular foods. Foods containing high amounts of fats such as butter, margarine, vegetable oil, mayonnaise, sour cream, and cream cheese can be liberally added to foods to boost calories (see box on the following

Tips to Boost Calories and Protein in Food

Fat. Add butter, margarine, and sour cream to baked goods, hot cereals, casseroles, soups, and as toppings on vegetables and potatoes.

Add heavy cream to puddings.

Add plenty of mayonnaise to sandwiches, salads, and salad dressings.

Cheese. Add to casseroles and as topping on vegetables and potatoes.

Use as a snack or in a sandwich.

Dried milk powder. Add powder to mashed potatoes, milk shakes, casseroles, creamed soups, scrambled eggs, macaroni and cheese, pancake batter, baked goods, and hot cereals.

"Instant breakfast" drink mixes. Add to puddings, custards, and milk shakes.

Eggs. Add extra eggs to pancake batter and to baked goods.

Chopped egg can be added to casseroles, sandwiches, soups, meat loaf, macaroni and cheese, and salads.

Gravies. Add plenty to meats, mashed potatoes, and rice.

---

page). While liberal use of fats in children with CF opposes current dietary guidelines in children who do not have CF, adequate caloric intake is the priority in children with CF. It should be noted that children with CF don't absorb all the fat they eat, even with appropriate enzyme replacement.

Snacks can also help children with CF to increase their caloric consumption, as it is difficult for them to obtain the high calorie requirement from only three meals. Some high-energy snacks are listed below.

Bagel with cream cheese	Muffins
	Nachos
Boiled eggs	Peanut butter
Cheese and crackers	sandwiches
Granola bars	Puddings
Milk and cookies	Seeds and nuts
Milk shakes	String cheese

Nutritious foods are preferred over "empty calorie" foods. Foods considered empty calories provide energy but are otherwise low in nutrient value. Examples include soft drinks and candy. These foods are permitted, but only occasionally. Low-calorie and reduced-fat products are not recommended.

Protein needs are increased in children with CF due to malabsorption. These children generally can meet their protein needs when calorie intake is sufficient, since the protein content of the typical American diet is quite high. Nevertheless, parents should monitor the type and amount of food that their children eat to ensure adequate intake of complete protein sources like meats, poultry, fish, dairy products, eggs, seeds, nuts, and legumes (beans and peas).

HIGH-CALORIE SUPPLEMENTS Some individuals with CF are unable to maintain their weight due to severe lung infections, gastrointestinal problems, and/or psychosocial factors. If weight loss or poor growth persists, oral supplements such as high-calorie milk shakes, prepared supplemental drinks and bars, and powder mixes are worked into the diet. A simple high-calorie milk shake can be made by blending whole milk and ice cream. Extra flavor and calories can be added with chocolate syrup, or by blending in canned fruits such as peaches. Dried milk powder or "instant breakfast" drink mixes can also be added. Several commercial supplements that are packaged in individual servings and do not need refrigeration can easily be carried to school or away from home. Some examples include Ensure, Sustacal, Scandi Shakes, and Calories Plus. Supplements should not be given in place of regular meals, as regular food intake should be encouraged as part of a normal lifestyle. When this type of nutritional intervention is unsuccessful, tube feedings (nasogastric or gastrostomy) may be required to improve the child's nutritional status. Tube feedings may be instituted temporarily or continued on a long-term basis, depending on the individual's need.

VITAMIN SUPPLEMENTS Supplements of fat-soluble vitamins (A, D, E, and K) are required in children with CF because of fat malabsorption owing to pancreatic insufficiency. Children with CF should faithfully take the prescribed doses of these vitamins, which perform important functions in the body. Water-soluble vitamins are often provided by a multivitamin, even though absorption of these vitamins is normal. This ensures adequate supply for the body's needs.

SODIUM AND FLUID NEEDS Children and adults with CF do not sweat more than anyone else, but their sweat contains significantly more salt than someone who does not have CF. This results in greater salt losses and increased salt requirements for those with CF. When salt loss surpasses intake, lethargy, vomiting, and dehydration may result. Most children and adults (including those with CF) take in plenty of salt in their diets and never have to worry about consuming too little. However, salt requirements are higher during periods of fever, hot weather, and intense physical activity. During these times parents of children with CF should give extra attention to ensuring adequate salt intake. Fever, which usually accompanies an illness, may hamper the appetite. Salty and easily tolerated foods such as broth, soup, sports drinks, and saltine crackers can help keep salt intake adequate. In hot weather and during exercise, salty snacks are recommended, and high-sodium foods should be chosen at mealtimes. Some examples are pretzels, cheese and crackers, processed meats, chips and dip, pickles, canned and frozen dinners, and convenience foods in general. Also, using the salt shaker at the table adds considerable salt to the diet.

Infants with CF may require extra salt due to the low sodium content of breast milk, baby formula, and infant foods. The addition of ⅛ to ¼ teaspoon per day is usually sufficient; however, this should be determined by a physician.

Resources

Cunningham, J. C., and L. M. Taussig. *An Introduction to Cystic Fibrosis for Patients and Families.* Bethesda, MD: Cystic Fibrosis Foundation, 1994.

Cystic Fibrosis Foundation, 6931 Arlington Road, Bethesda, MD 20814. (800) FIGHT CF (344-4823).

23

. . . .

Gastrointestinal Disorders

Children with gastrointestinal disorders often exhibit poor growth, poor weight gain, or other evidence of nutritional deficiencies. Such children often have specific nutritional needs, and their symptoms may improve with special dietary management. The first part of this chapter will focus on common, everyday problems in this area in children, and the latter part will discuss more serious chronic illnesses that can affect the gastrointestinal tract in children.

MYTH A glass of milk will minimize ulcer pain.
FACT Although milk temporarily neutralizes stomach acid, the protein in milk later stimulates acid production. As a general rule, it is best for each individual to determine which foods help minimize ulcer pain.

Common Gastrointestinal Problems

CONSTIPATION Constipation is a common problem in childhood and may be exacerbated by the tendency of younger children to withhold stool for fear that passing it will hurt. If stool is retained chronically, the colon stretches, losing tone and the sensation to have a bowel movement voluntarily. Treatment of chronic constipation requires an initial "clean out" with enemas

. . . .

Colston F. McEvoy ▪ Lisa Devine

or laxatives followed by maintenance medication (stool softeners, laxatives) for a period of time to be sure that the child completely and painlessly evacuates soft stools. Dietary management is helpful as an adjunct to treatment, and many children's conditions can eventually be controlled with diet alone. Increasing dietary fiber together with maintaining a good fluid intake keeps the stools soft (see chapter 34). Behavioral treatments may also be effective, such as having the child sit on the toilet at the same hour of the day at a time when the child is relaxed.

DIARRHEA Acute diarrhea owing to viral, bacterial, or parasitic causes is very common in infants and children. These children are able to absorb nutrients in their small bowel, but the loose and more frequent stools cause losses of water and electrolytes. During a viral or bacterial illness, many children can tolerate only clear liquids for one to three days. This does not provide adequate nutrients but does rehydrate the child by supplying the water and electrolytes lost through the bowel. The most effective rehydration fluids contain glucose as well as sodium, as these two nutrients together best promote absorption of water. However, fluids that contain too much glucose will actually increase the diarrhea by pulling water out of the body tissues into the intestinal lumen, where it is eliminated in the stools. Food or formula should be introduced early in the illness to provide calories. Early refeeding has been shown to increase the form of stools and decrease the volume lost.

In some cases infection may have slightly damaged the small intestinal lining causing a temporary lactose intolerance. For this reason pediatricians often recommend a short-term restriction of milk and milk products in older children or a lactose-free formula in infants (such as formulas based on soy, lactose-free milk, and protein hydrolysates). In some infants and toddlers, especially those with a family history of allergies, intestinal injury due to infection may result in the development of a gastrointestinal intolerance or allergy to cow's milk or soy proteins. In these cases the diarrhea persists and may have mucus or blood in it. These children may benefit from a dietary restriction of cow's milk protein and/or soy protein for several weeks to months. In a diet free of milk protein, all sources of milk—including the milk proteins casein and whey—are eliminated. If the child avoids milk, cheese, yogurt, ice cream, butter, and baked or processed foods containing milk derivatives, the immune system becomes desensitized to the milk protein. Cow's milk allergy is usually no longer a problem by age 3. If the child seems to be allergic to soy protein, as are many infants who are allergic to cow's milk, food items containing soy, soy flour, soy protein isolate, or tofu must also be eliminated.

There is a form of diarrhea seen in children 6 months to 5 years of age that is not due to infection or malabsorption. This is called toddler's diarrhea, "sloppy stool syndrome," or nonspecific diarrhea of childhood. These children have two to six watery bowel movements a day for more than two weeks, often following a viral infection. Growth and weight gain are normal, and the stool and blood tests show no evidence of infection or malabsorption. Treatment consists of dietary manipulations to minimize the diarrhea. Children with this condition often drink excessive quantities of fluids, particularly juices or juice drinks, which should be decreased. Fructose, a sugar found in fruit juice, may be contributing to the diarrhea and should be limited. Sorbitol, a nonabsorbable sugar alcohol used to sweeten sugarless gum and candies, may also cause loose stools and should be avoided. Increasing dietary fiber "normalizes" the intestinal transit time, thereby allowing time for absorption of water from the stools. Dietary fiber acts to give the stools more bulk. Most children will eventually outgrow this problem with no adverse consequences.

IRRITABLE BOWEL SYNDROME Irritable bowel syndrome or spastic colon is a chronic disorder of motility in the colon characterized by abdominal pain or cramping, gas, bloating, constipation, and/or diarrhea. The diagnosis is made after other more serious diseases of the bowel have been excluded. Irritable bowel syndrome does not lead to more serious diseases such as inflammatory bowel disease. Treatment is focused on a high-fiber diet, stress management, and occasionally antispasmodic medication.

Chronic Gastrointestinal Diseases

STOMACH DISORDERS Gastroesophageal reflux is the effortless regurgitation of stomach contents into the esophagus. A muscle at the end of the esophagus usually contracts to keep food and stomach acid from flowing back into the esophagus, and reflux occurs when this muscle doesn't contract as it should. Some reflux is common in infants and usually goes away by 1 year of age. A small percentage of infants and older children have pathologic reflux disease with complications such as esophagitis (inflammation of the esophagus), scarring or stricturing of the esophagus, lung disease, apnea (absence of breathing, usually only momentary), or failure to gain weight. The diagnosis is often based on symptoms of vomiting or irritability during or after feedings in infants. Older children can usually describe the sensation of regurgitation with reswallowing, heartburn, or pain located above the navel. Diagnostic tests such as a barium swallow or upper GI series may

be done to rule out other causes of vomiting. Continuous esophageal pH monitoring is done in certain children to diagnose and quantify the reflux. Medical treatment is aimed at decreasing the production of stomach acid regurgitated into the esophagus and at facilitating the forward propulsion of stomach contents through the digestive tract.

In infants with severe reflux, the vomiting may be significant enough to interfere with adequate intake of calories and result in poor weight gain. Thickening formula with rice cereal (1–2 teaspoons per ounce) adds calories and also appears to slow reflux, as thicker liquids are less easily regurgitated. It may be helpful to feed these infants smaller amounts of formula more frequently. In some instances further modification of the formula is necessary to increase the amount of calories the infant consumes. Some infants with reflux have an intolerance to cow's milk protein in formula or breast milk which exacerbates the vomiting. About 20–30 percent of these infants may also develop an intolerance to soy protein; in these cases there may be some benefit to switch to a protein hydrolysate-based formula (see chapter 19).

Peptic disease in children includes ulcers of the stomach or duodenum (small intestine), as well as gastritis, the diffuse inflammation of the lining of the stomach. The primary symptom of all of these disorders is abdominal pain usually located above the navel. The pain may awaken the child at night and may get better or worse after eating. Vomiting may occur and vomit may contain blood. The treatment is aimed at decreasing acid production in the stomach with medications that allow the injured stomach or duodenal lining to heal. While rare in children, gastritis caused by a bacteria, *Helicobacter pylori,* responds to antibiotics. Changes in diet may help decrease symptoms but are not necessary for healing. There is no good evidence that certain foods cause the injury. Avoidance of greasy or spicy foods is recommended if they exacerbate the child's pain. Highly acidic foods such as citrus fruit juices, vinegar, and tomato juice should also be avoided if they cause discomfort or pain. Other foods most often reported to cause pain are fried foods, coffee, red and black pepper, and alcohol, so it is often necessary to exclude these from the child's diet. Diet should be individualized according to the child's tolerance to various foods.

INTESTINAL DISORDERS Impaired absorption of nutrients can result from a variety of chronic intestinal disorders. Maldigestion implies the inability to break down nutrients and is usually related to deficiencies of pancreatic enzymes, which break down fats and proteins, or lactase, which breaks down milk sugar. Malabsorption occurs when the small intestine is unable to absorb previously broken down nutrients. This may be due to inflammation or infections, which decrease the total intestinal absorptive surface, or may result from surgical removal of part of the small bowel ("short gut syndrome"). Both maldigestion and malabsorption result in diarrhea, abdominal distention, and failure to gain weight. There are many causes of malabsorption and maldigestion, and the medical and nutritional treatments depend on the specific cause. In general, the goal is to supply adequate calories in an absorbable form, which may mean a special formula, supplemental enzymes, or larger quantities of food to compensate for the increased losses.

Celiac disease, also called celiac sprue or gluten-sensitive enteropathy, is a disorder of the small intestine caused by a permanent inability to tolerate gliadin, a protein component of gluten which is found in wheat, rye, barley, oats, buckwheat, and millet. Why this occurs is still unknown. There is a strong familial tendency, and this disease is seen more commonly in families living in or originally from European and Middle Eastern countries. Children usually exhibit poor weight gain, which becomes apparent after wheat is introduced into the diet. These children are characteristically irritable, have poor appetites, and usually have diarrhea, but constipation also occurs. They have distended abdomens and thin limbs with little muscle mass. Inflammation and destruction of the small intestinal villi, the site of nutrient absorption, is seen on intestinal biopsy. Blood tests for certain antibodies may be helpful in screening for the disease, but the intestinal biopsy is necessary to make a definitive diagnosis. A gluten-and gliadin-free diet (see chapter 19) is the treatment, as the absence of these proteins allows the intestinal villi to return to their normal state. The diet must be continued throughout life.

Carbohydrate malabsorption occurs in many gastrointestinal disorders that damage the lining of the small intestine. This damage results in a reduced ability to produce the enzymes needed to break down sugars and starches (see chapter 29). In carbohydrate malabsorption, undigested sugars pass through the intestinal tract, where they are normally absorbed, to the colon. In the colon, normal bowel bacteria break down the unabsorbed sugar and produce acid and gas. The result is bloating, gas, cramps, and diarrhea. Lactase, which breaks down the milk sugar lactose, is the enzyme most sensitive to intestinal injury; even transient viral infections can affect its activity. However, when the bowel heals, the enzyme function returns to normal. There is a form of permanent lactase deficiency that is common in adults, but can manifest itself as early as 3–5 years of age. This deficiency is more common in people of Asian, African, Arabic, Mediterranean, Jewish, and Native American ancestry. The diagnosis of lactose malabsorption can be made by performing a lactose tolerance test. This noninvasive test consists of an oral dose of lactose followed by serial measurements of hydrogen gas in the breath. If lactose is broken down by bacteria in the colon rather than absorbed in the small intestine, hydrogen gas is produced and then excreted by the lungs.

Lactose intolerance is treated by reduction or elimination of milk and milk products from the diet. The level of tolerance may vary from child to child and depends on the amount of lactose consumed. Some children can tolerate small amounts of lactose without symptoms, and this is learned by trial and error. Lactose is often better tolerated as part of a meal rather than taken separately as at snack time. Commercially available lactose-reduced milk and supplemental lactase enzyme tablets or drops taken with milk or milk products are often effective in diminishing symptoms. Aged cheeses (such as cheddar) have a rather low lactose content and therefore may be tolerated. Additionally, some yogurts contain ß-galactosidase, an enzyme in the bacterial culture which facilitates lactose absorption and is well tolerated. If milk must be restricted, a calcium supplement should be given daily to prevent calcium deficiency.

Inflammatory bowel disease (IBD), which includes the diagnoses of Crohn's disease and ulcerative colitis, is a chronic disease of the intestines that often begins in childhood. The cause is unknown, yet research is looking at the role of the immune system and the contribution of infectious organisms. There appears to be a genetic component to these diseases, as 20 percent of patients with IBD also have an affected family member. Symptoms may include diarrhea, rectal bleeding, abdominal pain, weight loss, poor growth, delayed sexual maturation, fevers, fatigue, joint pain, and mouth sores. Medical treatment consists of medi-

cations aimed at suppressing inflammation (immunosuppressive therapy) and occasionally antibiotics. Surgery is recommended only when medications fail or complications occur. Malnutrition is often associated with IBD to some degree and is related to decreased appetite, the fear that eating will exacerbate pain or nausea, increased caloric requirements due to inflammatory activity, anemia, or fevers, and poor intestinal absorption of nutrients.

In children with IBD, adequate nutrition is vital during their critical growth period. In general, dietary restrictions such as low-fiber or low-fat diets or limits on dairy products have been found to slow recovery rather than facilitate it. No specific foods cause IBD or make it worse. Unless a child has problems with a food, there is no need to routinely avoid any food. Some patients with IBD may have lactose intolerance, but it is no more frequent than in the general population. Rarely, an intolerance of cow's milk protein may occur in someone with IBD who experiences more diarrhea and bleeding after exposure to milk or milk products.

There may be a problem with the absorption of specific nutrients that is related to the location of inflammation in the bowel. Supplementation of certain nutrients may therefore be necessary. Iron may be poorly absorbed if the duodenum, the first section of the small intestine, is involved in Crohn's disease. Excessive iron loss and depletion of its stores may also occur from chronic bleeding anywhere in the small or large intestine. Disease that involves the jejunum, the mid-portion of small intestine, can result in malabsorption of folic acid and subsequent anemia. Folate absorption also decreases when the child is on anti-inflammatory medications commonly used to treat IBD. Vitamin B_{12} deficiency and anemia may occur if inflammation is in the ileum, the last section of small intestine, which is commonly involved in Crohn's disease. Vitamin B_{12} deficiency anemia is also seen if the ileum has been surgically removed or there is an overgrowth of intestinal bacteria in this region. Severe ileal inflammation can result in fat malabsorption similar to that seen in chronic liver disease.

LIVER DISEASE A number of viruses, toxins, and genetic disorders can result in damage to the liver. Chronic liver disease causes a special kind of malabsorption in which insufficient flow of bile from the liver into the intestines (known as cholestasis) occurs and is characterized by jaundice (yellowing of the eyes and skin) and relentless itching. Bile acids, which are produced by the liver, are necessary for the absorption of dietary fats in the intestine. When bile acids are lacking, fat is not well absorbed and the results are diarrhea and loss of calories. Fat absorption is also crucial for the absorption of fat-soluble vitamins (A, D, E, and K). If a child is diagnosed with this kind of liver disease—for example, biliary atresia—he or she will be started on supplemental fat-soluble vitamins and an infant formula or supplement which contains more easily absorbed fats (medium chain triglycerides). These smaller fats are directly absorbed by the intestine and don't require bile acids. Children with chronic liver disease have increased needs for calories, and every attempt should be made to maximize their caloric intake to achieve growth. Poor growth despite all of these efforts may be an indication that the liver disease has progressed to the point that liver transplantation is needed.

Resource

American Celiac Society, 45 Gifford Avenue, Jersey City, NJ 07324. (201) 432-2986.

PKU and Other Metabolic Disorders

What Are Inborn Errors of Metabolism?

The chemical processes that govern food use by the body are known collectively as metabolism. Inborn errors of metabolism are inherited conditions that affect the normal use of food by the body after the food has been digested and absorbed. These disorders can involve the production or breakdown of carbohydrate, fat, or protein, which results in accumulation of toxic compounds or a deficiency in a crucial compound (table 24.1). The liver, brain, kidneys, bone, and heart can be damaged as a con-

> **MYTH** Aspartame (for example, Equal) causes PKU.
>
> **FACT** PKU is a genetic disorder that impairs the body's use of the amino acid phenylalanine. Aspartame contains large amounts of phenylalanine, so individuals with PKU must avoid aspartame. However, aspartame does not cause PKU.

sequence. Fortunately, many of these conditions can be successfully treated with special diets that regulate the intake of the compound accumulated or deficient in the body or with drugs and vitamins to correct the abnormality. More than three hundred such inborn errors of metabolism are known. Each of these disorders is rare, but improvements in diagnostic techniques and the development of newborn screening programs have resulted in increased detection of these diseases. Phenylketonuria (PKU) is the most common of the inborn errors of metabolism.

. . . .

Margretta Reed Seashore ▪ Crystal Reil

TABLE 24.1
Some Inborn Errors of Metabolism

Disorder	Cannot metabolize	Diagnosis	Diet	Other treatments
Fatty acid disorders	Fatty acids of specific chain lengths, depending on specific disorder	Symptoms including hypoglycemia, muscle weakness. Sudden infant death	High-carbohydrate, low-fat diet, specific to each disorder	No prolonged fasting. Carnitine in some
Galactosemia	Galactose	Newborn screening	No galactose	
Hereditary fructose intolerance	Fructose	Symptoms after introduction of fruits and juices in diet	No fructose	
Homocystinuria	Methionine	Newborn screening in some states. Dislocated ocular lenses, skeletal abnormalities, vascular problems	Low methionine	Pyridoxine in some
Maple syrup urine disease (MSUD)	Leucine, isoleucine, valine	Newborn screening in some states. Acute metabolic illness in early infancy	Low leucine, isoleucine, and valine	Thiamine in some
Ornithine trans-carbamylase (OTC) deficiency	Ammonia	Coma, neurologic abnormalities	Low protein	Ammonia chelating agents
PKU	Phenylalanine	Newborn screening	Low phenylalanine	

The Role of Newborn Screening for Inborn Errors of Metabolism

Early detection of inborn errors of metabolism in the newborn infant is important, so that treatment can be started before the child becomes ill or is damaged by the toxic metabolites. Newborn screening began in 1961 when Dr. Robert Guthrie developed a test that could diagnose PKU from newborn infants' blood. This test could be done on a large number of blood samples in a timely and economical manner. More than thirty years of experience with newborn screening has proven that early diagnosis and treatment of PKU is effective in preventing the brain damage that results from untreated PKU. The newborn test consists of collecting blood from a newborn infant's heel onto filter paper, which is then sent to the laboratory for testing. Abnormal results are reported to the pediatrician for follow-up care and treatment of the affected infant.

All fifty states in the United States have a newborn screening program that tests for PKU and congenital hypothyroidism (underactive thyroid gland). Some also screen for one or more of the following disorders: galactosemia, maple syrup urine disease (MSUD), homocystinuria, biotinidase deficiency, sickle cell disease, toxoplasmosis, congenital adrenal hyperplasia, cystic fibrosis, and tyrosinemia. Such newborn screening is carried out throughout the developed world. Identifying these disorders in a newborn and beginning treatment at an early age can prevent many of the deleterious effects of these conditions. Early discharge of newborn infants from hospitals complicates newborn screening for some disorders. Tests that depend on the buildup of a toxic compound in the blood, such as the test for PKU, can be falsely reassuring when performed on the first day of life because the infant has just started eating. It is important that a second or follow-up blood test for PKU be done within two weeks on those infants who are tested on the first day of life.

Phenylketonuria

Phenylketonuria (PKU) is an inherited metabolic disorder in which the amino acid phenylalanine cannot be used properly. PKU is now considered to be part of a family of disorders of phenylalanine metabolism known as the hyperphenylalaninemias. Phenylalanine is one of the amino acids that makes up protein (see chapter 28). When dietary protein is digested and phenylalanine is absorbed into the bloodstream, either it is used to build up the body's protein or it is metabolized by the enzyme phenylalanine hydroxylase. When the activity of that enzyme is extremely low, the concentration of phenylalanine in the blood rises to levels that are five to ten times the normal concentration and the condition is called classical PKU. When the enzyme activity is higher, but less than 50 percent of the normal activity, the tolerance for phenylalanine is greater than in classical PKU, and the blood concentration of phenylalanine is not as high.

The discovery of PKU in the 1930s resulted from a Norwegian mother's concern for her two mentally retarded children. This mother took her children to many physicians seeking a reason for her children's odd, musty odor. Dr. Asbjörn Fölling, a physician and biochemist, tested the children's urine and discovered that the urine contained phenylpyruvic acid. The musty odor of the children was the result of this by-product of phenylalanine metabolism. Dr. Fölling tested other mentally retarded patients and in eight more cases found phenylpyruvic acid in their urine. He maintained that the mental retardation was inherited as an inborn error of metabolism, and went on to identify more affected children. Other characteristics of PKU were noted as more patients were found. Often the children were hyperactive and irritable and had seizures, along with mental retardation. Some were also observed to have fair hair and skin and could be afflicted with severe skin rashes. In 1953, a German physician, Dr. Horst Bickel, used a diet low in phenylalanine to lower the phenylalanine levels in the blood of a child with PKU. The child's improvement on this diet was encouraging, but identifying children with PKU early enough to prevent all the characteristics of PKU from developing was difficult. The development of newborn screening for PKU by Guthrie in 1961 marked the beginning of early treatment.

Diet for Children with PKU

Dietary treatment of PKU depends on the type of PKU the child has. A child with classical PKU has blood phenylalanine concentrations above 20 milligrams per deciliter when not treated. Children with hyperphenylalaninemia have lower blood phenylalanine levels than children with classical PKU. Dietary treatment for these children is not as restrictive as for children with classical PKU, and many do not require dietary treatment after infancy. Blood phenylalanine levels below 4 milligrams per deciliter are considered to be normal.

Dietary management of PKU requires balancing phenylalanine, protein, and caloric intake, depending on age and on the individual child (table 24.2). The artificial sweetener aspartame (Nutra-Sweet, Equal) contains phenylalanine and should not be consumed by individuals with PKU. All products that contain aspartame must be labeled with a warning that they contain phenylalanine. Foods containing large amounts of protein such as meats, legumes, eggs, and dairy products are omitted from the diet. Cereals and breads are restricted, and the amounts of fruits and vegetables eaten must be carefully monitored by weighing and measuring. To ensure an adequate intake of protein for growth, special medical foods (specially formulated to contain low amounts of phenylalanine) that contain all the amino acids but phenylalanine are prescribed. Also, an assortment of low-protein breads, pastas, and other foods is essential for making the PKU diet palatable and aid in long-term compliance. This is important since most experts recommend that children and adults with PKU maintain a low-phenylalanine diet for life.

An infant's low phenylalanine diet starts with combining regular baby formula or breast milk with a low-phenylalanine formula. When the infant is 4 to 6 months old, cereals and, later, fruits and vegetables can be introduced. The combination of formulas can be changed to accommodate the phenylalanine limits when foods are introduced. Adjustments are made to the diet based on the phenylalanine concentrations in the blood. The infant's diet is analyzed regularly to monitor the nutritional adequacy of the diet.

To maintain the desired blood phenylalanine level, the daily intake of phenylalanine must be calculated so that adjustments can be made to the diet. As the child grows, allowed amounts of table foods are introduced. It is necessary for a diet record to be kept daily in order to calculate the amount of phenylalanine ingested. Lists of foods and their phenylalanine content are available, as are low-protein cookbooks. As the child grows into adolescence and adulthood, the support of the physician and dietitian is essential in helping the person with PKU to follow his or her diet and maintain desirable phenylalanine blood levels.

Maternal PKU is a term used to describe the condition during pregnancy in women who have PKU. The placenta concentrates the maternal amino acids so that the fetus is exposed to higher than normal concentrations of amino acids. If the levels of phenylalanine in the mother's blood are kept at 2–6 milligrams per deciliter, the effect on the fetus seems minimal. However, higher maternal phenylalanine levels have been reported to cause low birth weight and a variety of other problems such as congenital heart disease and small head circumference, which can be associated with cerebral palsy and mental retardation. It is crucial that women with PKU maintain their blood phenylalanine concentration between 2 and 6 milligrams per deciliter before conception

TABLE 24.2

Typical Daily Diet for Children and Pregnant Women with PKU

Age	Breakfast	Snack	Lunch	Snack	Dinner	Snack
Newborn	Low-phenylalanine formula	Low-phenylalanine formula	Low-phenylalanine formula	Low-phenylalanine formula	Low-phenylalanine formula	Low-phenylalanine formula
6 months	Cereal, pureed fruit, low-phenylalanine formula	Low-phenylalanine formula	Pureed vegetable, low-phenylalanine formula	Low-phenylalanine formula	Pureed vegetable, low-phenylalanine formula	Low-phenylalanine formula
12 months	Cereal, fruit, low-phenylalanine formula	Fruit juice, low-protein crackers	Vegetable, fruit, low-phenylalanine formula	Fruit juice, low-protein crackers	Vegetables, low-protein bread, low-phenylalanine formula	Low-phenylalanine formula
2 years	Cereal, fruit juice, low-phenylalanine formula	Fruit	Low-protein bread, vegetable, low-phenylalanine formula	Fruit juice, low-protein cookies	Vegetables, low-protein pasta, low-phenylalanine formula	Fruit
6 years	Cereal, fruit, low-phenylalanine formula	Fruit juice, low-protein crackers	Salad, low-protein bread, low-phenylalanine formula	Fruit	Vegetables, low-protein pasta, low-phenylalanine formula	Low-protein cookies
16 years	Cereal, low-protein bread, low-phenylalanine formula	Fruit	Salad, low-protein bread, low-phenylalanine formula	Low-protein cookies, fruit juice	Vegetables, low-protein pasta, low-protein bread, low-phenylalanine formula	Low-protein cookies, fruit juice
Pregnant women	Cereal, low-protein bread, fruit, low-phenylalanine formula	Fruit, low-protein crackers	Salad, low-protein bread, low-phenylalanine formula	Fruit, low-protein crackers	Low-protein pasta, low-protein bread, vegetable, fruit, low-phenylalanine formula	Low-protein cookies, fruit

for the best outcome in pregnancy. High paternal phenylalanine concentrations have not been shown to affect the fetus.

Other Inborn Errors of Amino Acid Metabolism

Branched chain ketonuria (also called maple syrup urine disease or MSUD because of the smell of the urine) results from the child's inability to metabolize the branched chain amino acids leucine, isoleucine, and valine. In classical MSUD, damage to the central nervous system (CNS) and death can occur if dietary treatment is not started early. Infants become ill in the first days of life, with vomiting and acidosis. Treatment consists of a diet restricted in branched chain amino acids and supplemented with medical foods. Though the elevation of branched chain amino acids in the blood can be controlled by limiting intake, the exact mechanism that causes CNS damage is not understood. Several other forms of MSUD have been described. In addition to the early-onset severe form, MSUD can occur as an intermittent form, which is less severe and often includes difficulty with walking. Another form responds to large doses of thiamine, which enhances the activity of the affected enzyme.

Homocystinuria is a disorder which results from the inability to metabolize the amino acid methionine normally. With this deficit, homocystine, which is not normally identified in blood or urine, accumulates. Patients develop dislocated eye lenses, skeletal abnormalities, and clotting of blood within the blood vessels. Two forms are known, one of which responds to large doses of pyridoxine (vitamin B_6) and one of which responds only to dietary restriction of methionine. This is achieved through the use of a low-methionine formula and avoidance of high-protein foods.

Ornithine transcarbamylase (OTC) deficiency is an inborn error in the metabolic process that converts the excess nitrogen from protein metabolism to urea for excretion from the body. Malfunction of this process causes the accumulation of ammonia in the blood (hyperammonemia), which is toxic and can cause lethargy, vomiting, seizures, coma, and death. Treatment of OTC deficiency consists of restriction of dietary nitrogen and provision of alternative ways to rid the body of excess nitrogen. As the main source of dietary nitrogen is protein, dietary treatment consists of a low-protein diet. All diets that restrict amino acids or protein have to be carefully monitored to ensure that the child receives enough protein and calories for optimal growth and health. To achieve this, special medical foods need to be included in these diets. In addition to dietary therapy, several medications are used which combine with ammonia to allow the body to excrete the excess.

Inborn Errors of Carbohydrate Metabolism

Two inborn errors of metabolism involving carbohydrates are galactosemia and fructose intolerance. Both involve a defect in an enzyme necessary for their metabolism. The classical form of galactosemia is caused by a deficiency of the enzyme that converts galactose to glucose (see chapter 29); accumulation of excess galactose in the blood and body tissues results. Untreated, galactosemia causes cataracts, liver damage, and death from bleeding, liver failure, or infection. Early diagnosis and treatment are critical to survival. The treatment of galactosemia consists of a galactose-restricted diet. Galactose is a simple sugar found in all dairy foods, some fruits and vegetables, and processed foods and medications. Reading the labels of foods is important in following this diet.

Hereditary fructose intolerance is caused by a deficiency in an enzyme responsible for the utilization of fructose. Failure to thrive, vomiting, and kidney and liver damage characterize this condition. Children do not develop symptoms until they begin to eat foods which contain fructose, a simple sugar found in fruit, some vegetables and grains, and sucrose (table sugar). Symptoms commonly begin in infancy with the introduction of fruits and juices. The treatment for fructose intolerance is a diet that restricts fructose. Reading food labels is crucial to avoid foods that may contain high amounts of fructose.

Inborn Errors of Fat Metabolism

Some more recently discovered inborn errors of metabolism involve the oxidation of fatty acids. Fatty acids are the building blocks of the fats stored in the body and are used as a source of energy (see chapter 30). Specific enzymes and cofactors are involved and deficiencies can cause a fatty acid oxidation disorder. Symptoms of an acute episode are low blood sugar (hypoglycemia), coma, and sometimes muscle weakness and heart dysfunction. These disorders are often misdiagnosed as Reye's syndrome or sudden infant death syndrome. Recent developments in testing make the diagnosis of fatty acid oxidation deficiency easier. The treatment depends on the individual defect. Avoidance of fasting and consumption of a low-fat diet are keystones of treatment for this group of conditions.

Summary

Inborn errors of metabolism are rare inherited conditions which affect the ability to use important constituents of food. They may alter energy metabolism, affect utilization of protein, carbohydrate, or fat, or result in toxic effects from unused compounds or their metabolic products. Some of these are diagnosed in the newborn infant by mandatory screening programs. Others are not diagnosed until the child has symptoms. Newborn screening programs aim to identify affected children before the ravages of a disorder occur and cannot be reversed. Treatment in this group of conditions is designed to remove the offending compound, prevent its accumulation, or replace a deficient product. Dietary treatment is the mainstay of therapy in most of these conditions. Parents who understand the physiology of their child's condition can make a big difference in their child's care and his or her response. Manipulation of the diet should be undertaken with the supervision of a physician knowledgeable about these disorders and an experienced dietitian. The goal should be helping the parents and child to make wise food choices and to take the lead in dietary control. Programs which care for children with inborn errors of metabolism should always strive toward helping them to lead active and healthy lives.

Resources

National Institute of Child Health and Development. *Development of Medical Foods for Rare Diseases*. Life Sciences Research Office, Federation of American Societies; 1911 June 9, Bethesda, MD: Federation of American Societies, 1991.

Schuett, V. E. *Low Protein Cookery*. Madison: University of Wisconsin Press, 1988.

25

Feeding the Infant with Cleft Lip and Palate

Clefts of the palate are relatively common facial disorders which occur in approximately 1 in 1,000 children born in the United States. Clefts of the palate may be associated with other anomalies including cleft of the lip or the small lower jaw (mandible). Because the cleft involves distortion of the mouth structure, it can affect a child's ability to feed. Some babies have few feeding problems, whereas others experience significant difficulties, particularly when clefts are associated with an underdevelopment of the lower jaw. Children with clefts present a challenge to parents and health care professionals alike in achieving the goal of

> **MYTH** Babies with cleft palate cannot breastfeed.
> **FACT** Babies with cleft palate may require more attention, time, and special equipment to breastfeed successfully, but breastfeeding is possible for these infants.

adequate nutrition to support normal growth.

Anatomy

The palate is normally divided into two parts. The hard palate is in the front of the roof of the mouth, and the soft palate is in the back. Clefts may involve the soft palate, hard palate, or both (fig. 25.1). A cleft of the palate may also occur in combination with a cleft of the lip, and it may continue through the gums and affect growth and position of the teeth. The soft palate contains the muscles and soft tissues which normally close off the mouth from the nose during swallowing,

Mary Kuras ▪ Linda Gay ▪ John A. Persing

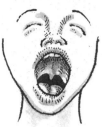

Normal palate

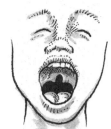

Soft palate cleft

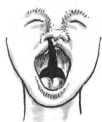

Unilateral complete cleft of the palate

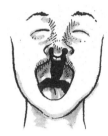

Bilateral complete cleft of the palate

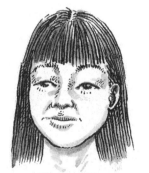

Normal lips

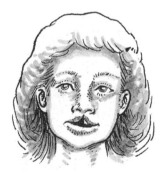

Unilateral incomplete cleft lip

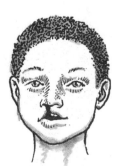

Unilateral complete cleft lip

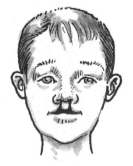

Bilateral complete cleft lip

FIGURE 25.1
Types of cleft lips and cleft palates.

drinking, and speaking. Two muscles in the back part of the palate are particularly important for the function of the palate in swallowing and speaking. When they contract they form a mobile platform which separates the mouth from the nasal cavity. They also open and close the eustachian tube, the channel between the middle ear and the mouth. Abnormalities of this movement may lead to repeated ear infections and loss of hearing. Surgical treatment of clefts is directed at establishing the normal barrier (the mobile platform) between the mouth and the nose so that it will effectively close the mouth off from the nose with swallowing and drinking, as well as assist in making certain speech sounds. The surgical repair is ordinarily performed between 9 and 18 months of age, at the beginning of speech development, and prior to the age where abnormal speech habits may become well established. The child needs to be in good nutritional status before surgery can be performed.

Feeding Difficulties

In order for an infant to suck from a bottle, negative pressure inside the mouth has to be achieved for the fluid to flow out. Negative pressure on a nipple is created by a good lip seal around a nipple and compression of the nipple between the tongue and the hard palate. The tongue's up and down motion creates suction. The role of the soft palate during sucking is twofold: it closes off the mouth from the nose, which allows an increase in the pressure achieved in the mouth, and it keeps food from going from the mouth up into the nose.

Infants with cleft palate alone usually are able to bottle- or breastfeed successfully. While feeding problems may arise due to the distorted anatomy, problems are more often due to feeding techniques that do not meet the infant's needs. Most infants with cleft palate will learn to eat effi-

ciently with modifications in feeding position and adjusted flow rate of the formula or breast milk, using adapted bottles and nipples.

When a child has a cleft palate and a cleft lip, lip seal around a nipple can be difficult. A cleft of the soft palate can cause feeding problems owing to the reduced ability to form sufficient suction. This is usually not an insurmountable problem, however, because the gum line can help to form a closed suction cavity. Clefts of the full palate, however, may create a greater obstacle for an infant. Without the hard surface of the palate for the tongue to compress a nipple against, effective sucking is quite difficult and, for some infants, not possible.

Infants with cleft palate should be fed in a semi-upright position. This is important because it helps prevent the movement of liquid into the nasal cavity or eustachian tubes. As noted above, movement of food or liquid into these tubes will increase the risk of ear infection.

Breastfeeding

Many infants with a cleft lip only are able to breastfeed successfully. The breast helps fill in the cleft site, which allows the infant to achieve a more effective lip seal around the nipple. If parents are interested in feeding their infant breast milk, but the infant is not a successful breastfeeder (as evidenced by poor weight gain), the breast milk may be pumped from the mother's breasts and fed to the infant in an adapted bottle.

Because the baby must usually empty both breasts in order to be adequately fed, the mother needs to hold the infant in a different position when feeding from each breast. For example, if the cleft is on the right side, she would use a cradle hold (cradling the baby in the crook of the left arm, with the baby lying across the lap) when nursing on the left breast. She would use a football hold (straddling the baby on the right arm with the baby's head in the mother's hand, and the baby's body alongside of hers) when nursing on the right breast (fig. 25.2).

Infants with cleft lip and palate on both sides will have greater difficulty achieving adequate suction for breastfeeding. However, supplemental nursing systems are available for mothers who wish to breastfeed. This equipment is manufactured by Medela and by Lact-Aid International and is available through La Leche League International.

Bottle-Feeding

Bottle-feeding is slower for the infant with cleft palate than for other infants, since the caregiver must help the baby to regulate the flow of liquid. Feeding smaller amounts at more frequent intervals during the day may help prevent fatigue in the infant. The feeding position and equipment for bottle-feeding can also be modified to make sucking easier for the infant. As shown in fig. 25.3, bottle-feeding an infant with a cleft in an upright rather than a horizontal position prevents back flow of formula. If these modifications are not made, the baby may tire and be unable or unwilling to suck long enough to obtain adequate formula or expressed breast milk.

There are many ways to compensate for the inability of the infant with cleft palate to generate sufficient suction to increase the flow of milk while sucking. Small adjustments to regular nipples and bottles or the use of special bottles made for babies with cleft palates are frequently effective. The type of bottle and nipple configuration which is easiest for an infant must be individualized, based on the response of the infant and the skill of the feeder. While it may be necessary to pur-

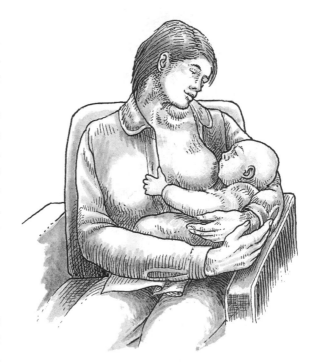

Regular hold

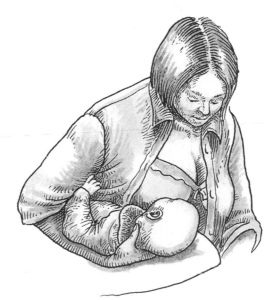

Football hold

FIGURE 25.2
Positions for holding an infant while breastfeeding.

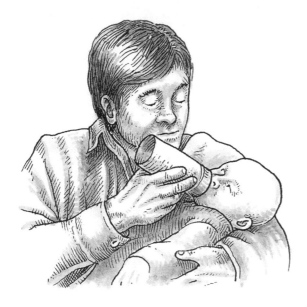

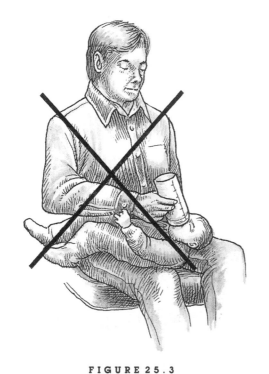

FIGURE 25.3
Correct position (top) and incorrect position
for holding bottle-fed infants with cleft palate.

chase specialized equipment, the caregiver should first try to adapt regular equipment by using different sizes or types of nipples. Some infants need only to have a regular nipple cross-cut at the top to provide for easier flow of the milk or formula. When the hole in a regular nipple is made slightly larger or cross-cut, gravity can assist in moving the liquid through the larger hole. Nipples with varying degrees of stiffness should be evaluated to determine the infant's ability to compress them.

If the infant does not feed effectively after the nipple has been adjusted, the next step would be to try using an adapted bottle such as the Haberman Feeder from Medela. This feeder relies on compression of the nipple alone (without suction) to release the formula or milk. Gravity assists the flow rate of the formula or breast milk into the infant's mouth. Flow rate levels can be adjusted to low, medium, or high, depending on the infant's needs.

If these methods of feeding are not successful, the next step is to use an adapted bottle that requires neither suction nor compression. One example is the Mead Johnson Cleft Palate Nurser, which allows the person feeding the baby to squeeze a reservoir of fluid (breast milk or formula) to release it into the infant's mouth. When assessing which feeding method is best for the infant, it is important to encourage the infant's oral motor development and ability. Choosing a feeding method that is too easy will not help the infant develop oral motor skills necessary for normal development.

Spoon-Feeding

A cleft lip is usually repaired at 3 months of age or less, before introduction of solid foods, but a cleft palate may be repaired as late as approximately

18 months of age. It is important that infants with cleft lip or palate develop feeding skills along the normal time line. Introducing lumpy foods at 10 to 11 months of age, as well as cup drinking, is just as important for children with cleft lip or palate as it is for other children. The timing of surgical repair should not interfere with feeding development. Delaying the introduction of cup drinking and presentation of lumpy foods may cause food refusal in the future, poor weight gain, and slower development.

Small amounts of semi-solid food should be presented slowly, to help minimize the risk of choking and loss of food through the nose. The infant will gradually learn to redirect the food around the cleft. Do not hurry the process. Let the infant decide when he or she is ready for the next bite.

Periodic coughing may occur as the infant learns to handle more challenging foods. This is seen in all children and is not an immediate cause for concern. Often, a child with a cleft palate is able to handle solid foods more easily than liquid foods. If a piece of food falls from the nose or gets caught in the palate, carefully remove it with a finger or swab.

Most infants with cleft lip or palate will learn to eat efficiently by using the modifications previously discussed. Infants whose central nervous system is functioning normally will be able to compensate for the problems caused by the cleft. If an infant continues to have difficulty feeding, a problem other than the cleft should be suspected, and the infant's level of development should be carefully monitored. Nutritional needs in these circumstances may need to be met by the placement of a feeding tube.

Post-Surgical Feeding Considerations

There are several ways to feed an infant after cleft surgery. Modifications in feeding style may be necessary to protect the newly repaired areas. Some surgeons recommend that no sucking (regular bottle- or breastfeeding or spoon-feeding) be done immediately following surgical repair of cleft lip so as not to introduce pressure on the suture lines. However, studies have shown that sucking does not interfere with the healing process of a newly repaired cleft lip, and infants are allowed to bottle- and breastfeed as early as 24 hours following cleft lip repair.

Feeding following cleft palate repair, however, is typically restricted in some form because of the greater stress on more fragile palatal tissues. As mentioned earlier, cleft palate repair typically takes place following the introduction of spoon-feeding. Following surgical repair, utensils are not to be placed in the mouth beyond the level of the gum line. Crunchy foods or foods that need to be chewed are restricted from the infant's diet to reduce the risk of palatal fistula (an opening in the palate created by breakdown of the suture line). Previously, syringe feeding had been recommended as the best feeding method following cleft palate repair. However, many infants are now encouraged to develop cup drinking skills prior to cleft palate repair so that they may still take liquids and purees after surgery. Bottle- or breastfeeding is still not recommended due to increased pressures in the oral cavity created by sucking and compression of the nipple against the newly repaired palate. Length of these adapted feedings, again, varies depending on the surgeon's preference, and ranges from 1 to 3 weeks following the cleft repair. Modified bottles have recently been introduced for use following cleft repair. The Soft-Cup, made by Medela, combines spoon-feeding and cup drinking skills in a bottle with a soft, bowl-shaped top. Liquids and purees can be dispensed into the child's mouth without making contact with the newly repaired palate.

In conclusion, a main goal for the child with cleft lip or palate is to feed successfully and efficiently. How this will be achieved and what feeding modifications are appropriate are determined by a team that includes the speech and language specialist, the surgeon, the parent or caregiver, and the dietitian. Establishment of the appropriate feeding modifications for each child facilitates successful feeding initially, which enhances the likelihood of uncomplicated healing following surgical repair and of overall growth necessary for development. If the infant continues to have difficulty feeding despite adapted equipment and positioning, a problem other than the cleft should be considered and investigated.

Attention Deficit Hyperactivity Disorder

Attention deficit hyperactivity disorder, or ADHD, is one of the most common neurobehavioral disorders that affect children. As many as 15–20 percent of children may be affected by ADHD, and four to five times as many boys as girls are affected by the disorder. ADHD's broad range of symptoms generally pertain to both learning and behavior. Symptoms related to learning problems include difficulties paying attention and concentrating, and a tendency to distractibility, particularly in group settings. Symptoms that reflect behavior problems include indications of hyperactivity, fidgetiness, and impulsivity. These are the children who are always in motion, cannot sit still,

> **MYTH** Sugar causes hyperactivity.
> **FACT** Sugar has not been shown to cause hyperactivity. A modest intake of sugar is acceptable in the context of a balanced, nutritious diet.

and often act before they think.

Historically, ADHD evolved from the disorder termed minimal brain dysfunction, or MBD, in the early 1960s. MBD represented a wide range of symptoms—including those relating to learning difficulties, neurologic abnormalities, and behavioral impairments. There were so many symptoms, in fact, that the disorder was found to be too unwieldy and eventually evolved into several more sharply focused conditions. Over time, the symptoms which comprised MBD and related to learning problems evolved into the group of disorders currently termed learning disabilities. The behavioral component became the forerunner of

· ·

Sally Shaywitz ▪ Bennett Shaywitz ▪ Ed Strenkowski

the disorder first termed the hyperactive child syndrome in 1980, and then attention deficit disorder (ADD) in 1982, and attention deficit hyperactivity disorder in 1987. In 1994 the diagnostic criteria for ADHD were further refined and now include symptoms of inattention and hyperactivity or impulsivity.

Inattention is defined as six (or more) of the following symptoms:

1. Doesn't pay close attention to tasks; makes careless mistakes.
2. Has difficulty in sustaining attention over time.
3. Doesn't seem to listen when spoken to.
4. Fails to finish work.
5. Has difficulty organizing work.
6. Avoids tasks that require sustained attention.
7. Loses belongings or work items.
8. Tends to get distracted from work at hand.
9. Tends to be forgetful.

Symptoms of hyperactivity and impulsivity are clustered together, and an individual should exhibit at least six of the following symptoms to be considered as having ADHD.

Hyperactivity
1. Tends to fidget or squirm.
2. Tends to get up out of his or her seat.
3. Tends to run about or climb at inappropriate times.
4. Has difficulty playing quietly.
5. Tends to be on the go as if "driven by a motor."
6. Tends to talk excessively.

Impulsivity
1. Tends to blurt out answers or call out in class.
2. Tends to have difficulty waiting for his or her turn.
3. Tends to interrupt others' conversations.

To qualify for a diagnosis of ADHD, a child must have the required number of symptoms for at least six months and they must result in some impairment at either home or school.

Attention deficit hyperactivity disorder may occur as one of three types:

1. *Combined type.* If symptoms of both inattention and hyperactivity or impulsivity are present.

2. *Predominantly inattentive type.* If the required number of symptoms of inattention are present, but not hyperactivity or impulsivity.

3. *Predominantly hyperactive-impulsive type.* If symptoms of hyperactivity or impulsivity, but not inattention, are present.

Adults who have had symptoms of ADHD as children, but who no longer meet the criteria, are considered to have ADHD "in partial remission." It is important to appreciate that the diagnosis of ADHD is currently made on the basis of behavior as reported by parents or teachers on rating scales. At the present time, there is no fully reliable or valid test to diagnose the disorder. The lack of a single laboratory test to determine whether an individual has ADHD reflects the fact that ADHD is not a single disorder, but rather a somewhat diverse group of disorders.

Research under way at the Yale Center for the Study of Learning and Attention is examining more than 700 boys and girls with ADHD to determine if different types of ADHD might have their own characteristics and respond to specific treatments. The disorder often co-occurs with learning disabilities, and any evaluation for ADHD should also include assessment for the possibility of an associated learning problem. The basic management of ADHD will include medications as well as educational and behavioral management strategies, if there is also a learning disability.

Parents have also sought more "natural" and unitary approaches to treatment of the disorder, including management through dietary restrictions. Over the past thirty years, one of the most widely debated issues about childhood nutrition has been whether table sugar, other dietary sweeteners, and food additives affect learning and behavior. Particularly during the 1960s and 1970s, high sugar intake was popularly thought to cause hyperactivity in schoolchildren. In 1975, a researcher named Dr. Benjamin Feingold hypothesized that certain food additives and colorings produced a syndrome of learning disability and hyperactivity in susceptible children. Many people immediately embraced his theory, since it confirmed their long-standing suspicions. Subsequently, Feingold Associations sprang up in a number of cities. Other scientific developments over the next several years encouraged the acceptance of Feingold's hypothesis.

Some studies suggested metabolic reasons for how the brain responds to the immediate intake of aspartame (NutraSweet) and other nonnutritive sweeteners. Aspartame was even thought to produce headaches, dizziness, mood alterations, and seizures. It is understandable that parents are concerned about table sugar (sucrose), aspartame, and other food additives, as they are common components of children's diets. Much of the nutritional information available to the general public does not focus on the inconclusive nature of popularized studies such as Feingold's, which have nonetheless had lasting effects on people's attitudes toward nutrition and behavior.

Two studies in fact have demonstrated that there are no grounds for believing that sugar or other sweeteners cause or intensify ADHD. In one study, children with histories of attention deficit disorder were given more than ten times the usual consumption of aspartame for four weeks. The study concluded that aspartame at greater than ten times the usual consumption level had no effect on the children's cognitive and behavioral function. The other study examined the effects of aspartame and refined sugar on the behavior of children who had been described by their parents as sensitive to sugar. Like the other study, this study was intended to provide definitive evidence about these sweeteners' long-term effects on children's behaviors, rather than the effects that were observed immediately after intake. The study, conducted for nine weeks on forty-eight children, revealed that even when intake far exceeded usual intake levels, neither dietary sucrose nor aspartame—when eaten as part of normal meals—affected the children's behavior or cognitive function.

Therefore, contrary to much popular belief within the past several decades, sugar and aspartame have not been proven to cause ADHD, and there are no specific diet recommendations to be made for the treatment of hyperactivity. Normal nutritional considerations for the child's age should be adhered to, with emphasis on maintaining good health and appropriate growth. Sweets are a part of everyone's diet and in reasonable quantities do not have any deleterious effects on cognition or behavior. However, when consumed in excess, they may lead to dental caries or excessive weight gain. If this is a concern, then low-calorie, readily available snacks should be incorporated into the child's diet. Snacks like fresh fruit, raw carrots, low-fat yogurt, and crackers are easily stored and require little preparation.

Apart from being diagnosed with ADHD, some children may have a proven allergy to a food or additive or even a dye; other chapters in this book discuss these considerations, including appropriate interventions. A child may react to caffeine, as some adults do, by feeling "edgy," or experience nighttime sleep difficulties. In cases like these the most appropriate step is to eliminate caffeine from the diet. A recent study done at Yale showed that a response very similar to that of caffeine can also be observed in some healthy non-ADHD children several hours after eating a large amount of sugar (equivalent to that in two cans of regular soda) without other food. Once again, a balanced diet is the key to preventing these problems.

If a child is being treated for ADHD, he or she may be placed on a stimulant medication, such as methylphenidate (Ritalin). Parents should be aware that some medications may initially decrease appetite, although with time, the child's appetite usually returns to premedication level. Parents should be aware of this potential effect and not be alarmed if the child's food intake or weight decreases slightly soon after medication is begun. The child's weight can be monitored once

a week and healthy snacks added to the diet to maintain normal weight. Food intake spread out over smaller and more frequent snacks may be easier for the child to handle than three large meals a day.

The relationship between what we eat and how we behave continues to represent a lively area of interest. Recent studies indicate very strongly that neither sugar nor sugar substitutes—in particular, aspartame—adversely affect children's behavior. However, as with any other growing and developing child, the child who has ADHD will benefit from an appealing, well-balanced diet that provides adequate calories.

Resource

National Center for Learning Disabilities, 381 Park Avenue South, Suite 1420, New York, NY 10016. (212) 545-7510.

Building Blocks for Good Nutrition

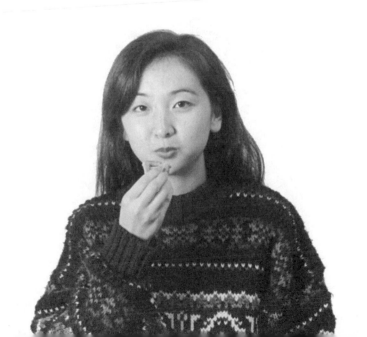

Calories: The Key to Energy Balance

Energy Intake

Food is the fuel the body uses to maintain its essential functions and to grow and perform physical activities. Food is converted into chemical energy for use by the body. Energy from food is expressed in kilocalories or, as they are more commonly called, calories. A calorie is a standard unit for measuring energy produced by food or energy expended by the body. Technically, it is the amount of heat energy required to raise the temperature of 1 gram of water by 1 degree Celsius.

Different foods provide differing amounts of energy (calories). All foods contain varying pro-

> **MYTH** You do not burn calories when you sleep.
>
> **FACT** Breathing and other metabolic functions require calories. Therefore, although calorie needs are lower during rest, they are not eliminated.

portions of the 3 major nutrients: protein, carbohydrate, and fat. Each of these macronutrients produces or provides energy for the body. One gram of protein and 1 gram of carbohydrate each provides approximately 4 calories. One gram of fat provides 9 calories, and 1 gram of alcohol provides 7 calories. Because 1 gram of fat contains more than twice as many calories as that of protein and carbohydrate, foods that are high in fat also tend to be high in calories. To see how calories are determined, look at the food components of a particular food. For example, 1 cup of skim milk contains the following:

. . . .

Nancy A. Held ▪ Rosa Hendler

8 grams protein × 4 calories/gram = 32 calories

12 grams carbohydrate × 4 calories/gram = 48 calories

1 gram fat × 9 calories/gram = 9 calories

Total = 89 calories

In comparison, 1 cup of whole milk contains:

8 grams protein × 4 calories/gram = 32 calories

12 grams carbohydrate × 4 calories/gram = 48 calories

8 grams fat × 9 calories/gram = 72 calories

Total = 152 calories

Thus, 1 cup of whole milk provides 63 more calories than an equal amount of skim milk solely because the whole milk has a higher fat content. Because any volume of whole milk has more calories than an equal volume of skim milk, whole milk is said to have greater "caloric density" than skim milk. Foods with a higher percentage of fat tend to have a high caloric density, whereas foods with high fiber and water content (which have no calories), such as vegetables, tend to have lower caloric density. For example, 2 cups of raw broccoli has approximately the same number of calories as 1 teaspoon of butter.

Energy Expenditure

The total energy expended by individuals to sustain normal bodily functions and activity can be divided into three parts: basal metabolic rate, physical activity, and thermogenesis.

The basal metabolic rate (BMR) is the energy an individual uses when at rest, such as before rising in the morning. This energy is needed for the heart to pump, for the respiratory system to breathe, for normal body temperature to be maintained, and for growth to occur. The BMR is highest during periods of rapid growth, such as in in-fancy and adolescence. In adults, the BMR usually accounts for almost two-thirds of the energy required each day. The BMR varies from person to person and seems to be genetically determined. Studies of families have shown that the BMR is quite similar among relatives in the same family but varies between families. Other factors also affect the basal metabolic rate, such as the endocrine glands, particularly the thyroid. An underactive or overactive thyroid respectively decreases or increases basal metabolism. Sleeping reduces the metabolic rate. Fever, emotional stress, caffeine, and cigarette smoking increase the metabolic rate. Climate also affects metabolism. In very hot temperatures individuals have a higher metabolic rate. The BMR even changes with a woman's menstrual cycle, increasing with the onset of a period and decreasing at midcycle.

The energy a child consumes through physical activity varies according to the type, intensity, and duration of the exercise, as well as the child's weight and level of fitness. An overweight child actually expends more energy than a thin child performing the same activity because he or she is carrying a heavier body. Obese children, however, tend to be less active than thin children, even when they engage in the same recreation. When in the swimming pool, for example, an overweight child is more likely to float in a tube, whereas a thin child will swim laps. During physical activity, most children use 1.7–2 times the energy they consume at rest, in contrast with adults, who use 1.5 times their resting energy during exercise.

A small amount of the energy required (or used) is contributed by processes related to the consumption of food. This is called thermogenesis, or the use of calories. After food is eaten, energy is used to digest, absorb, and store the food. This calorigenic effect of food depends on the amount and type of food consumed. Some re-

TABLE 27.1

Recommended Calorie Intake for Children

Age	Calories per pound	Calories per kilogram	Average per day
0–6 months	49	108	650
6 months–1 year	45	98	850
1–3 years	46	109	1,300
4–6 years	41	90	1,800
7–10 years	32	70	2,000
11–14 years (boys)	25	55	2,500
15–18 years (boys)	20	45	3,000
11–14 years (girls)	21	47	2,200
15–18 years (girls)	18	40	2,200

Source: Adapted from Food and Nutrition Board, National Academy of Sciences–National Research Council, *Recommended Dietary Allowances,* 10th ed. (Washington, DC: National Academy Press, 1989).

search has indicated that the calorigenic effect of food may be diminished in obese persons, thereby contributing to their degree of overweight. In other words, they use fewer calories to metabolize food. This theory remains controversial, however.

Striking a Balance

Normal growth and development in children depends on striking a balance between energy expenditure on one hand and energy intake on the other. Most children eat the right amount of food to meet their energy needs for growth and normal activity. Children who eat more food than their bodies need for growth and activity store the extra energy in their body as fat. Remember, humans did not always have refrigerators to turn to when they were hungry. Storing energy as fat during times of plenty helped people survive when food was scarce. However, a common problem in American children today is overeating and inactivity, which leads to excessive amounts of body fat, or obesity. Conversely, if children are

not taking in enough food, then all the calories are used to maintain the body's usual functions and there is not enough energy left over for normal growth.

Calories for growth vary depending on a child's stage of development. During rapid growth phases a greater proportion of calories are used for growth and a smaller proportion are used for activity and normal fuel requirements. For instance, newborns expend one-third of their energy for growth, and the rest to maintain bodily functions. Indeed, at this age, eating is the infant's main physical activity. In contrast, a 4-month-old baby uses just 10 percent of calories for growth because he or she uses more energy for physical activity. As children grow older, they need to consume a greater number of total calories because their bodies are larger, but their need for energy per pound of weight actually decreases.

Dietitians' tables list the number of calories usually required by children of different ages and body sizes. Energy intakes based on calories per kilogram of body weight recommended by the

Food and Nutrition Board of the National Academy of Sciences are provided here (see table 27.1). However, energy needs vary tremendously among individual children of the same age and sex, so a child's intake may fall below or above the recommendations and still be right for him or her. Other simple calculations can give a rough idea of how many calories a child usually needs. In the first year of life, a child needs about 1,000 calories per day, with an additional 100 calories for each year thereafter. Following this method, therefore, a 6-year-old might need to consume about 1,500 calories a day.

The best way to assess whether a child is getting the right amount of calories is to use growth charts and simple observation. If the child appears to be gaining too much weight, then energy intake is greater than energy expenditure. If the child is not gaining weight, then food intake is less than energy needs. Remember that there is a broad range of normal weights for any height. Your health-care provider has growth charts that can help evaluate your child's weight and overall growth (see growth charts appendix).

Without having to think about it, children carefully regulate their caloric intake through appetite and satiety centers in the brain. Scientists are studying these processes to learn more about how these appetite centers work. Keep in mind that although a child's average food intake is fairly steady, the quantity a child eats can vary considerably from day to day, particularly in young children. Even adults experience day-to-day variation in the amount they eat. If calorie needs are being met, then other nutrient needs, such as protein, vitamins, and minerals, are usually also being met.

Potential nutrient deficiencies can develop when the diet is high in calories but low in nutrients. Eating a lot of candy, for example, provides energy for normal activity but few or no other nutrients. Many adolescents who have poorly balanced diets manage to get enough nutrients only because they eat a large amount of food.

28
· · · · · · · ·

Protein: The Body's Building Blocks

Variety and moderation are the foundations of a well-balanced diet. In addition to adequate amounts of carbohydrate, fat, vitamins, and minerals, the body also needs protein. This chapter answers common questions about protein: what is protein, what does it do, and how much protein is enough for a young growing body?

amino acids, of which the body can manufacture only 13. The other 9 are called essential amino acids because they cannot be synthesized by the body and are therefore essential in the diet. Food proteins that contain all of the essential amino acids in the correct proportion for human needs are called "complete," whereas those that lack 1 or more essential amino acids are called "incomplete." Dietary sources of complete proteins in-

Proteins in the Body

Proteins are complex chemical compounds found in every living cell in the body. Human body proteins are built from 22 different units called clude such animal products as eggs, milk, meat, fish, and poultry. The proteins found in vegetables, grains, and beans are incomplete; however,

· ·

Lisa Tartamella ▪ Susan Boulware

they can be "complemented," or combined with each other, to provide all of the essential amino acids.

Protein is required for the synthesis of body tissues, such as muscle. In adults, protein synthesis is needed to maintain and repair existing tissue. During childhood, protein synthesis is necessary for growth in addition to maintenance and repair. Most of the body's protein is found in muscle; the rest is distributed in bone, cartilage, teeth, and other body tissues. In addition to providing the body's structural support (such as bone and muscle), protein is involved in a host of bodily functions. Examples of functional proteins include hemoglobin, which carries oxygen to cells; antibodies, which help fight infection; and enzymes and hormones, which perform a variety of important functions. Protein can be used as a source of energy, and amino acids can be converted to glucose to maintain blood glucose levels during times of fasting. These are not preferred uses of protein, however, because the proteins in the body are needed to serve many important non-fuel functions, and there is no protein storage "depot."

Dietary Requirements during the Growing Years

Daily protein requirements vary during each stage of the life cycle and are relatively higher for children than adults. This is crucial, because an adequate protein intake also ensures that the body has sufficient amounts of the essential amino acids during early stages of growth and development. Protein requirements per unit of weight decrease as the growth rate declines. During the first 2 months of life, 50 percent of protein is used for growth and 50 percent is used for the continuous repair processes mentioned earlier. By age 2 to 3 years, only about 11 percent of protein is used for growth, and after the growth spurt of adolescence, protein is used only for maintenance and repair. Sex, age, nutritional status, and the quality of protein in the diet must all be considered in estimating protein needs. Recommended daily protein allowances in childhood are provided in table 28.1. Adequate calories must be consumed with ample protein to ensure appropriate metabolism or use of the protein.

Consequences of Inadequate and Excessive Protein Intakes

Although protein deficiency is rare in the United States, it is observed more often in children than in adults because of children's relatively higher nutritional requirements. Children at highest risk for inadequate protein intake include those with severe medical illnesses or bowel disease (see chapter 23), those who have multiple food allergies (see chapter 19) or limited availability of food, or those who are vegan vegetarians. A vegan diet can be nutritionally adequate if proteins are combined correctly (see chapter 10).

A child can survive on a low protein intake depending on the quality of protein and amount of calories consumed. However, the body can compensate for a lack of protein for only a limited time. Protein deprivation eventually leads to malnutrition, which results in the stunting of growth, poor muscle tone, edema or puffiness of the skin because of fluid accumulation, thin and fragile hair, skin ulcers, decreased immune responses, and overall weakness and loss of energy. Low blood-protein stores and hormonal imbalances may also result.

Although inadequate protein intake can be det-

TABLE 28.1
Recommended Dietary Allowances during Childhood

Age	Representative weight (lbs)	(kg)	Protein (g) (per lb)	(per kg)	(per day)
0–6 months	13	6	1.00	2.2	13
6 months–1 year	20	9	0.72	1.6	14
1–3 years	29	13	0.54	1.2	16
4–6 years	44	20	0.49	1.1	22
7–10 years	61	28	0.45	1.0	28
11–14 years (boys)	99	44	0.45	1.0	45
15–18 years (boys)	145	66	0.41	0.9	59
11–14 years (girls)	101	46	0.45	1.0	46
15–18 years (girls)	121	55	0.36	0.8	44

Source: Adapted from Food and Nutrition Board, National Academy of Sciences–National Research Council, *Recommended Dietary Allowances,* 10th ed. (Washington, DC: National Academy Press, 1989).

rimental, excessive intake of protein is not desirable either. Eating more protein than necessary will not cause muscles to grow bigger or stronger, and excessive protein intake can actually harm infants with liver or kidney problems. Remember that high-protein foods such as meat and cheese are often high in fat. A well-balanced diet that includes moderate amounts of protein is the best bet.

It is relatively easy to meet children's dietary requirements for protein, and most young Americans consume amounts of protein well above recommended daily allowances. Given the wide variety of high-protein foods scattered throughout the Food Guide Pyramid (see chapter 4), it should not be difficult to build a protein-adequate diet for a healthy child. For example, a 4-year-old child weighing 44 pounds requires approximately 22 grams of protein each day (44 pounds × 0.49 gram/pound = 22 grams). This can be met by eating just one 3-ounce piece of meat. Other possible combinations include an 8-ounce glass of low-fat milk (12 grams), a slice of toast (3 grams), and 1 ounce of cheese (7 grams).

Best Bets for Protein

Protein intake can be assessed by evaluating the adequacy of a child's growth rate, quality of protein in the diet, and combination of foods that are providing the amino acids. Human milk or commercially prepared infant formula provides most of the protein needed during the first 12 months of life. Although prepared formulas supply slightly more protein than breast milk, the proteins provided by breast milk are believed to be used more completely, so both breast milk and formula are adequate for the first 6 months of life. Infants who do not drink cow's milk–based formulas are often fed soy-based formulas. Both formulations provide all of the appropriate nutrients in the right proportions. During the last 6 months of the first

TABLE 28.2
Protein Content of Selected Foods

Food	Portion size	Protein (g)
Breast milk	8 oz	2.4
Commercial formula	8 oz	4.0
Dry infant cereal	5 tbsp	2.0
Strained vegetables	4½-oz jar	2.0
Strained meats	3½-oz jar	14.0
Strained vegetables with meat	4½-oz jar	3.0
Whole milk	8 oz	8.0
Yogurt (whole milk)	½ cup	3.7
Cheddar cheese	1 oz	7.1
Hamburger patty	2 oz	15.4
Chicken drumstick	1 each	12.2
Peanut butter	1 tbsp	4.0
Egg, medium	1 each	5.7
Tuna	¼ cup	11.5
Bologna	1 slice	2.8
Hot dog, 5 × ¾ inches	1 each	5.6

Sources: P. L. Pipes, *Nutrition in Infancy and Childhood* (St. Louis, MO: Times Mirror, 1989); J. Pennington, *Bowes and Church's Food Values of Portions Commonly Used,* 16th ed. (Philadelphia: J. B. Lippincott, 1994).

year of life, infants should be introduced to other high-quality proteins, such as cereal, egg yolk, and strained meats. Once table foods are tolerated, a wide variety of foods can contribute protein to the diet. Common sources of protein and portion sizes for infants and children are provided in table 28.2.

Adolescents can use the Food Guide Pyramid to plan a diet that includes a wide variety of high-protein foods. High-protein food sources can be found throughout the pyramid. Remember that animal food sources provide complete proteins. Proteins from vegetables, grains, and beans are incomplete and need to be combined appropriately to ensure their adequacy as sources of protein.

29
· · · · · · · ·

Cash in on Carbohydrates

Foods are composed of 3 major nutrients: carbohydrates, protein, and fat. Of these, carbohydrates, which are found in grains, vegetables, fruits, and milk, provide the major source of energy in most diets throughout the world. By weight, each gram of carbohydrate (regardless of type) contains 4 calories of energy. For example, a teaspoon of refined sugar, weighing about 5 grams, provides 20 calories of energy. Protein also provides 4 calories per gram, whereas fat provides 9 calories per gram. Carbohydrates give sweetness, texture, thickness, and emulsifying properties to food.

> **MYTH** If you are watching your weight, skip the potatoes and bread.
>
> **FACT** Potatoes and bread are good sources of complex carbohydrates and are an important part of a balanced diet. Ounce for ounce, carbohydrates provide the same number of calories as protein and fewer than half the calories of fat.

Authorities generally agree that carbohydrates should comprise a large proportion of the diet. The Food Guide Pyramid recommends that individuals eat an abundance of grains, vegetables, and fruits (see chapter 4). At the base of the pyramid is the bread, rice, cereal, and pasta group; these foods, which are made up primarily of complex carbohydrates, should make up a larger portion of the diet than meats and fats.

There is no Recommended Dietary Allowance (RDA) for carbohydrates, but a good general guideline is that 50 percent of calories should be

· ·

Nancy A. Held ▪ William V. Tamborlane

TABLE 29.1
Understanding Carbohydrates

Type	Name	Food sources
Monosaccharides (single sugar molecules; simple)	Glucose	Dextrose in prepared foods
	Fructose	Fruits and honey
	Galactose	Not free in nature
Disaccharides (two monosaccharides joined together; simple)	Sucrose (glucose and fructose)	Cane and beet sugar, molasses, maple syrup
	Lactose (glucose and galactose)	Milk, milk products
	Maltose (glucose and glucose)	Barley malt, some breakfast foods
Polysaccharides (many monosaccharides joined together; complex)	Starch	Grains, legumes, tubers
	Dextrin	Produced from the breakdown of starch; used in prepared foods
	Glycogen	Meat, fish, shellfish
	Cellulose	Stalks and leaves of vegetables
	Hemicellulose	Fruits, vegetables, grains, nuts, seeds
	Pectin	Apples, citrus fruits, strawberries
	Gums and mucilages	Plant secretions and seeds
	Algal polysaccharides	Seaweeds and algae, carrageenan

derived from carbohydrates in children after infancy. If children are eating a lower percentage of carbohydrates, then they may be eating too much meat, cheese, butter, and other foods rich in protein or fat. Many people eat excessive amounts of protein and fat, and current recommendations are intended to correct this problem. When fat intake is high, the risk for heart disease increases. Fortunately, many children prefer starchy foods such as breads, cereals, and pasta. Fat content is increased, however, when fat is added in preparing foods, such as adding butter to bread or noodles. In years past, parents encouraged children to eat the meat portion of the meal more than the bread or potato portion. We now understand that only a small amount of protein is necessary for a healthy body and that foods high in carbohydrate are an important part of a normal diet.

Understanding Carbohydrates

MONOSACCHARIDES Carbohydrates are subdivided into 3 main categories: monosaccharides, disaccharides, and polysaccharides, depending on the number of sugar molecules they contain (table 29.1). Monosaccharides are single-sugar molecules, and they are the basic building blocks of all the other kinds of carbohydrates. Each monosaccharide molecule is made up of 6 carbon atoms, 12 hydrogen atoms, and 6 oxygen atoms in a ring structure. These rings are connected like beads in a chain to make disaccharides and polysaccharides.

The 3 most important monosaccharides are fructose, glucose, and galactose. Fructose commonly occurs in its monosaccharide form in unprocessed foods. It is often called "fruit sugar," because it is found primarily in fruits and honey. Fructose is also a component of a processed sweetener, high-fructose corn syrup (HFCS). HFCS contains fructose in amounts of 42 percent, 55 percent, or 90 percent, depending on the extent of processing. HFCS is used commercially in breads, jellies, ice creams, dairy products, and beverages.

Glucose is the main form of monosaccharide in the body. Poly- and disaccharides are digested in the stomach and intestines, broken down to the monosaccharides glucose, fructose, and galactose, and then absorbed into the bloodstream. Fructose and galactose are then converted to glucose in the body to be used for energy. When doctors speak about blood-sugar levels, they are really referring to blood glucose levels. The body (that is, the liver) can also produce glucose in order to keep blood glucose levels from falling too low when a person is not eating. Only a small amount of glucose (also called dextrose) occurs naturally in foods. Some glucose is added to processed foods and beverages and is listed on the label as dextrose. Galactose is not found free in nature, but it is produced when lactose (milk sugar) breaks down during digestion. Once galactose is absorbed into the blood, an enzyme in the liver rapidly converts it to glucose; deficiency of this enzyme causes the disease galactosemia.

Sorbitol, mannitol, and xylitol, known as sugar alcohols, are formed from glucose, mannose, and xylose, respectively. They have a sweet taste and are found free in nature. Plums, prunes, berries, apples, and cherries contain sorbitol. Pineapple, olives, asparagus, sweet potatoes, and carrots contain mannitol. Strawberries, raspberries, and cauliflower contain xylitol. Sorbitol and mannitol are about half as sweet as sucrose (table sugar), and xylitol is almost as sweet. Sugar alcohols are common ingredients in dietetic and reduced-calorie foods, including candies and gums. They are viewed as desirable sweetening agents because they produce a smaller rise in blood glucose levels than does sucrose. Sugar alcohols are also used as bulking agents, fillers that give form and volume to food and beverages. Caloric savings from the use of sugar alcohols over sugar are minimal: sugar alcohols contain 2 to 3 calories per gram, in comparison with sugar's 4 calories. A major drawback of sugar alcohols is that excess consumption usually causes flatulence, diarrhea, or bloating. In young children, as little as 5–10 grams of sorbitol may produce diarrhea. One piece of sorbitol-sweetened hard candy contains about 3 grams of sorbitol.

DISACCHARIDES As the name implies, disaccharides are made up of 2 monosaccharides (glucose, fructose, or galactose) joined together. The most important disaccharide is sucrose (refined sugar), which is composed of 1 glucose and 1 fructose molecule. Sucrose is found in sugar cane, sugar beets, maple syrup, and maple sugar. Cane sugar and sugar beets are refined to make table sugar. In addition to providing sweetness to foods, sugar provides bulk to ice cream, inhibits spoilage in jams and jellies, promotes fermentation in sausage products, provides tenderness in baked goods, and is food for yeast in raised baked goods. Sucrose also occurs naturally in many foods, particularly fruits and vegetables.

In the early stages of the sugar refining process, crystals of sucrose retain a coating of liquid known as molasses. Depending on the method of processing, the crystals produced in early stages of refining form dark and light brown sugar and raw sugar. Although these sugars may impart different flavor characteristics to recipes, they are all sucrose. Sugar can be treated with acid (in a process known as inversion), which breaks the sugar down into fructose and glucose. Invert sugar, as this product is known, is used in candies and commercially baked goods.

Lactose is another important disaccharide and is the principal sugar found in milk. Only about ⅙ as sweet-tasting as sucrose, lactose is a combination of the two monosaccharides galactose and glucose.

Maltose, or malt sugar, is composed of two glucose molecules that are a product of the digestion of starch. When a grain such as barley sprouts, its enzymes convert the grain starch to maltose. Barley malt is occasionally used as a sweetener in commercial food products.

POLYSACCHARIDES Polysaccharides are more commonly known as complex carbohydrates. They are composed of chains of monosaccharide molecules and include starch, glycogen, and cellulose. These polysaccharides may contain thousands of linked glucose units. Starch is the storage form of glucose in plants and the major constituent of grains, such as wheat, rice, oats, corn, millet, rye, and barley. Other sources of starch are legumes, such as peanuts, kidney beans, black-eyed peas, chick peas, and soy beans, which are also high in protein. Tubers such as potatoes, yams, and cassavas are other good sources of starch. The partial breakdown of starch into smaller chains produces dextrin. Dextrins taste sweeter than starch and are often used in the manufacture of corn syrup.

Glycogen is the storage form of carbohydrate in both animals and humans and is stored in the liver and muscle. It is a readily available source of glucose. Little glycogen is actually consumed from meat products, because only small amounts are stored in animal tissue.

Fruits, vegetables, and some grains contain a group of polysaccharides that cannot be broken down by the human body because humans lack the enzymes needed to digest them. These polysaccharides do not provide energy, but rather they provide fiber to the diet. Examples of polysaccharide fibers are cellulose, hemicellulose, pectins, gums, and mucilages. The importance of dietary fiber is discussed in detail in chapter 34.

Why Are Complex Carbohydrates (Polysaccharides) Better for Children Than Simple Sugars (Mono- and Disaccharides)?

If complex carbohydrates are broken down to monosaccharides in the intestines before they are absorbed into the blood stream, why are they any better than refined sugar or other di- or monosaccharides? To a great extent it has to do with the processes of digestion and absorption. Simple sugars require little digestion, and when a child eats a sweet food, such as a candy bar or can of soda, the glucose level in the blood rises rapidly. In response, the pancreas secretes a large amount of insulin to keep blood glucose levels from rising too high. This large insulin response in turn tends to make the blood sugar fall to levels that are too low 3 to 5 hours after the candy bar or can of soda has been consumed. This tendency of blood glucose levels to fall may then lead to an adrenaline surge, which in turn can cause nervousness and irritability. This process is not the same as attention deficit hyperactivity disorder (see chapter 26). The same roller-coaster ride of glucose and hormone levels is not experienced after eating complex carbohydrates or after eating a balanced meal because the digestion and absorption processes are much slower. In addition, when children eat a lot of complex carbohydrates in the form of grains and vegetables, they are also getting important sources of vitamins and minerals as well as fiber. When they eat refined sugar, syrups, and candies, that's all they get: "empty calories."

A large intake of sugar also increases problems with dental caries (see chapter 16). Eating sugary, sticky foods, especially between meals, increases the chance of developing cavities. Other factors, such as heredity, also play a role in the development of cavities. Behaviors that help to prevent caries are good dental hygiene, limiting the number of snacks between meals, taking fluoride supplements, and avoiding sugary, sticky foods.

How Much Sugar?

Having said all of the above, there isn't anything inherently bad about simple sugars as long as they are a reasonable component of a balanced meal plan. About 20 percent of calories in the average American diet come from simple sugars, both naturally occurring and added. Added sugars provide about 11 percent of the calories for adults and 13–14 percent for children. It has been suggested, however, that no more than 10 percent of calories should be derived from added sugars. Check the labels of packaged foods to see how much sugar they contain. Food labels list the total carbohydrate content, which includes both simple and complex carbohydrates. The simple carbohydrates (that is, mono- and disaccharides) are listed separately as "sugars." Keep in mind, however, that food labels do not distinguish between natural and added sugars. For instance, naturally occurring lactose (a disaccharide) in milk

is listed as sugar in the Nutrition Facts section of a milk carton label, but the ingredients section does not list any added sugar. In contrast, packaged cookies, which contain added sugar, list sugar both in the list of ingredients and in the Nutrition Facts section (see chapter 36).

With infants and toddlers, there is no reason to add sugar to foods or to offer very sweet snacks and desserts. Although their caloric needs are high in proportion to their size, so are their nutritional needs. With older children, strict avoidance of added sugar often causes children to search out these "forbidden" foods elsewhere. During periods of rapid growth (for example, adolescence), some sugar can supply extra calorie needs once nutritional needs are met. Children (and adults) like the taste of sweets, and some sugar is reasonable in a balanced diet, but not to the exclusion of more nutritious foods. Parents should also limit their intake of sweets because they should model as well as teach good eating behaviors.

Alternative Sweeteners

NUTRITIVE Alternative sweeteners are often categorized based on whether they have calories or not. Many simple sugars that are used to sweeten food have already been discussed. Consumers sometimes choose fructose, honey, or fruit juice sweeteners because they view these sweeteners as "healthier" sugars than sucrose (refined sugar). In fact, there is little difference in nutritional value among honey, fruit juice, and sucrose when they are used as added sweeteners. Although honey and fruit juice contain fructose, it comprises less than half of the total sugar content; sucrose provides the remaining sugar. Honey contains trace amounts of vitamins and minerals that are not present in refined sugar, but the amounts are too small to be significant. Fruit juice may sound nutritious, but it has the same amount of carbohydrates that sucrose does and affects the blood sugar in a similar way. In addition, refined sugar (sucrose) is half fructose and half glucose. In sum, there are no nutritional advantages to be gained by using honey or fruit juice rather than sugar as sweeteners. In fact, honey should not be given to infants less than 1 year old because their immature digestive tracts may permit the growth of botulism spores commonly found in honey. For its part, fructose seems to raise the blood glucose level less high than sucrose and may be useful in people with diabetes.

NON-NUTRITIVE SWEETENERS One of the many results of consumers' demand for lower-calorie foods has been the development of alternative, noncaloric sweeteners. Obviously, the main purpose of alternative sweeteners is to meet the craving for sweets without adding calories to the diet. Such sweeteners may also help to reduce swings in blood-sugar levels in conditions such as diabetes. Three alternative sweeteners currently have U.S. Food and Drug Administration approval and are in widespread use: saccharin, aspartame, and acesulfame-K. These sweeteners are discussed in detail in chapter 35.

Food Bulking Agents

Carbohydrates have been used for many years as ingredients in the food industry. One common product is modified food starch, starch that has been chemically treated for use as a thickening agent. It is used in commercial salad dressings, gravies, puddings, and canned soups. The added starch in commercial foods generally increases the total amount of calories compared with a similar homemade food. Dextrins are also used commercially as thickening agents. Newly developed products derived from carbohydrates are now also being used as bulking agents, giving form and satiety to foods. One of these is polydextrose. It is used as a partial substitute for fat and can be found in baked goods, chewing gum, frostings, frozen desserts, salad dressings, gelatins, puddings, and candy. Polydextrose is a polymer, or chain, of dextrose molecules and provides 1 calorie per gram.

30

·······

What's the Skinny on Fats and Cholesterol?

Introduction

In contemporary times, dietary fat has been viewed as the cause of many ills. Yet we need to remember that fat in the diet is both an essential nutrient and adds to the enjoyment of eating. Without fat, many foods would not be as tasty and would lack texture, satiety, and structure. In the body, fats are necessary for cell membrane structure and important blood-clotting functions. Once fats are digested and absorbed, they become carriers for the fat-soluble vitamins A, D, E, and K. Cholesterol is a necessary component of various hormones that the body must produce for good health. Fat is also an efficient way for the body to store energy because it is the most calorically dense nutrient. One gram of fat provides 9 calories, whereas protein and carbohydrates supply only 4 calories per gram.

Because fat is calorically dense, however, eating a diet that is high in fat may lead to excessive weight gain. High-fat and high-cholesterol diets may also lead to high blood cholesterol levels. This contributes in adulthood to hardening of the arteries, or atherosclerosis (see chapter 20). Blockage of the arteries from atherosclerosis causes heart attacks, strokes, and circulation

> **MYTH** Don't eat fat and you won't get fat.
>
> **FACT** Although fat contains more calories per gram than protein or carbohydrates, fat in and of itself does not cause weight gain. Excess calories from any food source cause weight gain.

·····················

Nancy A. Held ▪ Ellen Liskov

problems in the lower extremities. In addition, certain kinds of dietary fat have been associated with certain cancers. Thus, as with other nutrients, the right amount and kinds of fat in the diet are essential, and too little or too much fat can be harmful.

Basics

CHOLESTEROL It is important to distinguish between the cholesterol that circulates in the bloodstream and the cholesterol that we eat. In addition, cholesterol in the diet and fat in the diet are two separate things, although many foods that are high in cholesterol are also high in fat (such as hot dogs and prime rib of beef).

Cholesterol is a waxy, soft substance that has a number of important functions in the body. Cholesterol is transported in the bloodstream on carriers called lipoproteins, which are made of fats (triglycerides) and proteins. There are three main types: very low-density lipoprotein (VLDL), low-density lipoprotein (LDL), and high-density lipoprotein (HDL). One's risk of heart disease is usually assessed in terms of what types and amounts of cholesterol carriers are present in the bloodstream, since not all types are desirable. For instance, HDL transports cholesterol back to the liver, so it is not deposited in the arteries. HDL is therefore often referred to as a "good" or "protective" cholesterol, because high HDL levels are associated with less atherosclerosis. Conversely, because LDL carries cholesterol to the arteries and increases the risk of atherosclerosis, it is known as "bad" or "undesirable" cholesterol. VLDL is composed primarily of triglycerides, and its role in heart disease is controversial. A very high VLDL or triglyceride level may represent a risk for heart disease, particularly in adult women.

Cholesterol is only found in foods of animal origin, never in vegetable foods. The most concentrated sources of dietary cholesterol are listed below.

Egg yolks	Poultry (especially
Butter	duck and goose)
Lard	Beef
Whole milk dairy	Veal
products	Lamb
Organ meats (liver,	Pork
kidney, sweet-	Fish
breads)	Shrimp

In comparing the food values of red meats to poultry and fish, it is interesting to note that the cholesterol content per ounce portion does not differ vastly. However, the saturated fat content (see below) of most poultry and fish is a fraction of that in most cuts of red meat; thus, it is recommended that people eat more poultry and fish than red meat. Yet any diet that includes too many animal foods, even chicken or fish, is likely to be higher in dietary cholesterol content than is desirable.

FAT When food labels indicate fat content, they are referring to the amount of triglycerides, not cholesterol. Triglycerides are compounds that consist of a molecule of glycerol (which contains 3 carbon atoms) combined with 3 fatty acid side chains. Each fatty acid side chain consists of between 12 and 16 carbon atoms. Triglycerides may be completely bound with hydrogen atoms (saturated) or have 1 or more sites that are not bound with hydrogen (unsaturated). This distinction is important because saturated and unsaturated fats have different effects on the body.

SATURATED FAT Saturated fats are fats that are

solid at room temperature. Foods high in saturated fat include:

Beef
Lamb
Spareribs
Organ meats
Regular cold cuts
Sausage
Regular hot dogs
Bacon
Whole milk
Whole milk yogurt
Cream
Half and half
2 percent milk
Nondairy creamer

Whipped topping
Whole milk cottage
  cheese
Whole milk cheese
Ice cream
Coconut oil
Butter
Palm oil
Lard
Cocoa butter/chocolate
Doughnuts
Cookies
Cake

Saturated fat supplies the body with energy, but no one saturated fat is essential in the diet, because the body can convert one type of saturated fat to another. Large amounts of saturated fat in the diet are undesirable because there is a direct relation between the amount of saturated fat in the diet and levels of low-density lipoprotein levels in the blood. As stated above, high LDL levels in the blood are associated with an increased risk of heart disease. The effects of high levels of dietary saturated fats are illustrated by studies that looked at changes in cholesterol levels when people migrated from one country to another. For instance, when people from Japan (where saturated fat intake was low) migrated to America and adopted the high saturated fat intake of the typical American diet, their blood LDL levels increased. It also appears that diets with too much saturated fat depress the body's production of HDL, the lipid fraction that protects against heart disease. Authorities generally agree that saturated fats should

be kept to less than 10 percent of daily calories for children who are over 2 years old.

MONOUNSATURATED FAT Monounsaturated fat is one of 2 types of unsaturated fat. The other is polyunsaturated fat (see below). In monounsaturated fat all carbons but one are paired with hydrogens. Monounsaturated fatty acids are liquid at room temperature. Foods that are high in monounsaturated fats include:

Olive oil
Peanut oil
Canola oil
Macadamia nuts

Peanuts
Peanut butter
Pecans
Almonds

POLYUNSATURATED FAT In polyunsaturated fats, 2 or more carbon atoms are not fully bound by hydrogen atoms. Polyunsaturated fats are essential in the diet because the human body cannot make them. The major polyunsaturated fatty acids are linoleic and linolenic. Linoleic acid intake must be at least 2 percent of calories to prevent essential fatty acid deficiency. Vegetable oils, margarine, mayonnaise, and salad dressing provide linoleic acid. Corn oil and peanut oil contain linolenic acid. Other polyunsaturated fats are the omega-3 fats, which are found in high concentrations in fish oils. Darker, oily fish, such as bluefish, herring, rainbow trout, mackerel, salmon, and sardines, are most abundant in natural fish oils.

Polyunsaturated fats, when used to replace saturated fat in the diet, are known to reduce blood LDL levels. Safflower, sunflower, corn, and soybean oils are also high in polyunsaturates and are liquid at room temperature. Cottonseed oil, which is frequently used in commercially baked products, contains approximately 50 percent polyunsaturated fat and 25 percent saturated fat. So, if a child typically uses a few teaspoons of butter per day on foods, changing to a tub of soft corn-oil margarine would reduce saturated fat intake and likely have a positive effect on LDL cholesterol. However, a diet that is too high in polyunsaturated fat (more than 10 percent of daily calories) can suppress the production of desirable HDL. LDL levels are also improved when saturated fat is replaced with monounsaturated fat. In addition, monounsaturated fats do not negatively influence HDL values. The principle to remember is that, for children who are over 2 years old, all fats should be used in moderation (no more than 30 percent of daily calories). Monounsaturated fats may be better than polyunsaturated fats when a fat is called for in the diet.

TRANS FATTY ACIDS AND HYDROGENATED FAT
Food manufacturers commonly use hydrogenated fats in packaged food products. Hydrogenated fats are created through a process called hydrogenation, in which an oil that is largely unsaturated, such as corn oil or sunflower oil, has hydrogen added to it, causing the fat to become more solid at room temperature. Because solid fats are less likely to go rancid, hydrogenation extends the shelf life of products like crackers, cookies, and other packaged items. Margarines are hydrogenated to varying degrees, depending on the desired degree of hardness. During hydrogenation, the unsaturated fat becomes more saturated.

The more solid and hydrogenated the fat, the more trans fatty acids there are in the product. Therefore, a soft tub of margarine has fewer trans fatty acids than a stick of margarine or solid vegetable shortening. Studies have linked high use of stick margarine (4 or more teaspoons per day) with higher blood cholesterol levels and increased risk of heart disease. At this time, margarine still seems to be a better option than butter. Butter contains saturated fat, and saturated fat appears to be more detrimental than trans fatty acids. To keep both trans fatty acids and saturated fat content low, all fats should be used in moderation, with a preference toward using liquid oils or soft margarine.

How much fat and cholesterol and what types of cholesterol the liver manufactures varies significantly with an individual's behavior and habits. Although genetics plays an extremely strong role in determining blood cholesterol levels, so do physical activity, body weight, and the amount of saturated fat, total fat, cholesterol, and fiber consumed. Exercise helps the body manufacture more HDL, whereas soluble fiber, which is found in oats, oat bran, legumes, apples, citrus fruits, and barley, helps lower LDL cholesterol by binding bile salts, another cholesterol carrier. In adults, being overweight, particularly when the excess body fat is located in the abdomen (as opposed to the hips, legs, or buttocks), increases LDL and decreases HDL, again increasing the risk of heart disease (see chapter 20).

As far as fats are concerned, each has a unique effect on blood cholesterol levels. Believe it or not, it is not the amount of cholesterol but the amount of saturated fat in the diet that primarily determines levels of blood cholesterol.

NATIONAL CHOLESTEROL EDUCATION PROGRAM GUIDELINES The National Cholesterol Education Program of the National Institutes of Health has developed guidelines for interpreting blood cholesterol levels for adults and children. These recommendations are consistent with many other authorities, including the American Heart Association and the American Academy of Pediatrics. They are meant to provide pediatricians, health care practitioners, and parents with practical standards on how to interpret the scientific data regarding the importance of a low-fat diet.

The guidelines apply to children over 2 years of age.

1. Nutritional adequacy should be achieved by eating a wide variety of foods from all the food groups, since no single food or food group provides all the essential nutrients.
2. Calories should be adequate to support a child's growth and development and to reach a desirable weight (for a growing child) or maintain desirable weight (for a teenager who has reached adult height). Calorie needs will depend on height, weight, stage of development, gender, and activity level.
3. Saturated fat should be less than 10 percent of calories per day. Because saturated fats have such a potent effect on blood cholesterol levels, this goal is of primary importance.
4. Total fat should average no more than 30 percent of calories per day. A sufficiently low saturated fat intake usually can be achieved only if total fat intake does not exceed 30 percent of calories. The target of 30 percent of average daily calories from fat is a way to control saturated fat intake while providing sufficient fat for essential functions and calories for normal growth in children and adolescents. Fat intake may be more than 30 percent of calories on some days and less on others. An approximation of how many grams of fat a child should eat daily is given in table 30.1. This number is calculated by multiplying calorie intake by 0.3 (30 percent) and dividing by 9 (for example, 1,300 calories × 0.3 = 390 calories, 390 ÷ 9 = 43 grams of fat).
5. Dietary cholesterol should be less than 300 milligrams per day.

Most American children do not eat a low total fat or low saturated fat diet. Data from recent nationwide food consumption surveys show that

TABLE 30.1
Suggested Fat Allowance for Children

Age (years)	Average calories	Fat (g)	Saturated fat (g)
1–3	1,300	43	14
4–6	1,800	60	20
7–10	2,000	66	22
11–14 (boys)	2,500	83	28
15–18 (boys)	3,000	100	33
11 14 (girls)	2,200	73	24
15–18 (girls)	2,200	73	24

children get 35 percent of their calories from fat and 14–15 percent of their calories from saturated fat. Only 4 percent of children meet the goal of 10 percent of calories from saturated fat. Meats, dairy products, and eggs provide more than half of this fat and 75 percent of the saturated fat.

Lowering Fat Intake in Children

A low-fat diet is not appropriate for children under 2, but it is for those over 2. In the first 2 years of life, infants grow very rapidly. A calorically dense diet (or one high in fat) allows infants who have limited capacity for food to meet their high energy needs. Both breast milk and infant formulas provide about 50 percent of calories from fat. As growth rate slows in the second half of the first year of life, fat calories also decrease, as table food is introduced and partially replaces milk feedings. During this period, birth through age 2, children should not be fed skim milk (even if there is a positive family history of high cholesterol). Skim milk is concentrated with minerals and protein, and it can make infants vulnerable to dehydration.

At around 2 to 3 years of age, children's eating patterns begin to mirror those of the rest of the family. Toddlers are generally quite fussy about what they are willing to eat. During this period it is not critical to follow a strict low-fat diet; rather, there should be a gradual transition to a low saturated fat diet. Because children's nutritional needs, especially for zinc, iron, and calcium, are relatively high during this period, it is important to provide adequate foods with these nutrients. Lean meats and low-fat dairy products can supply the needed nutrients and reduce fat intake.

During the preschool period, children have lower caloric and nutritional needs per kilogram of body weight but have high absolute protein and other nutrient needs. Snacks help provide these nutrients and are a regular part of children's diets. In fact, children typically consume a sizable portion (10–22 percent) of their calories from snacks. Snacks that are low in saturated fat can be selected or prepared.

Potential areas of concern with extremely low-fat diets are that those diets may not supply enough calories for growth or such nutrients as protein, iron, and zinc. When fat provides 30 percent of the calories, calories are clearly sufficient for proper growth after age 2. However, more severe and prolonged restriction of fat can result in growth failure in children and adolescents. What exact level of fat poses a threat is difficult to state, but some studies indicate that a fat intake of 20 percent of calories inhibits growth.

Although total fat intake must be high enough to provide calories for growth, saturated fat and dietary cholesterol should still be kept low. Studies of cultures where children eat lower amounts of saturated fat and cholesterol than American children do show no impact on growth. In a practical sense, then, instead of focusing on providing a low-fat diet, it is reasonable to focus on limiting saturated fat. Eating lean meat and lower-fat dairy products, including milk and cheese—which are sources of protein, iron, zinc, and calcium—will go a long way toward lowering saturated fat intake.

Practical Tips to Lower Fat Intake

Changing the family diet can be easy, if one remembers a few basic things.

1. *Don't try to change everything at once.* This is often the path of most resistance, and good intentions may be short-lived. When changes are made gradually, they are more likely to be accepted and thus continued as part of a normal routine. Start by reviewing the optimal food choices, preparation methods, and recommended serving sizes listed in this chapter, and begin to identify where excess saturated fat, total fat, and cholesterol are coming from in the family diet. Each week, try to focus on making 1 or 2 positive changes.

2. *There is no one correct way of eating a heart-healthy diet.* After identifying the sources of fats and cholesterol, there are lots of choices for making improvements. Let's say that a child's favorite sandwich is bologna, which is a significant source of total fat, saturated fat, and cholesterol. Try some reduced-fat products that may have only a fraction of the total fat and saturated fat of the regular version. If this product is not palatable, try a different reduced-fat brand (not all taste the same) or a completely different alternative. Another approach is to continue with a tried-and-true brand of regular bologna but to alternate it with lower-fat luncheon meats, such as turkey or ham. Still another choice would be to use 1 slice of regular bologna instead of 2 and to add a slice of reduced-fat cheese.

3. *There are no "illegal" or bad foods.* There is room for favorite foods, such as bologna or pizza, because it's the average intake of saturated fat, total fat, and cholesterol that matters. Balance

foods that are high in fat with those that are low in fat. Refer to recommended serving information and the Food Guide Pyramid (chapter 4) for more ideas.

4. *Plan ahead and control what enters the house.* Shopping from a list, planning meals and snacks a week at a time, and buying the appropriate foods are all ways to improve the level of success with lowering the family's fat intake and eating healthier. Whenever possible, prepare enough for another meal and freeze it. There will always be occasions when there's not enough time to cook from scratch but there is enough time to reheat something!

5. *Involve children in food preparation.* When kids have a role in shopping for and preparing their own lunches, snacks, or part of dinner, they are often more willing to try new items (even vegetables) and to eat what is served. In addition, low-fat cooking skills can be taught for use in the years to come.

Fat Substitutes

Manufacturers are responding to consumer demand for foods that are low in fat but don't taste that way. To be successful, fat substitutes must impart the same properties to food that fat does, including satiety, taste, smooth texture, structure, and tenderness. Fat replacements can be classified as calorie-reduced substitutes, which are digested normally, and calorie-free substitutes, which are virtually unabsorbed. Ingredients used as calorie-reduced substitutes may be used to partially replace fat or to completely replace fat. They may be derived from protein or from carbohydrates.

The best-known fat substitute is Simplesse, which is currently approved for use in mayonnaise, sour cream, salad dressings, yogurt, ice cream, and cheese. It is made from milk and egg-white proteins and supplies 1 to 2 calories per gram. Other protein-based fat substitutes, called Trailblazer and Finesse, are making their way to the marketplace.

Calorie-reduced fat substitutes that are carbohydrate-based include polydextrose, maltodextrins, and hydrogenated starch hydrolysates. These ingredients are used to provide a number of characteristics, including satiety, bulk (adding form to food), and sweetness.

One calorie-free fat substitute is Olestra. It is actually a sucrose polyester, since it is composed of sucrose combined with 7 to 8 fatty acids. Olestra is a large molecule, and the body's digestive enzymes cannot break it down. Thus, it is not absorbed into the bloodstream, where it would otherwise be converted into calories. Olestra has been studied extensively and has been determined by the U.S. Food and Drug Administration to be safe. Olestra can currently be used in commercially prepared savory snack foods (potato chips, tortilla chips, and crackers) only.

The major issue, of course, for fat replacements in all populations is safety. Research has not shown any harmful effects of fat substitutes, but less information is available regarding the safety of fat substitutes in children specifically. Such products must be used carefully, especially in young children, because children need fat calories for growth and development. Yet small amounts of foods containing fat replacements may help control a typically high-fat diet. In overweight children these foods can help reduce total calories as long as the child or teen does not compensate by eating other foods. Sometimes these products can help ease parental guilt when buying treats. Of course, there are other ways to encourage and teach children to eat a lower-fat diet. These include eating less of such foods as cookies and chips, as well as less of dairy products made from whole milk, and emphasizing nutrient-rich foods, such as whole grains, fruits and vegetables, and lean meats.

Using the Food Guide Pyramid to Lower Dietary Fat

BREADS AND CEREALS As the base of the pyramid, this food group should be maximized, since the majority of the choices are low in fat and are sources of fiber.

FOOD SELECTIONS

- Buy more breads, pitas, and rolls (preferably wheat, rye, or pumpernickel), English muffins, tortillas, most cereals (oat, corn, wheat, rice, multigrain), pasta, rice, low-fat crackers, and pretzels.
- Go easy on low-fat baked goods (sources of sugar)—such as graham or animal crackers, vanilla wafers, fig bars, and angel food cake—home-prepared baked goods using standard ingredients, mixes for muffins and pancakes, reduced-fat granola cereals and bars, and other high-sugar cereals.
- Buy less of these: high-fat crackers (most butter or cheese types), croissants, egg noodles, commercial baked goods, packaged pastas or rice with creamy or cheese sauces, and regular granola cereals and bars.

SHOPPING AND LABEL READING HINTS

- Bread group servings should be fairly low in fat content at 0–2 grams of total fat per serving.
- Items labeled "fat free" have no fat and no saturated fat. However, "reduced fat" and "light" products simply contain less fat than the original or full-fat versions, so be sure to check the grams of fat per serving.

- Compare items that are equal in total fat content and select the one that is lowest in saturated fat content.
- Read the list of ingredients to see if the item uses more liquid oil as opposed to hydrogenated oil. The first ingredient is the most predominant by weight, with others listed in descending order.

FOOD PREPARATION IDEAS

- Use a small amount of tub margarine or, better yet, jam or marmalade on toast, breads, and English muffins.
- As a sandwich spread, use a thin coating of ketchup, mustard, reduced-fat mayonnaise, or low-fat salad dressing. Try a slice of fresh tomato!
- Use tomato sauce for pasta.
- Top potatoes with a small amount of tub margarine, reduced or nonfat sour cream or salad dressing, or salsa.
- When using mixes for rice, stuffing, or pasta, use 1 percent low-fat milk and tub margarine. But cut the amount of margarine called for by half and replace the difference with water or 1 percent milk. Or skip the margarine completely!
- When preparing pancakes, quick breads, muffins, or baked goods, use an egg substitute (¼ cup = 1 whole egg) or egg whites (2 whites = 1 whole egg). In addition, use liquid vegetable oil, preferably canola, in place of solid shortening or margarine. Experiment with reducing the amount of oil needed and replacing the difference with unsweetened applesauce, baby plums (for chocolate recipes), or nonfat sour cream. For example: When preparing brownies from a mix that calls for 1 whole egg and ½ cup oil (8 tablespoons), substitute 2 tablespoons of oil, 6 tablespoons of baby plums, and 2 egg whites. The fat saved per brownie is 4.6 grams.

- For any home baked goods that call for chocolate, substitute cocoa powder and vegetable oil as directed on the cocoa package to substantially reduce saturated fat.
- Make grains and beans the center of a meal instead of side dishes. Examples are pasta with marinara sauce and chili or casseroles that use smaller amounts of meat, poultry, or fish.

VEGETABLES With few exceptions (olives and avocados), vegetables have almost no fat or saturated fat and always have no cholesterol. Eat them liberally, but be sure that preparation methods don't boost the fat content.

FOOD SELECTIONS

- Buy more of these: fresh or plain frozen (no sauce) or plain canned (preferably with no salt added) vegetables and vegetable juices.
- Go easy on oven-baked French fries, mixes that use dehydrated potatoes or potato flakes, olives, and avocados.
- Choose less of these: fried vegetables, vegetables that are canned or frozen with butter, cheese, or cream sauces, and French fries.

SHOPPING AND LABEL READING HINTS

- Vegetable choices should have minimal fat content (less than 1 gram per serving). If you splurge on a fried vegetable or one with sauce, account for it in your fat gram allowance.

FOOD PREPARATION IDEAS

- Instead of butter, add lemon juice, butter-flavored granules, spices, salsa, or a splash of fat-free or reduced-fat Italian dressing, other fat-free dressing, or vinegar to cooked vegetables for taste.

- Prepare your own cream sauces by using spices, 1 percent low-fat milk, tub margarine, and a little flour or cornstarch. Or try a dollop of non-fat sour cream or yogurt instead.
- Stir-frying vegetables may require more oil than is desirable. Instead, steam the vegetables in some water or in the microwave until they are tender-crisp. Then use just a little oil to combine them on the stove.
- When making vegetable casseroles that call for condensed soups, buy the reduced-fat versions. If you cannot find a reduced-fat soup, use half the can and replace the other half with evaporated skim milk.
- When preparing mashed potatoes, use 1 percent low-fat milk, a small amount of tub margarine, and additional butter-flavored granules for flavor.
- If the family really enjoys French fries, use frozen steak fries and bake them in the oven.
- If the only way children will eat vegetables is with an accompanying dip, try mixing nonfat sour cream or yogurt with a reduced-fat salad dressing or salsa. Salsa and reduced-fat salad dressings can also be used alone.
- Keep on introducing vegetables. Don't be frustrated if children refuse to try a new vegetable the first several times it is served. The more they see it prepared and offered, the more likely they will be to try it. Serve a new vegetable along with a favorite family meal.

FRUITS Like vegetables, fruits have almost no fat and saturated fat and never have cholesterol. Some desserts, such as fruit in cream or whipped cream, can contain a lot of fat.

FOOD SELECTIONS

- Buy more of these: all fresh, canned, jarred, dried, or plain frozen fruit, and 100 percent fruit juices.
- Go easy on sugar-sweetened juices.
- Choose less of these: fried fruit chips (banana, for example) and fruits in cream sauce.

SHOPPING AND LABEL READING HINTS

- Fruit choices should have minimal fat content (less than 1 gram per serving). If you splurge, account for it in your fat gram allowance.

FOOD PREPARATION IDEAS

- Offer fruits as snacks and for dessert.
- Top homemade pancakes or waffles with chopped fruit.
- Put fruit in hot and cold cereals.
- Blend fruit with 1 percent low-fat milk and serve over ice for a sweet treat.
- Top off low-fat frozen desserts with chopped fruit or stir fruit into low-fat or nonfat yogurt.
- Combine dried fruits with cereals, unsalted pretzels, and a small amount of nuts or seeds for a healthy snack.
- Use a little low-fat yogurt or honey as a dip for freshly cut fruit.
- Incorporate fruit into main dishes, such as pineapple with chicken.
- Add canned or fresh fruit to gelatin and top with a small dollop of nondairy whipped topping or low-fat yogurt.

DAIRY PRODUCTS Dairy products are important sources of protein, calcium, and phosphorus. Low-fat and nonfat items have equal if not greater quantities of these nutrients than their full-fat counterparts. Full-fat dairy products are a major source of fat, saturated fat, and cholesterol in the diets of most children. If children are currently using whole milk products, try cutting down to 2 percent fat products for children over 2 years of age. In several weeks try 1 percent milk and maybe eventually even skim milk. Again, cutting back gradually may be more palatable to the family. Try the same approach for low-fat cheeses. Full-fat cheese has about 10 grams of fat per ounce. When embarking on a lower-fat way of life, try cheeses that have about 5 or 6 grams of fat per ounce and then move to those that have no more than 3 grams of fat per ounce.

FOOD SELECTIONS

- Buy more of these: 1 percent low-fat milk, nonfat and low-fat yogurt, low-fat cottage cheese, low-fat and nonfat frozen desserts (no more than 3 grams of fat per ½ cup), and cheese with no more than 3 grams of fat per ounce.
- Go easy on light cream cheese, 2 percent low-fat milk, frozen desserts with 3–5 grams of fat per ½ cup, and cheese with 4–6 grams of fat per ounce.
- Choose less of these: whole milk, ice cream, and frozen desserts with more than 5 grams of fat per ½ cup, full-fat cheese and cottage cheese, regular cream cheese, cream, half and half, whipped cream, and whole-milk or custard-style yogurt.

SHOPPING AND LABEL READING HINTS

- Optimally, the milk group should have no more than 2–3 grams of fat per serving. One serving is ½ cup of frozen desserts, 1 cup of milk or yogurt, ½ cup of cottage cheese, or 1½ ounces of full-fat cheese.

- Use 1 percent low-fat milk in place of cream or half and half in recipes.
- Use 1 percent low-fat milk when making puddings.
- If your children won't drink plain milk, a small amount of chocolate syrup is an acceptable addition. Better yet, blend the milk with fruit or a little low-fat flavored yogurt.
- Serve cubes of low-fat cheese and low-fat crackers as a snack.
- Purchase string cheeses instead of full-fat cheese; most are low in fat, but do check labels.
- Instead of buying ice cream and frozen yogurt with mixed-in foods that are high in fat, add to low-fat frozen desserts such items as crumbled reduced-fat cookies, low-fat granola cereal, dried fruit, or candy sprinkles.
- When ordering pizza, either ask for half the amount of cheese or inquire if part-skim cheese is available. Or get cheese only on half the pizza, with the other half topped only by vegetables and tomato sauce.

MEAT, POULTRY, FISH, AND ALTERNATIVES This group provides protein, B vitamins, iron, and zinc, so it is an important part of a heart-healthy diet. Do be aware, however, that most foods from this group contain fat, saturated fat, and cholesterol. Choices in this food group vary greatly in fat content. A good low-fat choice typically has 3–5 grams of fat per ounce. Some foods, such as eggs and liver, though not high in total fat, have a tremendous amount of cholesterol. For this reason, moderation in this food group is important.

- Buy more of these: legumes (peas and beans); fish (fresh or frozen, canned tuna, salmon, and sardines in water); poultry (all skinless types, deli turkey and chicken breast, turkey pastrami, ground turkey and chicken); beef (90 percent lean ground beef, flank steak, deli roast beef, London broil, top round, eye round roast, sirloin, filet mignon); pork (center, loin, tenderloin, ham, Canadian bacon); lamb (leg, shoulder chop); shellfish (crab, clams, oysters, mussels, scallops, lobster, and shrimp); and other meat products, such as low-fat sausage, hot dogs, deli meats, and bacon, that have no more than 3 grams of fat per ounce.
- Go easy on deli meats, hot dogs, sausage, and bacon with 4–6 grams of fat per ounce, eggs (no more than 3–4 per week), organ meats (once a month is okay), ground beef with 15 percent fat content, peanut butter (preferably natural, because it is low in hydrogenated fat) and nuts and seeds.
- Choose fewer of these: fried fish, seafood, and chicken, poultry with skin, regular bacon, spareribs, regular bologna, salami, liverwurst, and similar deli meats, regular ground beef, meat or poultry pot pies.

SHOPPING AND LABEL READING HINTS

- Optimally, food choices from the meat group should have no more than 3–5 grams of fat per serving.
- If your family enjoys frozen entrées, purchase those with no more than 10 grams of fat per serving.
- Ask for nutrition information pamphlets at fast food restaurants. Major chains have pamphlets available to assist customers in making appropriate food choices.

FOOD PREPARATION IDEAS

- Use "meal extenders," such as rice, pasta, legumes, and vegetables in ground beef dishes.
- Trim off all visible fat before preparing. Remove skin from poultry before cooking.
- To incorporate ground turkey into menus, begin by mixing half turkey with half lean ground beef to get used to the different taste. Be sure to use ground turkey breast without skin.
- Bake, broil, grill, and poach meat, poultry, fish, and shellfish. Refrain from frying in oil or pan-frying because the fat cooks back into the food.
- If your family likes fried foods, try oven-frying in place of pan-frying. Coat pieces of chicken, fish, or pork in 1 percent low-fat milk or egg whites and dip them in flavored dry bread crumbs. Place the pieces on a cookie sheet coated with nonstick spray and again spray the top of the meat. Bake until the bread crumbs are golden brown and crisp. Turn halfway through baking.
- Buy a meat loaf rack so that fat drips out while the meat loaf is baking. Use a rack when roasting meats or poultry to drain away fat.
- Eliminate additional fat from ground beef recipes by rinsing the sautéed ground beef under hot water before adding the remaining ingredients.
- Remove fat from gravies by using a gravy separator. This inexpensive device looks like a watering can with a spout that pours from the bottom. Fat rises to the top, so the juice can be poured out while leaving the fat behind.
- Remember to control portion sizes. No more than 6 ounces of cooked meats a day are needed, less for younger children. To the eye, this amount of meat looks like two decks of cards.
- Use reduced-fat salad dressings when making chicken or tuna salad.
- When eating at fast food restaurants and menu choices are limited, the best option is a grilled chicken sandwich, with a roast beef sandwich in second place. Believe it or not, a hamburger is lower in fat than a fried fish or fried chicken sandwich. Instead of ordering French fries to accompany the meat, choose a salad with reduced-fat dressing or a baked potato (with sauces on the side).
- At a deli-style restaurant, the best choices for meat are roast beef, turkey, and ham with mustard or a small touch of mayonnaise. Sandwiches that already have mayonnaise mixed in are almost always high in fat.

FATS AND SWEETS

- Servings from this food group should be chosen in the context of a child's overall fat allotment.
- Use in moderation liquid oils (preferably canola or olive, though corn, sunflower, safflower, sesame, and soybean are also okay), regular or light tub or squeeze margarine made from liquid vegetable oil, salad dressing made from acceptable oils (preferably reduced-fat or nonfat), and candies such as jelly beans and hard candies.
- Use infrequently butter, lard, bacon fat, coconut, stick margarine, shortening, products with palm or coconut oil, potato and corn chips, doughnuts, and high-fat pies, cakes, and cookies.

SHOPPING AND LABEL READING HINTS

- Read the Nutrition Facts section of food labels to see the grams of total fat and saturated fat or vegetable fats. Purchase foods with the lowest total and saturated fat.
- Read the list of ingredients on packaged foods and choose those containing liquid vegetable oils and margarine over those that contain hydrogenated or partially hydrogenated oils. Avoid palm or coconut oils.

FOOD PREPARATION IDEAS

- Use nonstick or cast-iron skillets and nonstick sprays.
- Try oven-frying instead of pan-frying or deep-frying (see above, under the meat, poultry, fish, and shellfish group).
- Learn to flavor foods with nonfat items, such as butter-flavored granules, spices, and lemon or lime juice.
- To reduce the amount of oil or fat needed when sautéing, keep a lid on the skillet to retain the moisture from the food.

A Practical Example

Let's take an older child's typical eating pattern and demonstrate how a few simple changes can really reduce the saturated fat, total fat, and cholesterol content of his or her diet. This also demonstrates once again that moderation and balance are most important and that favorite foods need not be eliminated.

Breakfast
½ cup orange juice
1 cup sweetened cereal
1 cup whole milk
½ banana
1 slice white toast
1 teaspoon butter

Snack
4 peanut-butter-filled snack crackers
4-ounce box apple-grape juice

Lunch
Bologna sandwich
   2 slices white bread
   2 ounces bologna
   2 teaspoons mayonnaise

1-ounce bag corn chips
1 cup chocolate milk (2 percent fat)

Snack
3 chocolate sandwich cookies
1 cup whole milk

Dinner
Fast food meal
   8 pieces chicken nuggets with barbecue sauce
   1 small order fries
   apple pie
   1 cup soft drink

Snack
3 cups microwave popcorn
½ cup cranberry juice

Nutritional Analysis
40 percent fat calories (exceeds 30 percent calories)
15 percent saturated fat calories (exceeds 10 percent calories)
222 milligrams cholesterol (acceptable)

   Now, looking at this menu, try to identify the sources of excessive saturated fat and total fat. They are whole milk, bologna, cookies, and fried foods. Is it necessary to eliminate all of these foods? Certainly not! In the modified diet, the items that have been changed are printed in italics.

Breakfast
½ cup orange juice
1 cup sweetened cereal
1 cup 1 percent low-fat milk
½ banana
1 slice wheat toast
1 teaspoon tub margarine

Snack
4 peanut-butter-filled snack crackers
4-ounce box apple-grape juice

Lunch
Turkey sandwich
  2 slices rye bread
  2 ounces turkey breast
  2 teaspoons mayonnaise
  ½ tomato
1 carrot, cut into sticks
1-ounce bag corn chips
1 cup chocolate milk (2 percent fat)

Snack
3 fig bar cookies
1 cup 1 percent low-fat milk

Dinner
Fast food meal
  1 hamburger
  1 small order fries
  Side salad with 1 packet reduced-fat dressing
  1 frozen yogurt sundae with strawberry topping
  1 cup cola-type drink

Snack
3 cups microwave popcorn
½ cup cranberry juice

Nutritional Analysis
25 percent fat calories (acceptable, even a little
  low on this day)
7 percent saturated fat calories (acceptable)
70 milligrams cholesterol (even better)

As the second meal plan shows, only a few changes are necessary to substantially reduce the total fat, saturated fat, and cholesterol content of a child's diet. Much to the relief of many children and their parents, such foods as French fries, corn chips, peanut-butter snack crackers, and microwave popcorn can be still eaten without guilt or worry! It's all about moderation and being attentive to healthy eating habits. Although some foods do provide a lot of calories from fat, other healthy choices don't, and overall balance is achieved.

Facts and Myths about Vitamins and Minerals

Vitamin Facts

Although vitamins do not provide energy to the body, they are essential nutrients that allow critical metabolic processes to occur. Vitamins are essential in the diet because the human body usually cannot manufacture them. Over the years functions have been ascribed to vitamins by observing what happens in various states of vitamin deficiency. Vitamins are grouped into two major classes: fat-soluble vitamins, including vitamins A, D, E, and K, and water-soluble vitamins, including the B complex vitamins and vitamin C.

> **MYTH** Vitamins give you energy.
> **FACT** Protein, fat, and carbohydrate provide energy (calories) to the body. Vitamins, minerals, and water are essential to the body but provide no energy.

FAT-SOLUBLE VITAMINS Vitamin A was discovered in the early twentieth century. Investigators discovered a fat-soluble substance that, when deficient, appeared to result in various diseases of the eye. That substance was found to be retinol, or vitamin A, and some of its chemically related compounds. Many fish are rich in vitamin A, and one form of vitamin A is the primary component of cod-liver oil. Yellow- and orange-colored foods, such as sweet potatoes, carrots, and squash, are rich in carotene, which is converted to retinol in the body. (Food sources and recommended

Tara Prather Liskov ▪ Jane Kerstetter ▪ Robert S. Baltimore ▪ Thomas Carpenter

TABLE 31.1

Fat-Soluble Vitamins

Vitamin	Food sources	Recommended intake	
Vitamin A	Liver, sweet potatoes, carrots, spinach, cantaloupe, winter squash	0–1 year	375 µg
		1–3 years	400 µg
		4–6 years	500 µg
		7–10 years	700 µg
		11–18 years (boys)	1000 µg
		11–18 years (girls)	800 µg
Vitamin D	Herring, salmon, sardines, milk, liver	0–6 months	7.5 µg cholecalciferol
		6 months–18 years	10 µg cholecalciferol
Vitamin E	Wheat-germ oil, corn oil, soybean oil, sunflower oil, milk, avocado	0–6 months	3 mg TE[a]
		6 months–1 year	4 mg TE
		1–3 years	6 mg TE
		4–10 years	7 mg TE
		11–18 years (boys)	10 mg TE
		11–18 years (girls)	8 mg TE
Vitamin K	Leafy green vegetables	0–6 months	5 µg
		6 months–1 year	10 µg
		1–3 years	15 µg
		4–6 years	20 µg
		7–10 years	30 µg
		11–14 years	45 µg
		15–18 years (boys)	65 µg
		15–18 years (girls)	55 µg

[a] TE = tocopherol equivalent

intakes of fat-soluble vitamins are provided in table 31.1.) Beta-carotene is currently being studied for its antioxidant properties, which may be protective against heart disease and some forms of cancer.

Deficiency of vitamin A is associated with night blindness. In countries where poor nutrition is common, vitamin A deficiency in children can mean a poor prognosis for the common infection measles. Like all fat-soluble vitamins, vitamin A can be stored in the body's fat tissue, so excessive intake can cause vitamin-toxicity or undesirable side effects. High doses of vitamin A can cause a potentially fatal condition known as retinoid toxicity, in which the bones begin to lose minerals rapidly, blood calcium levels become dangerously elevated, and hair and skin are shed.

Vitamin D was discovered shortly after "fat-soluble A" was isolated. This compound cured the bone disease known as rickets, which can develop when individuals are deprived of sunlight. It was eventually determined that the body can in fact make its own vitamin D, but ultraviolet rays of direct sunlight must be present for this to occur. It was also discovered that in order to function properly, vitamin D must be converted to more active compounds by the liver and kidney. The observation of repeated outbreaks of rickets in winter in northern climes led in the 1950s to the supplementation of vitamin D in cow's milk in the United States (see table 31.1). Although vitamin D deficiency may still occur, it is not common. The exclusively breastfed baby who does not go out-of-doors is at risk for the development of vitamin D deficiency rickets. However, because infant formula and cow's milk are supplemented with vitamin D, further vitamin D supplementation is necessary today only in specialized or unusual circumstances. As with vitamin A, vitamin D intoxication can occur, and it results in high levels of calcium in the blood.

Vitamin K was discovered in the late 1920s. It plays a role in the activation of clotting factors in the blood. For this reason, all newborns are given vitamin K to prevent bleeding disorders specific to low stores of vitamin K at birth. The bacteria that normally live in the human intestine synthesize some of the vitamin K that the body needs. Leafy green vegetables are the best sources of vitamin K (see table 31.1). Vitamin K deficiency occurs in severe liver disease and in fat malabsorptive states, such as cystic fibrosis, but otherwise it is relatively uncommon. Supplementation, if needed, is usually given by intramuscular injection.

Vitamin E is a fat-soluble vitamin that is actually a combination of several compounds called tocopherols and tocotrienols. The tocopherols, primarily alpha-tocopherol, provide most of the vitamin E activity. Vitamin E's most important function is as an antioxidant, which means it pro-tects other compounds from being oxidized. Oxidation of cells and other compounds in the body leads to their destruction through the production of damaging free radicals. Although vitamin C is also an antioxidant, it differs in its antioxidant properties from vitamin E because it is soluble in water. The fat solubility of vitamin E allows it to function within cell membranes, which are rich in fat-containing substances. The antioxidant properties of vitamins E and C, as well as beta-carotene, may help protect against heart disease and cancer in humans.

Vitamin E is found in a variety of foods but is most abundant in seed oils and nuts (see table 31.1). Vitamin E deficiency is rare in the United States but, when present, is associated with neuromuscular problems, such as loss of muscle coordination and reflexes, as well as with impaired vision and speech. Although vitamin E toxicity has not been proven, excessive intake is not recommended.

WATER-SOLUBLE VITAMINS Water-soluble vitamins function primarily as components of essential enzyme systems and are involved in energy metabolism. Because they are not usually stored in the body, they are best supplied daily, and vitamin toxicity is less of a concern. Water-soluble vitamins include the vitamin B complex and vitamin C. The vitamin B complex includes thiamine, riboflavin, niacin, vitamin B_6 (pyridoxine), folic acid, vitamin B_{12}, pantothenic acid, and biotin. Thiamine, riboflavin, niacin, and vitamin B_6 are widely distributed in foods. Healthy children usually obtain an adequate intake of these vitamins. Vitamin B_{12} is obtained from foods of animal origin only, so it would need to be supplemented to vegan vegetarians (see chapter 10). See table 31.2 for food sources and recommended intakes of the vitamin B complex.

TABLE 31.2

Water-Soluble Vitamins

Vitamin	Food sources	Recommended intake	
Thiamine	Pork, wheat germ, organ meats, legumes, whole-grain and enriched breads	0–6 months	0.3 mg
		6 months–1 year	0.4 mg
		1–3 years	0.7 mg
		4–6 years	0.9 mg
		7–10 years	1.0 mg
		11–14 years (boys)	1.3 mg
		15–18 years (boys)	1.5 mg
		11–18 years (girls)	1.1 mg
Riboflavin	Milk and milk products, liver, green leafy vegetables, eggs	0–6 months	0.4 mg
		6 months–1 year	0.5 mg
		1–3 years	0.8 mg
		4–6 years	1.1 mg
		7–10 years	1.2 mg
		11–14 years (boys)	1.5 mg
		15–18 years (boys)	1.8 mg
		11–18 years (girls)	1.3 mg
Niacin	Lean meats, poultry, fish, peanuts, brewer's yeast	0–6 months	5 mg NE[a]
		6 months–1 year	6 mg NE
		1–3 years	9 mg NE
		4–6 years	12 mg NE
		7–10 years	13 mg NE
		11–14 years (boys)	17 mg NE
		15–18 years (boys)	20 mg NE
		11–18 years (girls)	15 mg NE
Vitamin B_6 (pyridoxine)	Yeast, wheat germ, pork, liver, whole-grain cereals, legumes, potatoes, bananas, oatmeal	0–6 months	0.3 mg
		6 months–1 year	0.6 mg
		1–3 years	1.0 mg
		4–6 years	1.1 mg
		7–10 years	1.4 mg
		11–14 years (boys)	1.7 mg
		15–18 years (boys)	2.0 mg
		11–14 years (girls)	1.4 mg
		15–18 years (girls)	1.5 mg

TABLE 31.2
Continued

Vitamin	Food sources	Recommended intake	
Folic acid	Brewer's yeast, liver, green leafy vegetables, wheat germ	0–6 months	25 µg
		6 months–1 year	35 µg
		1–3 years	50 µg
		4–6 years	75 µg
		7–10 years	100 µg
		11–14 years	150 µg
		15–18 years (boys)	200 µg
		15–18 years (girls)	180 µg
Vitamin B$_{12}$	Liver, shellfish, milk, eggs, fish, yogurt	0–6 months	0.3 µg
		6 months–1 year	0.5 µg
		1–3 years	0.7 µg
		4–6 years	1.0 µg
		7–10 years	1.4 µg
		11–18 years	2.0 µg
Pantothenic acid	Liver, milk and milk products, egg yolk, yeast, beef, sweet potatoes	0–6 months	2 mg
		6 months–1 year	3 mg
		1–3 years	3 mg
		4–6 years	3–4 mg
		7–10 years	4–5 mg
		11–18 years	4–7 mg
Biotin	Organ meats, egg yolk, soybeans, yeast, milk, fish, nuts, oatmeal	0–6 months	10 µg
		6 months–1 year	15 µg
		1–3 years	20 µg
		4–6 years	25 µg
		7–10 years	30 µg
		11–18 years	30–100 µg
Vitamin C	Citrus fruits, tomatoes, raw leafy vegetables, strawberries, cantaloupe, cabbage, green peppers, potatoes	0–6 months	30 mg
		6 months–1 year	35 mg
		1–3 years	40 mg
		4–10 years	45 mg
		11–14 years	50 mg
		15–18 years	60 mg

[a] NE = niacin equivalent

Vitamin C, also called ascorbic acid, has many functions in the body. It is an antioxidant, is involved in the formation of collagen (an important component of connective tissue), helps in healing wounds, enhances the absorption of iron, and promotes resistance to infection. Vitamin C is abundant in citrus fruits, raw leafy vegetables, strawberries, and potatoes (see table 31.2). Scurvy is the deficiency disease associated with vitamin C that before the 1800s commonly afflicted sailors who were deprived of fresh fruits and vegetables for long periods. Although scurvy is now rare in developed countries, alcoholics, people with diets devoid of fruits and vegetables, and infants fed exclusively on cow's milk are groups at highest risk for vitamin C deficiency. Excesses of vitamin C are usually eliminated in the urine, but excessive intake can cause diarrhea. Also, "rebound scurvy" has occurred in people who suddenly stop taking large doses of vitamin C. The use of vitamin C as a cure for the common cold is controversial.

Mineral Facts

A mineral is an inorganic element (meaning that it does not contain carbon) obtained from water and soil. Minerals are incorporated into plants that thrive on water and soil. Animals obtain minerals from eating plants and drinking water, and humans obtain minerals from mineral-rich animal and plant foods. Minerals are essential for hundreds of life-sustaining body processes. They perform three basic functions. Some minerals (calcium, phosphorus, magnesium) are part of the structural integrity of such tissues as bone, teeth, and muscles. Many minerals are required for enzymes to function, and enzymes are needed for chemical reactions within the body. Other minerals called electrolytes (sodium, potassium, chloride) are involved in balancing fluids in the body and regulating the acid-base content of the blood.

The body loses minerals every day via the skin, urine, and the gastrointestinal tract. A well-balanced and varied diet generally provides adequate minerals to replace what has been lost and to support growth in children. Except for iron and possibly zinc, overt mineral deficiencies in healthy children in the United States are rare. Mineral deficiency generally results from poor dietary intake, increased mineral requirements (for growth or to heal wounds), or increased mineral losses (via the gastrointestinal tract or kidneys).

CALCIUM AND BONE HEALTH Calcium and phosphorus are important structural components of bones and teeth. In conjunction with magnesium, they regulate metabolic function in muscle and other body tissues (see table 31.1). Infants are born with about 200–250 grams of calcium in their immature skeleton, and the skeleton immediately develops rapidly in length, diameter, and composition. As bone grows, its porous matrix of protein strands retain calcium and phosphorus, making the bones strong and rigid. Babies derive these minerals from breast milk or infant formula.

Between ages 1 and 10, bone growth continues at a slower pace than in infancy. From age 10 to about 18, bones grow visibly longer, as the adolescent grows taller. Less obvious is the continued growth in density and thickness of the bones after they have reached their final length. In these years, large amounts of calcium are deposited daily in the skeleton. By the twentieth year of life, adult peak bone mass is almost fully attained. The adult skeleton contains about 1,000–1,200 grams of calcium, most of it deposited during adolescence (fig. 31.1). This amount is true for both males and females.

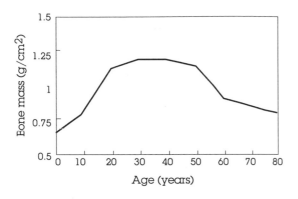

The condition known as osteoporosis ("porous bones"), in which bone mass decreases in density, making bones more porous and fragile, is a life-threatening epidemic, particularly in older women. Because osteoporosis is essentially irreversible, lifelong prevention strategies, including nutrition and physical activity, are essential. The most effective strategy for preventing osteoporosis is to maximize peak bone mass during childhood and adolescence. The higher the peak bone mass in early adulthood, the less likely an osteoporotic bone fracture will occur in late adulthood.

How much calcium should children consume? Guided by recent research, scientists at the National Institutes of Health (NIH) suggest a level that is higher than the 1989 Recommended Dietary Allowances (RDAs) for children (see table 31.3). The most recent nutritional surveys in the United States indicate that the average calcium intake of teenage girls and young adult women is critically low, far below NIH's recommendations. Although boys have a slightly higher level than girls, the calcium intake for most boys is still less than recommended by NIH.

The best sources of calcium are dairy products. Foods that are good sources of calcium are listed in table 31.3. A typical serving of a dairy food contains about 300 milligrams of calcium, so 3 to 4 servings of dairy products, in addition to a regular diet, are needed to achieve NIH's suggested level of intake for children. If children will not consume dairy products, parents should consider giving them a calcium supplement.

IRON-DEFICIENCY ANEMIA Low red blood cell counts, known as anemia, may originate from deficiencies in vitamin B_{12}, folic acid, and iron because all of these nutrients are involved in the development of red blood cells. Long-standing deficiencies in one, two, or all three of these important nutrients can cause anemia.

Of the three nutrients, iron deficiency is the most common. The highest incidence of iron deficiency appears in infants, young children, and menstruating adolescent girls and young women. Iron is the most important mineral in hemoglobin, which red blood cells use to carry oxygen to all living cells and tissues. Without adequate iron, all of the body's cells are deprived of oxygen and will malfunction to some degree. Iron-deficiency anemia, then, is really a systemic disorder.

A full-term infant is born with approximately 250–300 milligrams of iron, most in the form of hemoglobin in red blood cells. This natural endowment of iron is used for growth and will keep the infant healthy during the first 6 months of life. Iron supplementation from one or more foods (iron-fortified formula, iron-fortified cereal) should start between 4 and 6 months of age and should continue through the first year of life.

Iron-deficiency anemia is a worldwide health problem in children. Although improvements have been made in the past decade, iron-deficiency anemia remains the most prevalent nutri-

TABLE 31.3

Important Bone Minerals

Mineral	Basic functions	Deficiency signs	Food sources	Recommended intake
Calcium	Bone and tooth structure; important physiologic functions, including hormone release, muscle contraction, blood clotting, enzyme systems	*Mild:* no sign *Severe:* rickets, osteomalacia, osteoporosis, poor growth, muscle cramps, seizures	All dairy products, including milk, cheese, yogurt; other isolated foods including canned fish with bones, tofu (calcium set), turnip and mustard greens, broccoli, legumes, dried fruit	*0–6 months,* 400 mg *6 months–1 year,* 600 mg *1–5 years,* 800 mg *6–10 years,* 800–1,200 mg *11–24 years,* 1,200–1,500 mg
Phosphorus	Bone and tooth structure, cell membranes, energy metabolism	Bone loss, rickets, muscle weakness, neurologic problems	All protein foods, including meat, poultry, fish, eggs, milk, cheese, legumes; whole-grain products, soft drinks	*1–10 years,* 800 mg *11–18 years,* 1,200 mg
Magnesium	Component of bones, nerve transmission, protein synthesis, enzyme systems	Growth failure, muscle weakness, twitching or cramps, apathy; similar to acute manifestations of calcium deficiency	Legumes, nuts, whole-grain products, green leafy vegetables, seafood; processing substantially reduces magnesium levels in foods	*1–3 years,* 80 mg *4–6 years,* 120 mg *7–10 years,* 170 mg *Boys 11–14 years,* 270 mg *Boys 15–18 years,* 400 mg *Girls 11–14 years,* 280 mg *Girls 15–18 years,* 300 mg

ent deficiency in children in the United States and Canada. A U.S. public health directive for the year 2000 known as Healthy People 2000 has set a goal of reducing the prevalence of iron-deficiency anemia in children ages 1 to 4 to less than 3 percent.

The body's ability to absorb iron varies depending on the source of the iron. Heme iron, found in meats, poultry, and fish, is better absorbed than non-heme iron, which is found in vegetables, fruits, and grain products (table 31.4). On average, 10 to 16 percent of ingested iron is absorbed. Other factors in the diet also influence iron absorption. Vitamin C, meats, and gastric acid enhance iron absorption, whereas fiber, phytates, calcium, and tannins (found in tea and coffee) decrease the absorption of iron. Interestingly, for unknown reasons, iron from human milk is absorbed better than iron from cow's milk or infant

TABLE 31.4
Ensuring Adequate Iron Intake

Recommended Dietary Allowances (RDAs)

    All children 1–10 years: 10 mg

    Boys 11–18 years: 12 mg

    Girls 11–18 years: 15 mg

Food sources

    Liver, shellfish, meat, poultry, fish, egg yolk,

      legumes, enriched cereals, dark green vegetables

Absorption enhancers

    Vitamin C, meat, fish, poultry

Absorption inhibitors

    Fiber, phytates, calcium, tannins, oxalic acid

---

formula, though neither human nor cow's milk is a good source of iron.

If a child is iron-deficient, an iron-rich diet, a multivitamin with iron, or an iron supplement may be prescribed. Abdominal discomfort and constipation can be a side effect of iron supplementation. A common hazard in childhood is iron poisoning from the accidental over-ingestion of supplements. This type of poisoning is second in frequency to aspirin poisoning, with approximately 2,000 cases reported each year in the United States. Chronic overuse of iron supplements when not medically warranted can also damage the liver, pancreas, and heart.

ZINC Zinc is widely distributed in both plants and animals. In humans, this mineral is concentrated in the liver, pancreas, bones, kidneys, and some muscles. Many metabolic enzymes contain zinc. Zinc also helps to maintain structural integrity of materials inside cells. Zinc deficiency in children may contribute to poor growth and leads to anemia, impaired ability to heal wounds, and altered taste perception.

The body absorbs about 20 percent of ingested

zinc. Absorption is enhanced by concurrent protein intake, as well as by glucose and lactose. Zinc from breast milk is absorbed better than zinc from cow's milk. In contrast, fiber decreases the body's absorption of zinc, while iron and zinc compete for absorption. For this reason, mineral supplements that contain high doses of zinc, iron, or both are not recommended. High intake of calcium can also decrease zinc (and iron) absorption.

The RDAs for zinc in infants through adolescents is between 5 and 15 milligrams per day. Good sources of zinc are meat, fish, poultry, and dairy products. Shellfish, whole-grain cereal, dry beans, and nuts also contain substantial amounts of zinc.

TRACE MINERALS A number of trace minerals are important for metabolic function in the body, including copper, selenium, iodine, chromium, manganese, and molybdenum. These minerals are key components of enzyme systems and often interact with other minerals. For instance, copper aids iron absorption, whereas excessive zinc can impair copper absorption. Iron and zinc, as mentioned above, can each inhibit the absorption of the other. The body needs very small amounts of these minerals, and a well-balanced diet will ensure adequate intake. The basic functions, food sources, and recommended intakes of important trace minerals are summarized in table 31.5.

Vitamin and Mineral Supplementation

There is considerable scientific information regarding the sources, functions, and need for intake of vitamins and minerals and the role they play in maintaining good health in children. Nevertheless, various aspects of the actions of these micronutrients continue to be topics of medical research.

TABLE 31.5
Selected Trace Minerals

Mineral	Basic function	Food sources	Recommended intake
Copper	Enzyme systems; hemoglobin synthesis; normal iron metabolism; connective and nerve tissue function	Shellfish, organ meats, nuts, legumes, cereals, poultry, dried fruits, hard water and copper piping	1–3 years, 0.7–1.0 mg 4–6 years, 1.0–1.5 mg 7–10 years, 1.0–2.0 mg 11+ years, 1.5–2.5 mg
Chromium	Glucose metabolism	Brewer's yeast, oysters, liver, potatoes, corn oil, whole grains	1–3 years, 20–80 μg 4–6 years, 30–120 mg 7+ years, 50–200 mg
Selenium	Critical for glutathione, peroxidase (an important antioxidant enzyme)	Brazil nuts, seafoods, organ meats, meat, poultry, garlic; dependent upon amount present in water and soil	1–6 years, 20 mg 7–10 years, 10–20 mg Boys 11–14 years, 40 mg Boys 15–18 years, 50 mg Girls 11–14 years, 45 mg Girls 15–18 years, 50 mg
Iodine	Part of the thyroid hormones	Iodized salt, seafood, vegetables grown in iodine-rich soil	1–3 years, 70 μg 4–6 years, 90 μg 7–10 years, 120 μg Boys 11–18 years, 150 μg Girls 11–18 years, 150 μg

Scientific knowledge of vitamins and minerals is constantly being refined and revised, so speculation on actual needs continues to occur.

A common fallacy is that if a vitamin or mineral is good, then more of that vitamin or mineral must be better. The use of vitamins and minerals in doses far above officially recommended amounts now forms part of a number of commercial dietary supplements and fad diets. Often these doses, termed "mega doses," are ten to hundreds of times the RDA. A well-balanced American diet provides at least the recommended quantities of all known vitamins and minerals, and the intake of vitamins and minerals in excess of the minimum daily requirements has no known benefits for *normal* individuals. The RDAs ensure sufficient vitamin and mineral intake to provide for even unusual stresses and physical activities.

There are, of course, exceptions, and in some cases high-calorie, vitamin- and mineral-enriched supplements may help people with certain well-defined diseases and abnormal metabolic states. People who have been starved, those who have had a long convalescence from surgery, those with certain chronic diseases, such as cystic fibrosis, other intestinal malabsorption diseases, some cancers, and chronic infections may be aided by high protein and calorie supplements with added vitamins and minerals. But there is no scientific evidence or even logic to suggest that similar products will enhance the performance of normal healthy people.

Oversupplementation is not harmless. There are cases of children who have been severely harmed by ingestion of huge quantities of vitamins; their parents were usually responding to claims reported in the media or the advice of nutritionists who were not following usual medical practice. Reports of occasional poisoning by megadoses of vitamin A or D have been published in the medical literature, and megadoses of vitamin C have been shown to cause kidney stones. Another notorious example of the harm diet supplements can cause occurred in 1989, when many people were poisoned, some fatally, by the amino acid L-tryptophan. Many health food stores sold L-tryptophan—which was claimed to be helpful in treating insomnia, pain, depression, premenstrual syndrome, and weight gain—even though it had no demonstrated health benefits. The ensuing outbreak of the eosinophilia-myalgia syndrome, a painful and dangerous disease, resulted in a number of deaths.

Although mineral and vitamin supplementation may help ensure adequate intake of these nutrients, it will not correct an inherently bad diet. Vitamin and mineral supplementation will not help a diet that is too high in total calories, total and saturated fat, cholesterol, or protein, low in fiber, or high in simple sugars. Moreover, many of the foods we commonly consume are already supplemented or fortified with vitamins and minerals. Commercial bread products are enriched with niacin, riboflavin, thiamine, and iron. Milk is fortified with vitamin D and may have other added nutrients. Many breakfast cereals are enriched with a variety of minerals. Calcium-fortified juice is also available. Iron-fortified infant cereals, which are typically introduced around 4–6 months when the infant's iron stores are dwindling, are an excellent way to ensure adequate iron intake in infancy.

Recommendations

There is substantial evidence that the type of diet advocated by the U.S. Department of Agriculture and presented in the Food Guide Pyramid (see chapter 4) provides more than an adequate amount of essential vitamins and minerals and that the RDAs for vitamins and minerals are well in excess of the minimum requirements. Even when children eat poorly balanced diets, vitamin and mineral deficiency is rare in the United States.

A key population to which vitamin and mineral supplementation is marketed is healthy children. Many families consider a daily vitamin and mineral supplement for each member to be appropriate in their diet. Though probably unnecessary, taking such a supplement as "insurance" against possible dietary deficiencies is acceptable, as long as it is not used in place of a healthy diet. Children in strict vegetarian households, exclusively breastfed older infants, and children with certain medical illnesses may benefit from a daily supplement. If a supplement is taken, it should not supply more than the RDA for any individual nutrient. Generic and store-brand supplements are chemically identical to more expensive "natural" or name-brand supplements, so their use is perfectly acceptable and usually less expensive.

Water: Drinking for the Health of It

This chapter is about water—the soup stock of life. It explains why water is important and what happens when too little or too much water is consumed. Water is even more essential to the body than food. A person can live without food for several weeks, but a person can survive without water for only several days. Water is by far the largest component of the body, as well as the most plentiful substance in the diet. The body of a baby is 70–85 percent water, whereas the body of an average adult is 60–70 percent water. Without water survival is not possible because water is needed in nearly every chemical re-

> **MYTH** Drinking water is the only way to fulfill your daily fluid needs.
>
> **FACT** Although we get most of our fluids from drinking, foods also provide some water. Some foods, like watermelon, are high in water content. In addition, all liquids provide fluid to the body.

action that occurs in the body. Water plays vital roles in digestion, absorption of nutrients, growth and repair of tissues, removal of waste products through urine, and temperature control. Without water, the body would not be able to harvest energy from food or even use energy to work or play or think.

A Natural Balancing Act

The body contains water in three places: in the bloodstream, in tissues, and in cells. These compartments are interconnected and water can move back and forth between them. For example, when

· ·

Elahna Paul ▪ Lisa Devine ▪ Norman Siegel

food and drink are consumed water moves from the intestines to the bloodstream for distribution to all tissues of the body. The tissues and organs use water for metabolic reactions, structural support, and suspension of nutrients. Water bathes the cells on the inside and outside and keeps them moist. Water provides cells with nutrients from the bloodstream and washes away waste products.

Dehydration occurs when the body does not have enough water. Try to imagine what might happen if there wasn't enough water in the body. Fluid in the bloodstream would be low, and blood flow would be so sluggish that nutrients wouldn't be delivered properly to cells. And then, adding insult to injury, the undernourished cells would accumulate metabolic waste products (that are normally washed away), poisoning cells that are already starving. Minor dehydration is easily corrected by drinking fluids; severe dehydration can permanently damage organs through the build-up of natural metabolic waste products.

Now try to imagine what could happen if there was too much water in the body. Think of an elderly woman with heart problems and swollen feet, or a little boy who has had complicated surgery and looks puffy around the eyes. The swelling in these examples is called edema, and it happens when extra fluid and salt are pushed out of the bloodstream and into the tissues of the body. As long as this extra water in the tissue spaces of the body remains outside the cells, edema is not usually dangerous. In rare circumstances, however, edema can become a problem if the extra water begins to fill the lungs with fluid and impairs breathing or if it moves inside the cells and builds pressure. Too much water in brain cells, for example, can increase the pressure inside the skull enough to induce seizures or a coma. Another disorder, water intoxication, occurs when too much water is combined with not enough salt. Thus, not only is the amount of water in the body important, but the balance of water and other nutrients is critical to keep people well nourished and water distributed safely between cells, tissues, and the bloodstream.

Maintaining the Balance

In older children and adults, water is balanced by the kidneys and by the thirst center in the brain. These regulators help replace the water that is lost naturally every day. These continuous water losses are called insensible losses. Breathing is one natural way that water is lost from the tissues of the body because the exhaled air has moisture in it. In the cold weather this moisture can be seen as mist in the breath. A second source of water loss that is difficult to perceive and measure is the moisture that evaporates from the surface of the skin. Babies lose relatively more water through their skin than older children because their surface area (amount of skin) is large in proportion to their weight. The risk of dehydration through water evaporation is an important reason to protect babies from the sun and heat and to make sure that they drink sufficient fluids in hot weather. The most obvious daily water loss occurs through elimination in urine. The kidneys require a minimum supply of water in order to make enough urine to eliminate the body's daily metabolic waste products. Water is also lost in stools and in tears.

Eating and drinking are the only natural ways to replenish fluid in the body. It may be a surprise to learn that water is found not only in liquids but also in most foods. Fruits and vegetables are composed of 80–95 percent water, meats contain about 50 percent water, and even breads and grains contain 25–35 percent water. People regulate their water balance without realizing it. After a heavy workout or after eating salty food, for example, a person will become very thirsty and drink extra water. Excessive water losses and salt overload stimulate the thirst center in the brain, triggering the sensation of thirst. When the person consumes enough water to correct these imbalances, a normal salt and water equilibrium is restored. Because the water requirement varies day to day (and varies person to person), there is no set Recommended Dietary Allowance (RDA).

In general, healthy older children and adults can drink as much fluid as they like without negative consequences. They are incapable of drinking too much water to dangerously dilute their bloodstream. Normally functioning, fully matured kidneys can remove excess water and conserve water as needed. A person with abnormal kidney function, however, may have impaired excretion of water and may need to limit the intake of fluids to avoid overloading the body and causing water intoxication. People with medical conditions that cause excessive salt loss are similarly at risk.

The kidneys of infants and younger children are less efficient. Even a perfectly healthy baby has immature kidney function and therefore has problems excreting large amounts of water. Because their kidneys aren't fully developed, babies are vulnerable to water imbalance. For this reason, it is important to mix infant formula properly and not feed a baby formula that is too concentrated or too diluted. Breast milk and properly mixed infant formula contain a constant balance of salt, water, and other nutrients that a baby's kidneys can handle. Under normal conditions, infants do not require extra water.

The "naturally" impaired kidney function of very young children is the reason doctors advise using one of the commercially available oral electrolyte solutions when a baby is sick and unable to take breast milk or formula (see chapter 11). These solutions contain the appropriate amount of minerals and water. A sick infant who receives only plain water, fruit juices, or overdiluted formula for several days may become at risk for water intoxication. Symptoms of water intoxication are lethargy or extreme fatigue. If the water intoxication is not treated, a lethargic child can lapse into a coma or develop seizures. Doctors can measure the balance of salt and water in the blood (serum electrolytes) to determine whether a child has water intoxication.

Dehydration: Too Much Water down the Tubes

Babies and young children must depend on others to provide them with fluids to replace natural water losses. It is important, therefore, to understand how water is lost, what happens when water is lost, and what needs to be done about dehydration. A newborn's average fluid requirements range from 16 to 24 ounces per day, increasing to 32 to 40 ounces per day by age 1. As children grow, they learn to communicate and ask for beverages when they become thirsty. Water balance then becomes automatic, just as in adults, and water imbalance problems become likely only during episodes of vomiting, diarrhea, or fever.

As described above, everyone loses water all the time and replaces it on a daily basis. If the daily diet completely lacks water, then normal ongoing insensible water losses will result in dehydration within several days. Moreover, the amount of fluid lost changes with one's level of activity and state of health. Anything that increases metabolic rate (exercise, pain, illness, stress) also increases water losses and therefore increases daily water requirements. With a fever, for example, evaporation from the skin is increased in an attempt to reduce the temperature of the body through sweat. With a cold or other respiratory illness, children

TABLE 32.1
Dehydration: What to Look For

Dehydration	What to do
Mild dehydration causes decreased amounts and/or frequency of urine; urine is more concentrated, with a deeper amber color and a stronger smell than usual. Saliva may be decreased.	Give fluids[a] and contact your doctor
Moderate dehydration produces even less urine, along with dry mouth and dry eyes; the fontanel (baby's soft spot) and eyes may be sunken. The skin starts to feel abnormal and the heart starts to race.	Give fluids and see your doctor
Severe dehydration is like moderate dehydration without any urine; the child may be lethargic (too sleepy) or irritable (too cranky) or just too sick (vomiting, diarrhea) to drink enough.	See your doctor or go to the emergency room
Shock is severe dehydration so bad that the skin color is an abnormal blue-gray and the skin temperature is cool to the touch (because the blood pressure is too low).	Go to the emergency room immediately!

[a] Diluted juice, flat soda, or commercially prepared rehydration solutions

breathe faster than usual and therefore lose more water than they normally would through the lungs. These increased needs for water explain why a sick child can become dehydrated faster than a healthy child and why a sick child needs to drink more fluids than a healthy one (see chapter 11).

In addition to water losses through skin and respiratory evaporation and urine, large amounts of water can be lost in the gastrointestinal tract. For example, children with vomiting and diarrhea (gastroenteritis) can lose amounts of fluid that exceed their daily maintenance requirements. To avoid dehydration, a child with gastroenteritis needs daily maintenance fluid plus replacement of the volume of stool and vomitus. If the child cannot drink enough to keep up with losses or is vomiting and unable to keep anything down, parents should seek medical attention from a qualified health care provider who will assess the

situation and offer guidance for preventing severe dehydration.

Kidneys, as noted above, are important regulators of fluid status. When the body has an adequate amount of water, a child will produce normal amounts of urine. As a child becomes dehydrated, the kidneys conserve water and urine output gradually decreases. A decrease in the frequency and amount of urine that a child is making is an early warning of dehydration (signs of dehydration are listed in table 32.1). Parents can prevent serious problems from developing by giving extra fluids. Because kidneys of infants and young children are unable to conserve water as well as adults', these groups are particularly susceptible to dehydration. Anyone who is too ill to drink enough fluids to replenish their ongoing losses should seek medical attention.

Salt: The Spice of Life or the Taste of Doom?

In the past three decades a number of divergent and often contradictory trends have surfaced in the dietary habits of Americans, especially regarding the intake of salt. These diverse trends have led to such extreme manifestations as, on the one hand, the practice of salt loading in athletes, and on the other, the production of salt-deficient formula for infants. The contribution of a high-salt diet to high blood pressure and heart disease has led some to pursue a low-salt diet with near religious zeal. For certain people, this is quite appropriate, but the application of this approach to everyone, especially to growing children, can be harmful. The predominant American habit, however, is the unconscious consumption of high-salt foods, especially fast and convenient foods. Clearly, the best approach would be to seek a balance between these extremes. Where this balance exists, though, is often obscured by the confounding practices of alarmist media reports, misleading advertising, and confusing product labeling. For a clearer understanding of dietary salt, it is useful to have some knowledge of what salt does in the body and how having either too much or

> **MYTH** If children eat a low-salt diet, they will not have high blood pressure.
>
> **FACT** It is reasonable to reduce an unnecessarily high salt intake, especially if there is a family history of high blood pressure or heart disease. In healthy children, though, moderate salt intake is acceptable.

· · · · · · · · · · · · · · · · · · · ·

Scott Van Why ▪ Lisa Devine

too little of this good thing can be harmful. An important caveat to bear in mind throughout this chapter is that any divergence from an average salt intake, whether an increase or a restriction, should be undertaken only with the guidance of a physician and the assistance of a dietitian.

What Is Salt?

Salt is an ionic compound consisting of positive and negative ions that form a crystalline solid at room temperature. Because many varied ions exist in nature, there are thousands of different salts. For example, common dietary "salt substitutes" are actually salts that contain potassium rather than sodium. Common table salt is composed of two ions, sodium (Na^+) and chloride (Cl^-); both are important in a variety of biological functions. However, most nutritional concerns focus on sodium. Thus, a "low-salt diet" is more precisely termed a low-sodium diet. This distinction is important because sodium can be consumed in forms other than table salt. It is also found, for example, as sodium bicarbonate in baking soda, as sodium benzoate in lunch meat, and as sodium caseinate in coffee creamer.

Why do we have such a taste for the substance? An understanding of the historical and biological roles of salt may answer this question and explain why it is often called the "spice of life."

Historical Perspective

For the greatest part of human history, salt was a precious commodity in areas geographically remote from the sea. This, in part, can be explained by the general requirement for a certain amount of salt for growth and overall health. The biological need for salt, then, may be responsible for our taste for salt (see chapter 3). Contrary to modern views, in earlier ages, a high-salt diet contributed to health through multiple effects. For example, the ready availability of salt would have improved survival from epidemic diarrheal illnesses, in which large quantities of salt and water are lost from the body. In addition, salt as a food preservative ensured a steady, regular supply of food to reduce malnourishment and starvation. Before the development of refrigeration, the preservation of meats was limited to a few techniques, such as smoking or curing. Salt curing was an effective and efficient method of preserving meat that persists to this day. And although salt pork is not widely consumed today, hams are still cured with salt, as are some kosher foods. Certain terms that persist echo past practices of preserving meat: "corned beef" refers not to the presence of corn but to the kernels or "corns" of salt used to cure the beef. Americans have a strong tradition of high salt consumption that reinforces the taste for salt. Lest the power of taste be underestimated, it should be recalled that the desire for spices to supplement salt spurred the Europeans to explore regions of the world unknown to them and to trade with East Asian cultures for many spices. Today, of course, a wide variety of spices to supplant salt is available to us at far less cost or effort than in previous eras. Yet salt remains plentiful in convenience or fast foods and processed foods.

In *From Fish to Philosopher* (1961), the great physiologist Homer Smith wrote, "The most important constituents in the body fluid of all vertebrates are water and sodium chloride—ordinary table salt, the primary salt of the sea and of plants and animals. One cannot, in connection with living organisms, think of water without salt or salt without water." From this he argues convincingly that it was the evolution of the kidney, and its ability to regulate the composition of the internal environment with respect to both water and salt, that was responsible for our evolutionary ancestors' movement from the sea to a free and independent life in a variety of land environments. His bold thesis becomes readily apparent and reasonable when we understand the various and essential roles these simple ions play in the complex working of independent organisms, especially one so intricate as a human being.

Functions of Salt

Many functions within the body depend on separation of the internal environment into specific compartments. The most important separation is between the inside of cells and the fluid that bathes the outside of cells, known as the intracellular and extracellular compartments, respectively. A special pump system on the surface of the cell propels potassium into the cell and sodium out of the cell. This makes potassium salts the main intracellular ions and sodium salts the main extracellular ions. The partitioning of these two salts across the cell surface allows the body to absorb nutrients and eliminate waste without loss of essential substances. It sets up the electrical potential necessary for contraction of every type of muscle, including the heart. It is essential for the conduction of nerve impulses for movement and sensation. Partitioning of the salts is responsible also for regulation of cell volume, extracellular fluid volume, and total body fluid volume. Therefore, tight regulation of salt balance both within body compartments and relative to the external environment is crucial for life.

To accomplish these marvelous feats, the body requires a surprisingly small amount of salt. An average 154-pound (70-kilogram) adult contains 2½ ounces (70 grams) of sodium, equal to 6⅔ ounces (175 grams) of table salt. Salt can be lost through skin, the intestinal tract, and urine. The skin is an effective barrier that prevents excessive loss of salt and water to the external environment. Under normal circumstances, small quantities of salt are lost in sweat and are readily replaced by the diet. The loss of water and salt through the skin can increase significantly, however, with excessive heat, fever, or exercise. This can be a particular problem in children with cystic fibrosis, who have excessive amounts of salt in their sweat and may require sodium supplementation. The upper intestinal tract (see chapter 2) secretes one-seventh of the total body of sodium each day to assist in the absorption of digested nutrients. Under normal conditions, along with that which is eaten, essentially all of the sodium in the intestinal tract is subsequently reabsorbed. However, in cases of severe diarrhea in which intestinal secretions are lost, significant amounts of sodium salts can be lost along with water. The kidneys perform an even more amazing task of filtering and handling more than 9 times the total body of sodium each day. The kidneys are able, on the one hand, to eliminate excess salt that is consumed and, on the other, to reabsorb essentially all of the sodium presented to them when the body is salt-depleted. Kidney disease can damage these abilities and can require significant alterations in diet—in some cases severe restriction of sodium intake, in others actual salt supplementation. Because of the potential for wide variation present in the disease states mentioned above, any alterations from a typical diet in these conditions should be undertaken only with the guidance of a physician.

Sodium and Children

Although most adolescents and adults would benefit from less salt in their diet, it would be inappropriate to restrict salt sharply in the infant and growing child. It has been established that infants and children require a minimum of 50–70 milligrams of sodium and 70–100 milligrams of chloride per 100 calories for health and adequate growth. Infant formula production is carefully regulated and monitored to provide sufficient salt for healthy growth. In addition, a well-balanced diet of readily available foods provides sufficient salt for growth and health in children.

Sodium and High Blood Pressure

If salt plays such important roles in the body and if the kidneys are able to remove excess salt, why is there such concern about sodium intake? With social, technological, and medical advances, people are living longer. Modern methods of food storage depend less on salt for effective preservation and distribution. In developed nations, public health practices, including sanitation and safe water supplies, have largely removed the specter of vast segments of the population dying young from such epidemics as typhoid and bubonic plague. With the absence of cholera and with access to medical care for other diarrheal illnesses, the advantages of a high-salt diet disappear. And as longevity has increased, other diseases have taken on greater importance for the population. By the middle of the twentieth century it was apparent that cardiovascular disease, in particular heart attacks, stroke, and kidney disease, was claiming an increasing number of people. Researchers have discovered that a number of factors contribute to a person's risk of developing cardiovascular disease. Two of the most important are smoking and the presence of high blood pressure, or hypertension. Subsequent studies have shown that cessation of smoking and good control of blood pressure significantly reduces a person's risk for cardiovascular disease.

The importance of salt in this whole picture is in its effect on blood pressure. One determinant of blood pressure is extracellular fluid volume, and as mentioned above, the main determinant of extracellular fluid volume is the quantity of sodium in the body. Sodium is thus an important determinant of blood pressure. Too much sodium in the body can cause high blood pressure. For this reason, a salt-restricted diet is an important part of therapy for many patients with high blood pressure. Is a low-salt diet in the adolescent or adult without high blood pressure of any benefit? The answer to this question, as yet not definitive, is very important because it would be better to prevent high blood pressure than to treat it with medication. As outlined earlier, a healthy person can eliminate excessive amounts of salt through the kidneys. This is accomplished in part by a slight, transient rise in blood pressure. It appears that in many people who are prone to develop the most common type of high blood pressure, called essential hypertension, this delicate balance is upset. In such individuals, the slight blood pressure elevations appear to become persistent rather than remaining transient. If not treated, mild, persistent elevation in blood pressure then progresses to more severe elevations in blood pressure. Many people who have essential hypertension are salt-sensitive and often require only a salt-restricted diet to improve or normalize blood pressure. Once high blood pressure is well-established, however, medication is frequently required. The hope is that early dietary intervention could prevent the development of established high blood pressure in salt-sensitive individuals.

It is not yet known why certain individuals are salt-sensitive and prone to develop high blood pressure. It is also not yet possible to identify these salt-sensitive individuals before the time that high blood pressure is established. Until these at-risk individuals can be reliably identified, a more gen-

TABLE 33.1

Foods with Low to Moderate Sodium Content (0–349 mg/serving)

Foods	Serving size
Beverages, all types (except vegetable juice)	8 oz
Breads, rolls, bagels, all types; no visible salt	1 piece
Breakfast cereals, several types (check labels)	1 cup
Butter, margarines, vegetable oils	1 tsp
Cooked cereals, regular or quick (no salt added)	1 cup
Crackers, several types (check labels)	varies
Eggs (cooked without added salt)	1
Fresh or fresh frozen meats, poultry, fish	3 oz
Fresh, frozen, or canned fruits and fruit juices	½ cup
Fresh or frozen vegetables (no added sauces)	½ cup
Ice cream, ice milk (plain varieties)	½ cup
Milk, all types; milk beverage mixes	8 oz
Natural cheeses (cheddar, mozzarella, ricotta, etc.)	1 oz
Natural grains (wheat, rice, oats, barley, etc.)	½ cup
Pasta, all types (cooked without added salt)	1 cup
Peas and beans, dried (cooked without added salt)	½ cup
Peanut butter	1 tbsp
Pepper, herbs, and spices	varies
Potatoes, fresh or frozen (frozen—check labels)	½ cup
Tuna and salmon, canned (rinsed)	3 oz
Yogurt, all types, including frozen	½ cup

eral approach to preventing high blood pressure is prudent. Because salt-sensitive essential hypertension is common and contributes to the high incidence of cardiovascular disease, a general reduction in the unnecessarily high salt intake of adolescents and adults is advisable. The imperative to reduce salt intake is even greater for those who have a family member who has suffered from high blood pressure or cardiovascular disease.

Dietary Sodium

Breast milk and infant formula provide sufficient salt for normal growth and development of healthy infants. When table foods are introduced, a balanced diet will continue to provide the necessary salt. Provision of salt-rich food is not necessary for growth and development through childhood, but no systematic effort should be made to restrict salt intake in otherwise healthy children. Lifelong dietary habits are often formed before adulthood, so it is best to promote moderation in salt consumption beginning in the school-age years. Many adolescents seem to have a particular taste for high-salt foods; modifying this habit is important because essential hypertension begins to appear in adolescence and young adulthood.

The estimated minimum requirement for so-

TABLE 33.2
Foods with High Sodium Content (350 or more mg/serving)

Foods	Serving size
Bouillon, canned broths[a]	8 oz
Breakfast cereals, several types (check labels)	1 cup
Canned vegetables, regular[a]	½ cup
Commercial cheese sauce or cream sauce	2 oz
Cottage cheese	½ cup
Cured, smoked, and salted meats, poultry, fish	3 oz
Deli salads (macaroni, potato salad, coleslaw)	½ cup
Fast foods, pizza	varies
Frozen breaded meats, poultry, and fish	3 oz
Frozen pancakes, waffles, French toast	2 pieces
Frozen dinners and entrées[a]	varies
Instant pudding	½ cup
Ketchup, mustard, soy sauce, barbecue sauce[a]	2 tbsp
Pancake and waffle mix	¼ cup
Pickles, green olives, vegetables in brine	varies
Pre-prepared pies, cakes, pastries (check labels)	1 piece
Preseasoned rice, potato, or noodle mixes	½ cup
Processed cheeses (American, cheese spreads, etc.)[a]	1 oz
Processed meats (hot dogs, bologna, salami, etc.)[a]	2 oz
Salad dressings, bottled or dry[a]	2 tbsp
Soups, canned or dehydrated (regular)[a]	8 oz
Table salt, seasoned salts, MSG	¼ tsp
Tomato sauces, pizza sauces[a]	½ cup
Vegetable juice (regular)[a]	8 oz

[a] Lower-sodium versions are available, but check labels carefully

dium in healthy children ranges from about 200 milligrams per day in a 1-year-old to about 500 milligrams per day in children age 6 and up. Adults, too, require a minimum of 500 milligrams of sodium per day. Because diets rarely lack sodium, nutrition experts emphasize moderation in sodium consumption. Moderation is defined as no more than 6 grams of salt or 2,400 milligrams of sodium per day.

Most Americans consume excessive amounts of sodium. Adults average 4,000–6,000 milligrams of sodium per day, while school-age children average 3,000–4,000 milligrams per day. Overconsumption of sodium usually occurs from salt added during cooking and at the table, along with the frequent use of convenience and processed foods. A few simple changes in shopping and cooking habits can reduce a family's consumption of sodium.

Sodium is found in almost all food. In tables 33.1 and 33.2, common foods are categorized by their sodium content. Foods that contain less than

TABLE 33.3

Sodium Claim Guide

Sodium	*Sodium free:* less than 5 mg per serving
	Very low sodium: 35 mg or less per serving
	Low-sodium: 140 mg or less per serving
	Note: If the food is not "low in sodium," the statement "not a low-sodium food" must appear on the same panel as the Nutrition Facts. Foods in the following categories may not actually be low in sodium:
	Light in sodium: At least 50% less sodium per serving than average reference amount for the same food with no sodium reduction
	Lightly salted: At least 50% less sodium per serving than reference amount
	Reduced or less sodium: At least 25% less per serving than reference food
Salt (sodium chloride)	*Salt-free:* Sodium free (see above definition)
	(If the food is not "sodium free," the statement "not a sodium-free food" or "not for control of sodium in the diet" must appear on the same panel as the Nutrition Facts.)
	Unsalted, without added salt, no salt added:
	• No salt added during processing, and the food it resembles and for which it substitutes is normally processed with salt.

Source: Adapted from 1990 Nutrition Labeling and Education Act, Food and Drug Administration, U.S. Department of Health and Human Services.

350 milligrams sodium per serving (low) are listed in table 33.1; foods that contain 350 milligrams or more sodium per serving are listed in table 33.2. The foods in both tables may be eaten in a well-balanced diet; however, caution is necessary when choosing items from table 33.2 because the sodium in these foods adds up quickly. Fortunately, the food industry is beginning to accommodate consumers by offering reduced-salt products; several foods listed in table 33.2, for example, are available in lower-sodium versions. Product labeling can be confusing, but sodium claims are defined by law. The Sodium Claim Guide (table 33.3) should be of assistance. Note that many of the definitions are not absolute but refer to similar products. Gradual changes in product choices and cooking methods can lead to a healthier family diet, perhaps even without much notice (or complaint) by family members.

Is My Child's Diet High in Sodium?

Not all children consume a high-sodium diet. To discover whether your child eats too much sodium, evaluate the child's intake over a period of several days. In a span of 5 or 6 days, does the child consume more foods from table 33.2 than table 33.1? Does the child eat several high-sodium foods 3 or more times per week? If so, it would be wise to eliminate gradually some of the foods from table 33.2 or buy lower-sodium versions. The child who uses the salt shaker should be encouraged to use it less and eventually not at all. Occasional high-salt meals or snacks are acceptable and expected in the diet of a healthy growing child. Again, moderation is the rule; striving for a very low sodium intake is inappropriate for young children.

Fast-Food Tips

Busy lives often force families to eat meals from fast food or take-out restaurants. Most fast food is high in sodium, but it is possible to eat fast food in moderation without compromising nutrition. What is ordered and how often it is eaten are the real issues to keep in mind (see chapter 39 for details on how to eat nutritiously at fast food restaurants).

Healthy Snack Ideas

Many parents are concerned about the snacks their children eat, especially after school when they may not be monitored. One solution is to stock the kitchen with lower-salt snacks such as those listed below.

CRUNCHY

Popcorn, plain or with butter (no salt added)
Unsalted pretzels
Reduced sodium crackers with natural cheeses
Granola bars
Tortilla chips with salsa (several brands are low in sodium)
Raw vegetables with peanut butter, natural cheeses, or cream cheese

SWEET

Animal or graham crackers (chocolate varieties, too)
Ginger snaps, vanilla wafers

Homemade cookies, breads, and muffins (made with half the salt)
Fruits, all kinds, fresh or canned

CHEWY

Raisins (yogurt or chocolate covered, too)
Granola bars
Dried fruits

FROZEN

Juice bars, popsicles, pudding pops
Frozen yogurt, ice cream, sherbet, and sorbet (even in a cone)
Fruited milkshakes

Summary Guidelines

A guide for achieving a moderate sodium intake in children follows.

- Decrease the amount of salt used in cooking; use herbs and spices instead.
- Do not put the salt shaker on the table.
- Read labels and compare sodium content.
- Choose fresh, frozen, or unsalted canned vegetables.
- Watch for high sodium content in condiments; use them in moderation.
- Parents are role models for their children; set a good example.
- If a food tastes salty, it probably is very high in sodium.
- For the child with a strong salt preference, reduce salt intake gradually.
- When possible, reduce salt by half or leave it out of recipes.
- Limit the use of convenience and processed foods.

Fantastic Fiber

Fiber is an essential part of the diet and has many beneficial characteristics, even though it is not digested or absorbed, and it does not provide any calories, vitamins, or minerals. Fiber influences the digestive system in many ways. It helps regulate the bowel and has been shown to have protective effects against the development of many diseases. A high-fiber diet is thus good for a child's health, both now and for the future.

> **MYTH** Tough and stringy meats are high in fiber.
> **FACT** Fiber is the indigestible parts of plants. Therefore, although some meats might look fibrous, they contain no fiber at all.

What Is Dietary Fiber?

Dietary fiber is the part of fruits and vegetables that cannot be digested by humans. It is also commonly referred to as "roughage." Only plants contain fiber. Some meat may look tough or stringy, but it does not contain fiber. Dietary fiber is divided into two groups: soluble and insoluble.

Soluble fiber includes gums, pectins, and some hemicellulose and is commonly found in oats, legumes (beans and peas), barley, apples, citrus fruits, and strawberries. In the digestive system, it forms a thick solution when mixed with food and can be fermented in the large intestine (colon) by bacteria that normally live there. It does not contribute significantly to stool bulk.

. . . .

Teresa Fung

Insoluble fiber includes cellulose and some hemicellulose and is commonly found in whole-grain products, vegetables, and bran. It is relatively resistant to bacterial fermentation. It increases stool weight and hastens the time it takes for digested material to pass through the colon.

The amount of fiber available in food is affected by how it is prepared. For example, fresh fruits have more fiber than canned fruits, because much of the fiber is in the peel, which is usually removed in processing.

What Does Fiber Do in the Digestive System?

Various types of fiber influence the digestive system (see chapter 2) in different ways. The effects are also related to the amount of fiber eaten. In the stomach, fiber contributes to bulk and may create a sense of satiety or fullness. It also thickens the food in the stomach. Soluble fiber has been shown to slow the emptying of food from the stomach to the small intestine.

In the small intestine, fiber binds with water, which increases the bulk of intestinal contents and may dilute toxins and carcinogens and bind cholesterol and other substances. Soluble fiber delays the absorption of both nutritive and non-nutritive substances. This delay is a result of increased viscosity and reduced mixing of intestinal contents. Fiber has the opposite effect on the large intestine (colon). Fiber shortens the time it takes for food to pass through the colon. This means a reduction in the time available for the colon to be exposed to carcinogens. The increased bulk also controls stool consistency. Fiber promotes the growth of harmless bacteria that normally live in the colon; these bacteria ferment the fiber and produce various gases.

Fiber and Disease

Fiber is known to have regulatory effects on the digestive system. It can help both constipation and diarrhea. It is also thought to have beneficial health effects in preventing colon cancer, coronary heart disease, and excessive weight gain. Although colon cancer and heart disease are not usually diseases one would worry about in a child, it is important to establish good eating habits at a young age because changes in later years may be harder to make. There is also evidence that hardening of the coronary arteries may be present by young adulthood, as autopsies of young soldiers killed in battle have demonstrated (see chapter 20).

Constipation, defined as decreased frequency of stooling in combination with the presence of hard stools, is a frequent parental concern (see chapter 23). A diet low in fluids and in fiber, especially cereal fiber, can aggravate or cause constipation. Fiber helps to relieve constipation by increasing stool bulk and by stimulating contraction of the colon to promote elimination. It also reduces passage time of the stool in the colon. Cereal fibers increase stool weight more than vegetable and fruit fibers and are thus more effective. Parents should encourage children to eat whole-grain cereals and breads or add bran to food for relief from or prevention of constipation.

Fiber is also beneficial in controlling diarrhea by the same property of increasing bulk and contributing to viscosity. In this case, soluble fiber is the better choice. Soluble fiber has been shown to decrease the duration of diarrhea, while also increasing stool consistency. Fruits and beans (legumes) are especially rich in soluble fiber.

Epidemiological studies have repeatedly demonstrated the protective effect of fiber on colon cancer. Cultural groups and countries with high fiber intake in their diets have been found to have fewer cases of colon cancer when compared with cultural groups and countries that have a low fiber intake. It is believed that fiber dilutes the concentration of carcinogens in the intestines and decreases their absorption by speeding passage of stool through the colon. Insoluble fiber, especially wheat bran, has been shown to have the most beneficial effect on lowering the risk of colon cancer.

Soluble fiber has been shown to reduce the risk of coronary heart disease by modestly reducing blood cholesterol levels. Pectin, a soluble fiber found in many fruits and vegetables, is known to decrease cholesterol, and oat bran has been shown to reduce levels of low-density lipoprotein (LDL), the type of cholesterol linked to higher risk of heart disease. The mechanism of action is believed to be the formation of gels by soluble fibers, which in turn bind bile salts (the carrier of cholesterol) in the small intestine and thus decrease cholesterol absorption. Also, fermentation of fiber in the colon by natural bacteria produces short-chain fatty acids that might decrease cholesterol synthesis in the liver. Oat bran may be the most effective soluble fiber in lowering cholesterol levels. Many early studies used very large doses of oat bran and the results were so dramatic that they generated a lot of media attention. The dosages that were used were often unrealistically large. Since then, however, other studies that involved moderate and realistic amounts of fiber intake have also shown cholesterol-lowering effects.

High-fiber diets can also have a beneficial effect on obesity. Fiber dilutes the caloric density of food (see chapter 27). It prolongs chewing, which may reduce food intake. The bulking effect in the stomach makes the eater feel full sooner, and at the same time, food enters the small intestine at a slower rate, which may prolong satiety.

Increasing Fiber in the Diet

Most children probably do not eat an adequate amount of fiber, since vegetables and beans are not particularly popular with children. Studies of adults show that Americans in general fall short of eating the recommended amount of fiber (11–22 grams per day versus the recommended amount of 20–35 grams per day). The American Health Foundation has recommended the following formula for calculating the fiber needs of 3- to 18-year-olds: the child's age (in years) + 5 = recommended daily fiber intake (in grams). For example, a 13-year-old should eat 13 + 5 = 18 grams of fiber. Maximum fiber intake should not exceed the child's age + 10; that is, a 13-year-old child should not eat more than 23 grams of fiber (13 + 10). The American Academy of Pediatrics uses a different formula to calculate recommended fiber intake for children: ½ gram per kilogram of the child's weight, with a maximum intake of no more than 35 grams a day.

In light of the many benefits of fiber, children should be introduced early to a diet with adequate fiber, both soluble and insoluble.

How to Increase Fiber in Your Child's Diet

In general, the less a fiber-containing food is processed, the more fiber it contains (see table 34.1). The simplest way to increase fiber intake is to eat more fruits, vegetables, dried beans, whole grains, and nuts.

The skins of fruits are good sources of fiber. Encourage children to eat fresh fruits. Raw fruits and vegetables can be appealing if presented in interesting ways, as in decorative fruit salads, or as colorful celery and carrot sticks served with a low-fat dip or peanut butter.

Unrefined and whole-grain products, such as whole wheat bread, pasta, and cereals, contain insoluble fiber. Choose higher fiber breads like rye, whole wheat, and pumpernickel. It is also possible to add fiber to home-baked goods by substituting whole wheat flour for part of the white flour in muffins, cookies, biscuits, and pie crusts. Adding a few spoonfuls of bran or wheat germ to casseroles increases fiber content without drastically changing the taste and texture. Although cereals made with wheat, oats, and bran are good sources of fiber, children might not like them because of their relatively bland flavor. Mixing a high-fiber with a low-fiber cereal or adding nuts and fruits to cereal adds both fiber and flavor.

Legumes (dried beans and peas) are a very good source of fiber. Kidney beans, lentils, garbanzo, and lima beans can be added to soups, casseroles, stews, and salads.

Because fiber binds water, it is important to drink more fluid with greater fiber intake. To avoid stomach discomfort, increase fiber intake slowly. Using the suggestions outlined above, a typical child's daily intake (table 34.2) can become higher in fiber (table 34.3) relatively easily.

Too Much Fiber?

Some studies have shown that fiber decreases the absorption or bioavailability of some minerals and vitamins, in particular calcium, magnesium, zinc, iron, vitamin B_{12}, and folic acid. Although information is limited, this effect is usually small and should not be a concern unless dietary intake of

TABLE 34.1
Fiber in Selected Foods

Food	Serving size	Fiber (g)
All bran cereal	⅓ cup	9.2
Baked acorn squash	½ cup	4.5
Apple with skin	1 medium	3.7
Shredded wheat	½ cup	2.0
Lima beans, cooked	½ cup	5.4
Whole wheat bread	1 slice	2.0
Banana	1 medium	2.7
Broccoli, cooked	½ cup	2.3
Kidney beans, cooked	½ cup	5.7
Cheerios	1 cup	2.0
Carrot, raw	1 large	2.2
Macaroni, cooked	1 cup	1.8
White bread	1 slice	0.8

TABLE 34.2
Typical Menu

Breakfast	Lunch	Dinner
Apple Jacks cereal (¾ cup)	Cheeseburger (1)	Meatloaf (3 oz)
Whole milk (8 oz)	French fries (small serving)	Green peas (½ cup)
	Cola (12 oz)	Mashed potato (½ cup)
		Whole milk (8 oz)
		Ice cream (½ cup)
	Afternoon snack	*Evening snack*
	Potato chips (1½ oz)	Sugar cookies (2 medium)
Total dietary fiber = 12 g		

TABLE 34.3
Higher-Fiber Menu

Breakfast	Lunch	Dinner
Cheerios (1¼ cup)	Cheeseburger (1)	Meatloaf (3 oz)
Whole milk (8 oz)	Medium apple (1)	Green peas (½ cup)
	Cola (12 oz)	Baked potato (1 medium)
		Whole milk (8 oz)
		Peach cobbler (3 × 3-inch slice)
	Afternoon snack	*Evening snack*
	Carrots and celery sticks with peanut butter (2 oz)	Oatmeal cookies (2 medium)

Total dietary fiber = 21 g

vitamins and minerals is marginal. Only in very high fiber diets (more than 35 grams a day) does the absorption of vitamins and minerals become a concern. Although fiber rarely dilutes calories to an extent to cause malnutrition or slow growth, parents are advised not to be overzealous in increasing their children's fiber intake.

Some stomach discomforts are associated with high fiber intake: bloating, stomach pain, and an increase in gas production. These discomforts are often temporary, but as stated above, the amount of fiber should be increased gradually and should be added to the diet with plenty of fluids. If symptoms persist, fiber intake should be reduced.

Fresh Facts about Pesticides
and Food Additives

Food additives are very important to our food supply, and without them, the wide variety of foods that are available today would not be possible. The use of pesticides has dramatically increased the production and year-round availability of fresh produce. Many people are concerned about pesticides and food additives, however, and they wonder if purchasing organically grown foods is a reliable way of ensuring that they are providing "safe" foods for their children. In this chapter we address these issues in an effort to allay fears and enlighten perspectives.

> **MYTH** Aspartame (such as Equal and NutraSweet) causes cancer.
>
> **FACT** Aspartame is the most widely tested sweetener available to consumers. It has been tested in adults, children, and pregnant women, and it has been found to be safe.

Pesticides in the Diets of Infants and Children

The use of pesticides in the agricultural industry has improved and increased the production of fresh vegetables and fruit, thereby improving public health and nutrition. As a result, however, people are exposed to pesticides through their diet. Pesticide residues—defined as the trace quantities of pesticides present in or on food—have become an important topic of discussion as consumers have expressed concern and fear over their potential for harmful effects. An assessment of the

· ·

Erica L. Liebelt ▪ Tara Prather Liskov

overall impact of pesticides in the diet must take into account their potential toxicity and effects on the nutritive values of foods, as well as their vital role in crop survival and in maintaining sufficient food production.

WHAT ARE PESTICIDES? Pesticides are chemicals used to kill insects, weeds, and fungus that can destroy plants. There are hundreds of types of pesticides, each possessing varying degrees of toxicity, depending on the specific chemical. Effects on the body can be acute or chronic and delayed depending on the type of pesticide and the amount and duration of exposure. Accidental exposure to large amounts of pesticides can cause severe reactions. The major concern for the general public, however, is whether lifelong dietary exposure to trace amounts of pesticides has adverse health effects. Specifically, it has been questioned whether such exposure leads to neurologic problems, abnormalities of the immune system, or cancer. Although these health problems have been linked to pesticides in scientific studies, most studies examined the effects of long-term exposure to large amounts of pesticides. The amounts used were far greater than would be obtained from the diet, so definitive conclusions cannot be drawn from these studies with regard to the effect of dietary intake of trace amounts of pesticides.

WHAT ACTION HAS THE GOVERNMENT TAKEN TO ENSURE THE SAFETY OF THE FOOD SUPPLY FOR CHILDREN? In the United States, pesticide use and pesticide residue on food are regulated by the Environmental Protection Agency (EPA) and the Food and Drug Administration (FDA). In 1988, Congress requested that the National Academy of Sciences establish a committee to study scientific and policy issues concerning pesticides in the diets of infants and children. Their findings and recommendations are found in the book *Pesticides in the Diets of Infants and Children* and are summarized below.

1. There are both quantitative and occasionally qualitative differences in toxicity of pesticides between children and adults.
2. Infants and children differ both qualitatively and quantitatively from adults in their exposure to pesticide residues in food. For example, infants and young children may consume much more of certain foods, especially processed foods, than adults. The committee concluded that differences in diet, and thus in dietary exposure to pesticide residues, account for most of the differences in pesticide-related health risk that were found to exist between children and adults.
3. Through innovative analytical procedures, the committee estimated that some children may be exposed to pesticides that exceed the tolerable limit and commented that exposures to pesticides early in life can lead to a greater risk of chronic effects that are seen only after long periods of exposure.

On the basis of its findings, the committee recommended changes in current regulatory practices of pesticide exposure. Specifically, they recommended that the EPA modify its decision-making process for setting tolerances (the legal limit of pesticide residue allowed in or on raw agricultural products and processed foods) to account for human health considerations rather than agricultural practices. Second, the committee felt it was essential to develop toxicity testing procedures for pesticide residues that specifically evaluate the vulnerability of infants and children.

This report should not cause panic, nor should

children stop consuming milk, fruits, and vegetables, which are needed for adequate nutrition. It represents a realization of the potential harmful effects of chemicals and an effort to make the food supply even safer for children. Pesticide residues exceed safe and acceptable levels in only 0.1 percent of conventionally grown foods, and then by very small margins. Children should be able to eat a healthful diet containing legal residues of pesticides without endangering their health.

The "Alar scare" of 1989 is an example of unnecessary hysteria surrounding the use of pesticides. Daminozide (marketed as Alar) is a pesticide used primarily to keep apples red and to slow the ripening process. Studies demonstrated that daminozide caused cancer in laboratory animals, but the EPA did not feel that enough evidence was available to warrant a ban on this product. In 1989, the Natural Resources Defense Council published a study that argued that children consume larger quantities of apples and apple products (and therefore pesticides) than adults, which therefore placed them at much higher risk for cancer from their greater exposure to the pesticide residue. After this study was widely reported in the media, people stopped buying apples and school cafeterias removed apples and applesauce from their menus. However, the EPA estimates that Alar is used on only a small percentage of the total apple crop and that the risk of not including apples in the diet outweighs the risk of exposure to daminozide. The lesson is that an evaluation of all available data should be completed before an entire foodstuff is removed from a child's diet.

PRACTICAL SOLUTIONS TO MINIMIZE PESTICIDE EXPOSURE Children should continue to eat a wide variety of fruits, vegetables, grains, and milk to get the vitamins and minerals they need.

Although pesticide application to some components of processed food is likely to occur at some point (for example, field applications to crops used as ingredients in infant formula), extensive testing of infant formula, infant cereal, and processed baby foods has failed to detect any pesticide residues. There has also been concern that infants may be exposed to pesticides through the mother's breast milk, depending on her exposure. However, major studies have failed to demonstrate that the small concentration of pesticides found in some women's breast milk has any adverse effects in exposed children. Thus, the significant benefits of breastfeeding outweigh the remote possibility of pesticide exposure unless there is a recent history of a significant maternal exposure to pesticides or a known chronic exposure in the past.

The following steps can be taken to lessen exposure to possible pesticide residues on fresh foods:

- Wash fresh fruits and vegetables thoroughly. Some fruits can be scrubbed with a brush under running water. It has been clearly shown that small pesticide residue concentrations on fruits and vegetables can be reduced by washing with water. Produce can be washed in water containing two drops of dishwashing liquid and then rinsed thoroughly.
- Discard the outer leaves and skin of some fruits and vegetables.
- Trim fat from meat because pesticides concentrate in fatty tissues.

The technology of genetic engineering has resulted in the ability to produce pest- and fungus-resistant vegetables and fruits through special DNA modifications. Perhaps this technology will eliminate the need to use pesticides in the future.

Organic Foods and Organic Gardening

Organically grown foods have been grown in soil enriched with manure and compost rather than with chemical or synthetic fertilizers and pesticides. Organically processed foods have not been treated with hormones, antibiotics, synthetic additives, preservatives, dyes, or waxes. Some consumers choose to buy organic foods to give themselves peace of mind in hopes of decreasing potential risk. However, consumers should keep a few things in mind.

- An organic food that is grown and processed properly is not necessarily free from pesticides. There may be cross-contamination from wind drifts, soil shifts, or groundwater.
- Organic foods do not necessarily have greater nutritional value than nonorganic foods, although vitamin contents of vegetables and fruits are sometimes decreased by pesticides. Several studies of herbicides used in wheat production have shown that vitamin content actually increases when herbicides are used.
- Organically grown foods are 20–100 percent more expensive than conventionally produced foods but do not necessarily look or taste better. In fact, the appearance of organically grown produce is often poor because it decays and spoils sooner than other produce.
- Organic fertilizers may sometimes be a source of pathogenic bacteria, since they are not sterilized.
- There are no federal regulations to govern the production of organic foods; regulations are left to the individual states. Be aware, therefore, of potentially false labeling and advertising.

Organic gardening and farming techniques are less harmful to the environment because they avoid the use of synthetic pesticides. They rely on natural fertilizers like compost and manure and natural pesticides like garlic juice, pepper, wood ash, and physical barriers. Other organic gardening techniques to control pests include biological pesticides (other insects and organisms), crop rotation, interplanting, and optimal timing, planting, and harvesting of plants.

Food Additives

Food additives are not a modern innovation. People discovered centuries ago that adding salt to meat would make the meat last longer. Today there are thousands of direct and indirect food additives in the diet. The purpose of additives is to enhance the quality, edibility, and appearance of food, to improve the safety of food by preventing microbiological contamination, to facilitate the preparation of foods, and to improve the nutritional value of food. Like pesticides, there is growing concern that many of these chemicals added to the food supply may be dangerous to the health of children. The role of food additives in children with behavioral disorders, particularly attention deficit hyperactivity disorder, has caused great concern among parents and is discussed in chapter 26.

Food additives may be divided into several categories—preservatives, flavorings, colorings, bleaching and maturing agents, irradiation, and nutritional supplements (table 35.1). Concern over the safety of certain food additives has surfaced over the years, so some specific additives are discussed in detail below.

NITRITES Nitrites are used as curing agents for bacon and such other pork products as ham and Vienna sausages. They protect food from the bacteria that cause botulism. After ingestion, some nitrites can be converted to nitrosamines, which are

TABLE 35.1
Food Additives

Preservatives	Nitrites
	Sulfites
	BHA (butylated hydroxyanisole)
	BHT (butylated hydroxytoluene)
	Benzoic acid
Flavorings	Monosodium glutamate (MSG)
	Saccharin
	Aspartame
	Acesulfame potassium
	Essential oils, spices, oleoresins
Colors Artificial	Red Dye No. 3 (Erythrosine)
	Yellow Dye No. 5 (Tartrazine)
	Citrus Red No. 2, Yellow Dye No. 6, Green Dye No. 3
	Blue Dye Nos. 1 and 2, Red No. 40
Natural	Beets, caramel, carotene, carrot oil
	Grape color extract, turmeric
Bleaching or maturing agents	Benzoyl peroxide
	Chlorine
	Nitrogen oxides
Nutrition supplements	Vitamins
	Minerals
	Amino acids
Irradiation	Ionizing radiation

potent carcinogens. The FDA has lowered the acceptable level of nitrites to the minimum required to prevent botulism and to minimize the risk of cancer from eating bacon and other pork products. The addition of such antioxidants as ascorbate (vitamin C) or alpha-tocopherol (vitamin E) retards the formation of nitrosamine in nitrite-containing foods.

SULFITES Sulfites are preservatives that protect foods from discoloration, overripening, and spoilage. They are found in such processed beverages and foods as fruit juices, soft drinks, wines, cider vinegar, potato chips, and dried fruits and vegetables. Until 1986, they were frequently used on restaurant salad bars to keep produce from browning and spoiling and were classified as GRAS (generally recognized as safe) by Congress. However, numerous allergic reactions (predominantly among asthmatics) and several deaths possibly associated with sulfites were reported in the early 1980s. These incidents forced the FDA to withdraw the GRAS status of sulfites as preservatives of fruits and vegetables. Reactions to sulfites may include wheezing, hives, flushing, swelling of the lips and throat, diarrhea, and, in severe cases, loss of consciousness and anaphylactic shock.

Sulfites must be listed on the labels of wine and packaged foods sold in supermarkets when they are added in excess of 10 parts per million. If a child has a history of asthma, eczema, or allergies, parents should question restaurants about preparation of food with this additive. Potato products and some canned foods served in restaurants could contain sulfites. Also, be cautious about "prepared" foods if the child is known to be sulfite-sensitive. If the child is not sensitive to sulfites, there should be no problems related to this additive.

BHA/BHT Butylated hydroxyanisole (BHA) and butylated hydroxytoluene (BHT) are 2 food additives that are widely used as preservatives in the food supply. Dry cereal, shortening, instant potatoes, active dry yeast, dry drink and dessert mixes, and food packaging often contain these preservatives. These preservatives have been in use for years. Although there is some evidence that they may cause cancer in animals fed very large amounts, there is no human evidence that demonstrates an increased cancer risk, and BHA and BHT are still recognized as safe.

MONOSODIUM GLUTAMATE Monosodium glutamate, or MSG, is used as a flavor enhancer in the brand-name seasoning Accent and some packaged foods, as well as in many restaurants that serve Asian cuisines. Adverse reactions to MSG include dizziness, nausea, vomiting, flushing, tingling, numbness, headache, and pressure in the face and chest. However, MSG still maintains its GRAS status with the FDA and no limitations are placed on its use as a food additive because there are no known adverse effects of MSG for individuals who are not sensitive to it.

SACCHARIN Saccharin is a sugar substitute that has been widely tested in humans. It is 300 times as sweet as sugar and occurs naturally in grapes. In 1977, the FDA banned saccharin as a food additive in the United States because it was weakly linked to bladder cancer in laboratory animals when given in extremely large doses. The ban met with intense public opposition, because at that time saccharin was the only approved sugar substitute on the market. In response, Congress passed the Saccharin Study and Labeling Act in 1977, which placed a moratorium on the ban and therefore permitted the use of saccharin in food. The moratorium has been extended 5 times since 1977, and in December 1991, the FDA withdrew its proposal to ban the use of saccharin in foods, primarily because the link between saccharin and cancer in humans has since been found to be remote at best. Saccharin is approved for use in more than 90 countries worldwide.

ASPARTAME Aspartame, sold under the brand names Equal and NutraSweet, is a sugar substitute that is 180 times as sweet as sugar. It has undergone more testing than any other food additive in the history of the FDA. Aspartame is the methyl ester of 2 amino acids, aspartic acid and phenylalanine. It is metabolized by the body to methanol, aspartic acid, and phenylalanine; these substances occur naturally in food. For example, ounce for ounce, milk has 6 times the phenylalanine and 13 times the aspartic acid as a diet soda sweetened with aspartame. Similarly, fruit juices have 2–3 times as much methanol and tomato juice has 6 times as much methanol as an equal amount of diet soda sweetened with aspartame.

Aspartame is safe for children, adults, pregnant and breastfeeding women, and children with diabetes. Only people with the rare genetic disorder phenylketonuria (PKU) should avoid aspartame, because those people are unable to metabolize phenylalanine properly. All NutraSweet products are labeled with a warning to parents of children with PKU (see chapter 24).

It has been questioned whether aspartame causes headaches, seizures, and behavioral changes in children. These reports have been thoroughly investigated, and aspartame has continued to be found remarkably safe. Aspartame has been found to have no detrimental effects on learning, behavior, or mood in children, nor is it a carcinogenic risk. Like saccharin, aspartame is approved for use in more than 90 countries.

ACESULFAME POTASSIUM (K) In 1988, the low-calorie sweetener acesulfame-K was approved by the FDA and is now marketed under the brand names Sunnette, Sweet One, and Swiss Sweet. It is 200 times as sweet as sugar and when mixed with other sweeteners tastes even sweeter. It can be used in cooking and baking, has no lingering aftertaste, and has a long shelf life. The FDA reviewed more than 90 safety studies and determined this sweetener to be safe.

YELLOW DYE NO. 5 (TARTRAZINE) Tartrazine, also known as FD&C Yellow No. 5, is a color used in a variety of foods, such as prepared breakfast cereals, imitation strawberry jelly, bottled soft drinks, gelatin desserts, ice cream, sherbets, dry drink powders, candy, confections, bakery products, spaghetti, and puddings. As many as 6 per 1,000 persons are sensitive to tartrazine. This is manifested as hives, runny nose, wheezing, eczema, and anaphylaxis. In addition, between 10

percent and 40 percent of people sensitive to aspirin are also sensitive to tartrazine. There have also been reports of an association of behavioral changes, such as irritability, restlessness, and sleep disturbances in children after the ingestion of tartrazine. However, these studies have been criticized for methodological flaws and dietary effects are unlikely to be the sole contributing factor to behavioral problems in children. Yellow No. 5 must be listed on the label of all food items that contain this coloring, so if a child is sensitive to this ingredient, it is easily avoided.

IRRADIATION The use of ionizing radiation for food processing is considered a food additive. Irradiation of food can reduce microbiological and insect contamination that causes spoilage and food-borne diseases. Acceptance of food irradiation has been slow because of the public's association of the process with fears of nuclear accidents and the toxic effects of radiation. These fears are misguided because the process of food irradiation does not make food radioactive, nor does it usually change food's color or texture. Indeed, irradiation may be less dangerous than other food additives. Food irradiation has been approved in the United States for wheat, flour, potatoes, spices, pork, and fresh foods available to the general public. Some have questioned whether food irradiation reduces the nutritional value of foods, but these fears also appear to be unfounded. The World Health Organization encourages the use of irradiation in food preservation because it would improve the world's overall food supply. The FDA requires a label and international logo on all foods that have been irradiated (fig. 35.1).

FOOD ADDITIVES AND CHILDREN'S BEHAVIOR Concern and debate continues over whether food

FIGURE
35.1
Logo for food
products
treated with
irradiation.

chemicals and artificial ingredients must be allayed through the provision of accurate information on the risks and benefits of food additives and alternative methods of ensuring food safety. Natural additives are not necessarily free from toxicity, and appropriate data should be required to test their safety in certain circumstances. Research methods must also be able to correlate animal data with human risks. In general, the benefits of food additives outweigh the risks.

additives, particularly food colorings and aspartame, cause behavioral changes in children. It is generally felt that the existing research data do not support this causal relationship and that food additives are not contributing factors in the majority of children. This topic is discussed in more detail in chapter 26.

Consumers' fears of the harmful effects of

Resources

Committee on Pesticides in the Diets of Infants and Children. *Pesticides in the Diets of Infants and Children.* Washington, DC: National Academy Press, 1993.

Ogden, S. *Step by Step Organic Vegetable Gardening.* New York: Harper Perennial, 1992.

Woteki, C. E., and P. R. Thomas. *Eating for Life.* Washington, DC: National Academy of Sciences, 1992.

Making Sense of Food Labels

In the United States, food labeling is regulated by two government agencies, the Food and Drug Administration (FDA) and the Food Safety and Inspection Service (FSIS) of the U.S. Department of Agriculture. The FDA regulates almost all food products with the exception of meat and poultry, which are regulated by the FSIS. Regulations for food labeling in the United States were first issued in 1906. Since then a number of additions and changes have been made in laws that regulate food labeling, but by far the most sweeping change was the Nutrition Labeling and Education Act (NLEA) of 1990. The NLEA mandated

MYTH You can't trust claims on food labels.
FACT Federal labeling laws enacted in 1994 require that claims on labels meet specific standards established by law. Therefore, food labels may not make false or misleading claims.

dated that all foods regulated by the FDA, with a few exceptions, must be labeled with nutrition information. In addition, the law mandated that nutrient claims, health claims, and serving sizes be defined. The NLEA came into effect on May 8, 1994, and it has greatly enhanced the ability of parents to provide their children with healthy, balanced diets.

Label Format

All nutrition labeling must follow the format presented in figure 36.1. Nutrition information is listed for 1 serving of the product, and serving

. . . .

Tara Prather Liskov

Nutrition Facts	
Serving Size 1 cup (228g)	
Servings Per Container 2	

Amount Per Serving	
Calories 90	Calories from Fat 30

	% Daily Value*
Total Fat 3g	5%
Saturated Fat 0g	0%
Cholesterol 0mg	0%
Sodium 300mg	13%
Total Carbohydrate 13g	4%
Dietary Fiber 3g	12%
Sugars 3g	
Protein 3g	

Vitamin A 80%	•	Vitamin C 60%
Calcium 4%	•	Iron 4%

*Percent Daily Values are based on a 2,000 calorie diet. Your daily values may be higher or lower depending on your calorie needs:

		Calories:	2,000	2,500
Total Fat	Less than		65g	80g
Sat Fat	Less than		20g	25g
Cholesterol	Less than		300mg	300mg
Sodium	Less than		2,400mg	2,400mg
Total Carbohydrate			300g	375g
Dietary Fiber			25g	30g

Calories per gram:
Fat 9 • Carbohydrate 4 • Protein 4

FIGURE 36.1
Standard format for nutrition labeling.

sizes are standardized and based on the average amount of food usually eaten at a sitting. Serving sizes must be listed in both common household (e.g., cup, tablespoon) and metric (e.g., milliliters, grams) measures. Calories, calories from fat, total fat, saturated fat, cholesterol, sodium, total carbohydrate, dietary fiber, sugars, protein, vitamin A, vitamin C, calcium, and iron content must be listed. These nutrients were chosen for inclusion on labels because they are related to health issues of importance today, such as heart disease, cancer, osteoporosis, and iron-deficiency anemia. Other nutrients are no longer a health concern; now that flour is fortified with B vitamins, for example, these vitamins are widely consumed and are therefore no longer required on food labels.

A small number of foods are exempt from nutrition labeling. Foods processed by small businesses ("small" is based on number of employees and the amount of product produced), foods in small packages (less than 2 square inches), foods served for immediate consumption (as at salad bars and food concessions), plain coffee and tea, some spices, and other foods that contain no significant amounts of any nutrient are all exempt from nutrition labeling. Nutrition labeling for raw fruits, vegetables, and fish remains voluntary. However, at least 60 percent of supermarkets must voluntarily label at least 90 percent of these products, or mandatory labeling will go into effect. Pamphlets, posters, booklets, and signs are acceptable forms of nutrition labeling for these foods.

Percent Daily Value

Percent Daily Values replace the U.S. Recommended Daily Allowances (USRDAs) as reference values on the revised nutrition label. Daily Values are based on a healthy, balanced diet of 2,000

TABLE 36.1
Percent Daily Value Conversion

Calorie level	Adjusted Percent Daily Value[a]
1,000	50
1,200	60
1,400	70
1,600	80
1,800	90
2,200	110
2,400	120

[a] The total Percent Daily Value for each individual nutrient should add up to the number in this column, not 100%, as for a 2,000 calorie diet

calories per day and include values for total fat, saturated fat, cholesterol, sodium, total carbohydrate, dietary fiber, protein, vitamin A, vitamin C, calcium, and iron, as required by the NLEA. Daily Values have also been established for 16 other vitamins and minerals, but their use on the label is optional. These Daily Values are used to calculate the Percent Daily Values. The Daily Values are intended to illustrate how a serving of the packaged food fits into the 2,000 calorie reference diet. For example, in the label illustrated here, 3 grams of fat is 5 percent of the Daily Value for a 2,000 calorie diet (3 grams is 5 percent of 65 grams). Over the course of the day, the Percent Daily Values of foods consumed should add up to about 100 percent for each nutrient. Because not everyone eats a 2,000 calorie diet, the notes at the bottom of the Nutrition Facts panel list Daily Values for both a 2,000 calorie diet and a 2,500 calorie diet. The higher calorie levels would be helpful for teenage boys, but most small children do not eat even 2,000 calories. For smaller children, the Percent Daily Value on the labeled food needs to be increased proportionally. For example, a serving of food listed as having 3 grams of fat equals 5 percent of the Daily Value for fat in the 2,000 calorie diet, but it is 10 percent of the Daily Value in a 1,000 calorie diet. Alternatively, the percentages could add to a number other than 100. For example, children who eat 1,200 calories a day are only eating 60 percent of a 2,000 calorie diet, and their total Percent Daily Value should add up to just 60 percent, not 100 percent (table 36.1).

Nutrient and Health Claims

Nutrient content claims, such as *sugar-free, low-fat,* and *reduced sodium,* are now governed by strict definitions and therefore cannot be used unless a serving of the product meets the definitions. These claims, therefore, are believable and can be used to compare similar products. Further, any package that bears a nutrient content claim must bear the statement, "See side/back panel for nutrition information." See table 36.2 for a list of approved claims and their definitions.

A health claim is any statement on a label that relates a food or substance in a food to a disease or health-related condition. Foods that bear health claims must meet specific, government-defined nutrient levels. For instance, there are upper limits on total fat, saturated fat, cholesterol, and sodium. There are eight health-related conditions that can currently be associated with food products. The number of these approved relations may increase in coming years, but at present only the associations listed in table 36.3 are approved. The federal government has developed model statements for each of the health claims in table 36.3. Food manufacturers may either use the model statement or develop their own, but the statements must be complete, truthful, and not misleading.

TABLE 36.2
Nutrient Claim Definitions

Claim	Definition
Calorie free	A product containing fewer than 5 calories per serving
Low calorie	A product containing 40 or fewer calories per serving
Reduced or fewer calories	A product containing at least 25% fewer calories per serving than the original
Lite	A product containing ⅓ fewer calories or 50% less fat than the original product
Fat free	A product containing less than 0.5 g of fat per serving
Low fat	A product containing 3 g of fat or less per serving
Reduced or less fat	A product containing 25% less fat than the original product
Cholesterol free	A product containing less than 2 mg of cholesterol and 2 g or less of saturated fat per serving
Reduced or less cholesterol	A product containing at least 25% less cholesterol than the original product and 2 g or less of saturated fat per serving
Sugar free	A product containing less than 0.5 g sugar per serving
Reduced or less sugar	A product containing at least 25% less sugar than the original product per serving
Sodium or salt free	A product containing less than 5 mg sodium per serving
Very low sodium	A product containing 35 mg or less sodium per serving
Low sodium	A product containing 140 mg or less sodium per serving
Reduced or less sodium	A product containing at least 25% less sodium than the original product per serving
Light in sodium	A product containing 50% less sodium than the original product
High fiber	A product containing at least 5 g of fiber per serving
Good source of fiber	A product containing 2.5 to 4.9 g of fiber per serving
More or added fiber	A product containing at least 2.5 g more fiber than the original product per serving
Healthy	A product containing, per serving, no more than 3 g fat, 1 g saturated fat, 480 mg sodium (350 mg by end of 1997), and 60 mg cholesterol and supplying at least 10% of the Daily Value for at least 1 of these 6 nutrients: vitamins A and C, calcium, iron, protein, and fiber

Infant and Toddler Foods

Foods intended for infants and children under 4 years of age have special labeling rules. Examples of such foods include infant cereals, infant strained fruits, vegetables, and meats, "junior" foods and juices, and teething biscuits. Because infant formula is regulated separately, it is not included in these rules.

For children under age 2, dietary fat is an important component of the diet and should not be limited. Therefore, foods intended for children less than 2 cannot list the amount of saturated fat, polyunsaturated fat, monounsaturated fat, cholesterol, calories from fat, or calories from saturated fat. These food labels are also not permitted to carry any nutrient or health claims other than *unsweetened* and *unsalted*.

TABLE 36.3
Approved Health Claims

Nutrient/Food source	Disease/Health-related condition
Calcium	Osteoporosis
Fiber-containing grain products, fruits and vegetables	Cancer
Fruits and vegetables	Cancer
Fiber-containing grain products, fruits and vegetables	Coronary heart disease
Fat	Cancer
Saturated fat and cholesterol	Coronary heart disease
Sodium (salt)	High blood pressure
Folic acid (in pregnancy)	Neural tube defects (in the fetus)

Labels on foods intended for children aged 2 to 4 must list cholesterol and saturated fat per serving. If the manufacturer desires, they can provide calories from fat and saturated fat, as well as the amount of polyunsaturated and monounsaturated fat per serving.

So, finally, the food label is both useful and believable. Nutrition information is available on almost all packaged foods, serving sizes reflect amounts that are typically eaten, and nutrient content and health claims are factual. It is now up to the consumer to understand and use the information on the food labels to develop a balanced and nutritious diet.

PART FIVE

Eating In, Eating Out

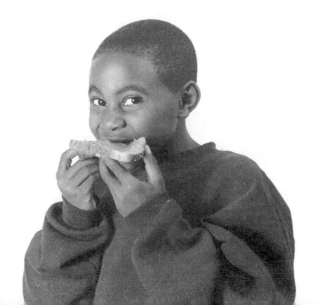

From the Grocery Store to the Home: Stocking the Kitchen

Equipment

Stocking a kitchen with children in mind can be challenging! But with a few key appliances, utensils, and some food staples, the job can be dramatically simplified. The first appliance that is particularly useful in a home with children is a food processor. Homemade baby food and breakfast shakes, as well as such snacks as vegetable pieces (carrot coins, pepper rings, celery discs), can be easily prepared in a food processor. Food processors are available in a variety of price ranges; an expensive model is not necessary. In fact, a small model is often more useful for preparing single portions.

> **MYTH** A food can never be refrozen once it has been defrosted.
>
> **FACT** If foods are thawed in the refrigerator, they can be refrozen. Refrozen foods are safe to eat, but the quality may be compromised.

If a food processor is unavailable, a blender can often be used instead.

Toasters or toaster ovens, sandwich makers, and waffle irons are also helpful in a home with children because they produce foods that children find appealing. A large kettle or pot is important, especially for homes with infants. Water may need to be boiled for formula preparation, and boiling water can be used to warm bottles of either formula or breast milk that have been previously refrigerated. A microwave oven can also be used to boil water and reheat food. Baby bottles should never be warmed in the microwave, however, because microwave

Tara Prather Liskov ▪ Donna Caseria

ovens can heat unevenly. The contents of the bottle might seem to be an appropriate temperature from the test drop, but the formula could be much hotter in other parts of the bottle and thus burn the baby. Children should never use kitchen equipment without adult supervision.

Age-appropriate dishes and utensils are of great importance in a home with children. For infants and toddlers, a good supply of bibs, safety spoons (plastic coated), sippy cups, and plastic dishware is essential. Older children may still use plastic dishware and cups as well as plastic placemats or tablecloths, since they minimize breakage and allow for easy cleanup of spills. Cabinets should be organized to allow young school-age children to reach plastic dishware without having to use a stool or climb on the kitchen counter. This will encourage self-reliance as well as help prevent accidents.

Food

Providing nutritious meals and snacks for growing children is much easier if the pantry and refrigerator are filled with a good variety of healthy foods. Frequent trips to the supermarket, grocery store, and produce market are unavoidable, and shopping with the children may often be a necessity. For tips on surviving shopping excursions with children, see box on the following page.

A number of pantry staples are important for a well-stocked kitchen. If there is a formula-fed infant in the house, at least a week's supply of formula should be on hand. A reasonable supply of other baby foods, such as dehydrated baby cereal, teething biscuits, and prepared baby foods (if these are used), is also necessary. For toddlers and older children, fresh bread, crackers, peanut butter, low-sugar cereal, canned fruit, pasta, rice, beans (either dry or canned), and soup are help-ful to have on hand. Children often need snacks, and a wide variety of foods will ensure that a nutritious snack is easily available. Flour (both white and whole wheat), oats, cornmeal, molasses, sugar, raisins and other dried fruit, and various spices are important if baking from scratch is common. Dry pantry staples (pasta, rice, flour, dry beans) are usually sold in boxes or bags. Always check to be sure packaging is intact, and store these foods in a sealed container after opening, as they are subject to insect contamination. Canned foods should be stored in a cool, dry location. Never buy swollen or dented cans, since the integrity of a dented can could be compromised and therefore allow bacterial contamination. Swelling could indicate bacterial growth within the can. Canned goods last much longer than fresh foods, but they are still subject to eventual deterioration. If canned goods are stored in a high moisture environment for long periods of time, they may rust.

A good supply of fresh fruits and vegetables, milk, cheese, and yogurt is a must for the well-stocked refrigerator. These items also make healthy snacks for children. When possible, prepare fresh vegetable sticks ahead of time, so that when a hungry child is looking for a snack, it will be ready to eat. To preserve vitamins and ensure both quality and flavor, proper storage is essential. Most fresh produce should be stored in the refrigerator, in the crisper section to prevent moisture loss. Exceptions include apples, avocados, bananas, citrus fruits, pears, potatoes, and onions, which are best stored in a cool, dry location. Neither fruits nor vegetables should be washed before storage since the extra moisture can contribute to the growth of mold.

When purchasing dairy products, always check the containers for leaks and other damage. The "sell-by" date is also important. Never buy a product if that date has already passed. It is safe to use

Surviving the Supermarket Excursion

A trip to the supermarket with children can be exhausting or exhilarating, depending on the age of the child and on the parent's approach to the experience. To turn an exhausting trip into an exhilarating one, try the following suggestions.

1. Never take hungry or tired children to the grocery store. If they are hungry, they may insist on having something to eat immediately, or they may request many favorite foods. In addition, tired or hungry children will be cranky and unable to tolerate waiting in line at the deli counter or at the checkout counter.

2. Use the grocery store as a classroom for toddlers and preschoolers. Have them identify the foods they eat regularly, and always tell them the names of foods that pique their interest.

3. Have older children help with the shopping. Provide them with a short list of items to collect, but be sure that the items are not breakable and are shelved within the children's reach.

4. Avoid conflicts over the purchase of particular food items by setting limits prior to arriving at the supermarket. If older children are allowed to choose snacks for their lunches, for example, let them know ahead that they must choose between two healthy snacks, for instance, pretzels and dried fruit. With toddlers and preschoolers, avoid the urge to purchase any item they request, just to avoid a conflict. If you refuse calmly and remain consistent, over time, they will learn what the limits are.

5. Occasionally allow the purchase of sweets or foods that are high in fat. On the way to the store, decide whether or not a treat will be purchased at that visit, and let the children know your decision. If a treat will not be purchased, state this and give a brief reason why ("We still have chips at home" or "You've had a lot of Halloween candy recently"). If they will be allowed a treat, set limitations before entering the store. If children get accustomed to knowing that they can have treats only occasionally, they are less likely to demand a treat on every visit. This reduces the likelihood of a tantrum in the store.

---

a product at home for a few days past the "sell by" date (remember it is a "sell by" date, not a "use by" date). Table 37.1 lists storage for various dairy products. Milk and cheese can be safely frozen, but the quality of the thawed product will be compromised. Previously frozen milk and cheese are thus best used in cooking.

Meat and poultry are also important dietary staples. Always choose fresh-looking meats and poultry and, as with dairy products, be sure that the "sell by" date has not yet passed. In addition, always check that the packaging material is intact. To avoid possible contamination of other foods by raw meat or poultry juice, fresh meat and poultry should be bagged separately from other foods. Table 37.2 lists storage conditions for various meat and poultry products. Refrigerated meats should be left in their original packaging, but frozen food should be wrapped in moisture- and vapor-proof packaging such as plastic bags, freezer paper, or

TABLE 37.1
Average Storage Time for Dairy Products

Food	Refrigerator storage time (40°F)
Milk (whole, low-fat, skim)	4–5 days
Yogurt	1–2 weeks
Cottage cheese	10–20 days
Cream cheese (opened)	2 weeks
Cheese slices	3 weeks
Hard cheese (cheddar, Swiss, etc.)	3–4 weeks
Sour cream	2–4 weeks
Eggs	3–5 weeks
Butter or margarine	1–2 months

TABLE 37.2
Average Storage Time for Meats and Poultry

Product	Refrigerator storage time (40°F)	Freezer storage time (0°F)
Fresh ground meat (all types)	1–2 days	3–4 months
Hot dogs, opened	1 week	1–2 months
Hot dogs, unopened	2 weeks	1–2 months
Lunch meat, opened	3–5 days	1–2 months
Lunch meat, unopened	2 weeks	1–2 months
Steaks or roasts, beef	3–5 days	6–12 months
Chops or roasts, pork	3–5 days	4–6 months
Chops or roasts, lamb	3–5 days	6–9 months
Chicken or turkey, whole	1–2 days	1 year
Chicken or turkey, pieces	1–2 days	9 months

aluminum foil (make sure all edges are carefully sealed). Freezer burn in meats is not harmful, but it does compromise taste and texture. If only one area of a product has a freezer burn, that section can be removed, and the taste and texture of the remaining portion will not be affected. It is safe to refreeze meats and poultry that have been thawed in the refrigerator, but the quality and taste will be compromised. Never thaw meats at room temperature.

Appropriate frozen foods can round out a well-stocked kitchen. Frozen vegetables are easily prepared and therefore extremely convenient for quick meals. Frozen fruits can be thawed for dessert or used to make frozen breakfast shakes. Fruit juice concentrates are the most economical way to purchase juice. Frozen fruits and vegetables are best if used within 2 to 3 months of purchase.

Resources

Brody, J. *Good Food Book.* New York: Norton, 1985.

Margen, S. *The Wellness Encyclopedia of Food and Nutrition.* New York: Health Letter Associates, distributed by Random House, 1992.

38
· · · · · · · ·

What's for Lunch?

The simple question, "What's for lunch?" can create quite a dilemma for parents who are trying to instill healthy eating habits in their children. The school lunches preferred by children are often higher in saturated fat, total fat, and sodium than is desirable, but at least children will eat them and not go hungry. Brown-bag lunches have the potential to be healthier, but not if children throw food away or trade healthy food for other items. When trying to ensure that children eat nutritious lunches, the principles to remember are variety, balance, and moderation. Keep in mind the following guidelines:

MYTH Children should take their lunch to school if they want a nutritious meal.
FACT If wise choices are made, school lunches can be healthy. Children should be encouraged to select a variety of foods.

1. Use the Food Guide Pyramid to plan a healthy lunch, whether purchased or brought from home (see fig. 4.1). Although including a majority of the food groups at lunch is a good idea, it is not necessary to eat a food from each group at lunch every day.

2. Involve children in planning their lunches. Using published cafeteria menus, jointly decide which lunches will be purchased and what the most desirable selections are. For brown-bag lunches, allow children to make choices and to assist in preparing some items; they may have more interest in eating what they themselves have fixed!

· · · · · · · · ·

Ellen Liskov

3. Include age-appropriate food items in bag lunches. For smaller children, plain foods, finger foods, and items with more interesting shapes (such as sandwiches cut with cookie cutters) may be most appealing.
4. Permit some favorite items (cookies, cupcakes), even if they are higher in fat, sodium, or sugar. Remember, it is the overall balance of the diet that matters, not one particular item.
5. Set limits and a budget for the purchase of less nutritious items from vending machines and snack bars.

No More "Brown-Bag Blues"

Packing a brown-bag lunch with a creative flair can help assure a varied, balanced diet that children will eat. For most school-age children, lunch should include at least two servings from the grain group, one fruit or vegetable, one or more servings from the meat or dairy group, and limited added fats and sweets.

GRAINS Sandwiches are popular with most children, and the occasional child enjoys a peanut-butter-and-jelly sandwich day in and day out, but for many children, sandwiches can get monotonous. Vary the style of breads used or, for a change of pace, use pita breads, rolls, English muffins, or tortillas. Younger children may prefer to eat crackers or a muffin rather than a sandwich. Whole-grain breads and rolls are good choices because they are high in fiber. Use biscuits, croissants, buttery-type crackers, and high-fat snack crackers less often.

Another lunchtime possibility is a pasta or rice salad, which may include small pieces of vegetables, cheese, beans, or meat, if they appeal to your child.

FRUITS Fresh fruit is the best choice, since it provides fiber and other nutrients. Fresh fruit can be served whole, or, for quick snacks, it can be cut up and stored. Fruits that are susceptible to browning when cut should be coated with orange or lemon juice. Dried fruits such as raisins, apricots, and apples are popular and may be readily accepted. Canned fruit packed in its own juice is another good alternative. Fruit juice is popular with children, but be sure to purchase drinks that are 100 percent juice rather than drinks with added sugar. Generally, 4 ounces of juice per day is sufficient.

VEGETABLES It is often a challenge to get children to eat vegetables, raw or cooked. As an enticement, dips like salsa, salad dressings made with unsaturated fats, and those made with reduced-fat sour cream can be used. Celery stuffed with reduced-fat cheese spread or peanut butter is an appealing way of combining the meat and vegetable groups. Lettuce and tomato add texture, moisture, and fiber to sandwiches, but these sandwich ingredients can make the bread soggy, so wrap them separately. Bits of raw or cooked vegetables can be mixed into pasta or rice salads as well. Finding a way to incorporate vegetables into the diet is important, since this food group provides many vitamins and minerals, as well as fiber.

MEATS All the items in this group are good sources of protein. Protein is an important dietary component, but the foods in this group also contribute a substantial amount of saturated fat, total fat, and cholesterol to most children's diets. Many older children need no more than 6 or 7 ounces from the meat group per day, and protein need not be included in every meal. Processed meats may be high in sodium and fat, but they are very convenient to use. Many sandwich meats are available in low-fat (about 5 grams of total fat per ounce) and nonfat varieties. Another option is to prepare extra meat or poultry at dinnertime for use in lunches. When making meat salads (such as tuna or chicken), the total amount of fat can be reduced by using low-fat mayonnaise.

Peanut butter is an all-round favorite for most children, but it is quite high in fat. The good news, however, is that most of the fat in peanut butter is unsaturated, especially when "natural" peanut butters are purchased. Reduced-fat peanut butter is also available.

DAIRY PRODUCTS Calcium and vitamin D are primarily obtained from this food group, which forms an essential part of a healthy diet. Many low-fat items are available: the chocolate milk sold in most schools is low-fat, reduced-fat cheese can be used for sandwiches, low-fat cheese can be spread on a celery stick, and many yogurts come in low-fat or nonfat varieties. By using a gel ice pack and an insulated lunch bag, yogurt can be safely chilled until lunchtime.

FATS AND SWEETS Fats should not be overly restricted in a child's diet unless medically advised, but, at the same time, reasonable limits should be set on the total amount of fat that a child eats, and saturated fats should be limited to no more than 10 percent of daily caloric needs. The most common sources of fat at lunch are mayonnaise, sandwich meats, peanut butter, whole-milk dairy products, snack foods, and bakery goods. Sweet treats are an enjoyable end to lunch, but the saturated fat and total fat content of these items should be closely monitored. Whenever possible, make baked goods at home using canola or other acceptable vegetable oils. Many low-fat recipes exist, or you can use your favorite recipes but reduce the amount of fat by between 25 and 50 percent by using applesauce instead of part of the oil. Muffins (corn, oatmeal, blueberry, apple, or pumpkin) and oatmeal raisin cookies are among favorite nutritious baked goods. When purchasing sweets, look for those that use unsaturated liquid oils and limit those prepared with hydrogenated or partially hydrogenated oil, shortening, butter, or lard. Candy is acceptable as an occasional treat; the best choices are those that are lowest in saturated and total fat, such as jelly beans, licorice, or hard candy.

POSSIBLE BROWN-BAG MENUS The lunch menus in the boxes are consistent with the dietary guidelines and use the Food Guide Pyramid for balance.

As these menus illustrate, it's possible to have a balanced diet and still pack interesting and tasty brown-bag lunches.

DID YOU PACK IT SAFELY? Food safety is an important consideration when packing a brown-bag lunch. Before preparing any food, of course, you need to wash your hands and any utensils you may be using. Any raw fruits or vegetables should also be thoroughly washed. To minimize the risk of food-borne illness, hot food should be kept hot and cold food should be kept cold. Store a prepared cold lunch in the refrigerator until the child leaves the house. Hot foods should be well heated (to a temperature in excess of 140°F) before being poured into an insulated bottle.

Here are some additional ideas for safely storing foods in brown-bag lunches.

1. If the lunch is usually a cold lunch, try using a thermal bag with a gel freezer pack to keep items cold.
2. Try freezing the sandwich. Plain sandwiches

Sample Lunch Menus

Menu 1

Turkey pita pocket sandwich		Calories:	560
Whole-wheat pita	(bread)	Fat (g):	17 (27 percent of calories)
2 slices turkey breast	(meat)	Saturated fat (g):	5 (8 percent of calories)
2 tsp mayonnaise	(fat)	Cholesterol (mg):	47
Lettuce and tomato	(vegetable)	Sodium (mg):	1400
8 oz carton 2 percent milk	(dairy)	Fiber (g):	5
Raisins	(fruit)	Calcium (mg):	345
3 gingersnap cookies	(sweets)		

Menu 2

Apple juice box (4 oz)	(fruit)	Calories:	430
2 oz low-fat cheese cubes and		Fat (g):	13 (26 percent of calories)
diced ham	(meat)	Saturated fat (g):	4 (7 percent of calories)
6 crackers	(bread)	Cholesterol (mg):	33
Carrot and celery sticks	(vegetable)	Sodium (mg):	1200
Low-fat pudding cup	(dairy)	Fiber (g):	2
		Calcium (mg):	373

Menu 3

Peanut butter (2 tbsp) and jelly	(bread,	Calories:	411
on wheat bread	meat, sweets)	Fat (g):	21 (44 percent of calories)
8 oz carton 2 percent milk	(dairy)	Saturated fat (g):	6 (13 percent of calories)
15 grapes	(fruit)	Cholesterol (mg):	18
		Sodium (mg):	280
		Fiber (g):	3
		Calcium (mg):	315

such as turkey, roast beef, or ham, if made the night before and then frozen, will defrost by lunchtime. Toppings such as lettuce or tomato will not freeze well, so they should be stored separately in the refrigerator.

3. Freeze juice boxes. The frozen box will act as an ice pack and chill other items in the lunch bag. By lunchtime, it will be thawed enough to drink.

4. Use an insulated bottle to keep yogurt or milk cold or to keep hot foods such as soup hot.

What Every Parent Should Know about School Lunches

In the past few years, school lunch programs have been criticized for providing meals that are not consistent with the principles of good nutrition.

Sample Lunch Menus (Continued)

Menu 4

Juice box (4 oz)	(fruit)	Calories:	540
Pasta salad		Fat (g):	14 (23 percent of calories)
½ cup cooked macaroni	(bread)	Saturated fat (g):	3 (15 percent of calories)
¼ cup tuna or 1 oz cubed		Cholesterol (mg):	17
low-fat cheese or chicken	(meat)	Sodium (mg):	650
¼ cup chopped tomato or		Fiber (g):	3
other raw vegetables	(vegetable)	Calcium (mg):	220
1½ tbsp reduced-fat salad			
dressing	(fat)		
1–2 Dutch pretzels	(bread)		
4 oz fruit yogurt	(dairy)		

Menu 5

Bologna sandwich		Calories:	660
2 slices turkey bologna	(meat)	Fat (g):	21 (29 percent of calories)
2 slices white bread	(bread)	Saturated fat (g):	9 (12 percent of calories)
2 tsp mustard	(misc)	Cholesterol (mg):	75
Lettuce	(vegetable)	Sodium (mg):	1140
2 percent chocolate milk	(dairy)	Fiber (g):	9
1 medium apple	(fruit)	Calcium (mg):	435
1 granola bar	(sweets)		

Week's Average

Calories:	527
Fat (g):	17 (29 percent of calories)
Saturated fat (g):	5 (9 percent of calories)
Cholesterol (mg):	38
Sodium (mg):	940
Fiber (g):	4
Calcium (mg)	340

Unfortunately, the foods that are made available at an extremely low cost to school systems are often high in fat, saturated fat, and sodium. Legislation was passed in 1995 that allows schools more flexibility in planning their menus but also requires federally subsidized school lunches to conform to current dietary guidelines. Therefore, meals must now contain no more than 30 percent of the total calories from fat and no more than 10 percent from saturated fat. However, à la carte items can still be high in fat, so planning remains necessary to ensure a child eats a healthy school lunch.

To make reasonable decisions about school lunches, start by having the children bring home cafeteria menus provided by the school. If the meal is high in fat or sodium, balance this in planning dinner meals or snacks for that day. On a day when a child chooses chicken nuggets (fried), French fries, cake, and milk, appropriate low-fat and healthy snacks—fruit, pretzels, or low-fat yogurt—should be selected to help achieve balance. A suitable dinner might include pasta with marinara sauce, salad with low-fat dressing, a vegetable, and fruit for dessert. Encourage children to choose low-fat milk and select fruit for desserts. Many schools have a salad bar that can be healthy if items are chosen carefully. Salad dressings and high-fat meat and pasta salads should be used in moderation.

Many parent teacher organizations (PTOs) have been instrumental in making school meals healthier, so consider getting involved. Food preparation methods and recipe modifications can be employed that will significantly lower the total fat and the saturated fat content of the foods offered.

Secrets behind the Glass

Vending machines and snack bars are found in many schools, and the choices they offer are often not as healthy as parents would like. Again, PTOs can be influential in deciding which items should be offered and which are not appropriate. Unfortunately, these decisions may be based on which items sell best (not which are most nutritious), because the income generated often benefits extra-curricular programs. Even in a vending machine packed with candies and chips, there are more acceptable food choices available. Some suggestions are given below.

Granola bars	Muffins
Pretzels	Bagels
Popcorn	Trail mix
Baked tortilla chips	Hard candy
Crackers	Fruit
Fruit juices made from 100 percent juice	Fig bars
	Frozen yogurt
Dried, canned, or fresh fruits	Frozen fruit bars
	Pudding pops
Low-fat milk	Sherbet
Low-fat yogurt	Italian ice

Discuss with your children the best vending machine choices and set limits and a budget for purchasing these items.

Fast Foods and Restaurants: Are You Speeding Past Good Nutrition?

The great diversity of ethnic cultures in the United States provides the opportunity to enjoy a variety of international foods as part of our daily diet. Pizza is often ordered by phone, or Chinese "take-out" is picked up on the way home from work. Fast foods are particularly popular because of their accessibility and convenience. Attractive television commercials and promotional ploys make them especially appealing to children.

Adults need to find their own way to obtain nutritious meals and to teach children to make healthy choices at fast food establishments. Fast

MYTH Fast food is junk food.
FACT Many fast foods are high in fat, calories, and sugar, but the occasional consumption of these foods can fit into a healthy diet. Moreover, many fast food restaurants offer healthier items, such as salads or reduced-fat sandwiches. Remember that moderation is the key.

foods have commonly been labeled unhealthy, but many fast food restaurants now offer items that are lower in fat and sodium. In this chapter, the characteristics of fast food and several common cuisines will be described and guidelines on menu selection will be given.

Fast Foods and Take-Out

THE PROBLEM The sample fast food meal presented in table 39.1 provides almost 1,000 calories and 40 grams (360 calories) of fat. The large number of calories may not by itself

TABLE 39.1
Typical Fast Food Meal

	Calories	Fat (g)	Fat (calories)	Cholesterol (mg)	Sodium (mg)	Calcium (mg)	Vitamin C (mg)
Cheeseburger	295	14	126	37	616	111	2
French fries	237	12	108	11	124	12	4
Soda (12 oz)	144	0	0	0	14	9	0
Apple pie (fried)	266	14	126	13	325	12	1
Total	942	40	360	61	1079	144	7

be a significant concern, since many active children require a large number of calories. One of the problems with this meal is that the fat content constitutes 38 percent of the total calories (30 percent of the total calories from fat is the recommended maximum). The sodium content (1,079 milligrams) of this single meal is almost half of the maximum recommended daily intake of 2,400 milligrams. Although calcium is very important for bone development, this meal provides only 144 milligrams, compared with the recommended daily allowance of 800 to 1,200 milligrams. The same trend is seen for vitamin C, iron, and vitamin A as well: the meal fails to provide a good amount of these important nutrients.

In general, fast food meals tend to provide an excess of fat, cholesterol, sodium, and possibly calories. These excesses are associated with an increased risk for hypertension, cardiovascular diseases, and obesity in future years. A typical fast food meal can easily derive 45 to 55 percent of its calories from fat. At the same time, fast foods are generally low in the vitamins and minerals that are important for normal growth and well-being. Moreover, servings are bigger than ever. In the past, there were small fries and large fries; now there are "super" fries. Soft drinks used

to come in small, medium, and large sizes; now there is also a "jumbo" drink. Teenagers often eat fast foods quickly without paying attention to the large amount they are consuming because they are doing something else at the same time, such as watching a movie.

THE SOLUTION Although most of the choices available at fast food restaurants tend to be too high in some nutrients and too low in others, it is possible to get a nutritionally sound meal, as shown in table 39.2.

This meal contains 35 percent fewer calories than the meal presented in table 39.1. Calories from fat are only 10 percent of the total for this meal, and the sodium content is substantially lower. Vitamin C content satisfies the Recommended Dietary Allowance (RDA) for the whole day, and the calcium content is also higher. This meal is much healthier than the one presented in table 39.1.

To make healthy choices in a fast food restaurant, one has to look at both the cooking method and the food itself. Select foods that are naturally nutritious (low in fat and sodium, and high in vitamins and minerals), and choose a cooking method that does not add a lot of fat and sodium

TABLE 39.2

Healthier Fast Food Meal

	Calories	Fat (g)	Fat (calories)	Cholesterol (mg)	Sodium (mg)	Calcium (mg)	Vitamin C (mg)
Grilled chicken sandwich	254	3	27	47	506	117	5
Strawberry frozen yogurt sundae	210	1	9	5	95	190	1
Orange juice (6 oz)	84	0	0	0	2	17	73
Side salad	60	3	27	41	85	76	7
Total	608	7	63	93	688	400	86

(baking, broiling, and grilling are wise choices, for example, whereas deep-fried or pan-fried foods should be avoided). For example, in the typical fast food meal presented in table 39.1, the combination of beef and cheese in the cheeseburger is inherently high in fat. In French fries, although potatoes are inherently low in fat, the frying process adds a large amount of fat to the food. In the healthier meal presented in table 39.2, the chicken in the grilled chicken sandwich is naturally low in fat and the cooking method (grilling) does not add extra fat. Table 39.3 summarizes some of the healthier food choices.

Restaurants

Trying to get children to eat a healthy meal at a restaurant need not be a nightmare if one knows what to choose. Almost all restaurants offer some healthy menu choices, since consumers are requesting meals with less fat and less sodium.

First of all, select a balanced meal that includes carbohydrate, protein, and vegetables. Order a side salad or vegetables if the main dish does not include vegetables. Make use of the Kids' Menu if the restaurant offers one. Encourage children to choose items prepared using a low-fat cook-

ing method like baking, broiling, poaching, steaming, or roasting. Methods of preparation that use more fat (au gratin, buttered, creamed, fried, or marinated in oil) should be selected infrequently. Dishes seasoned with herbs, spices, or lemon juice are good choices. Vegetarian dishes that are not prepared with cream or cheese sauce (Alfredo sauce, for example) are also a good idea. Note that some sauces like soy sauce, teriyaki sauce, tomato sauce, and barbecue sauce are high in sodium. Of course, in addition to the cooking method, choosing nutritious food is also important.

Many restaurants are happy to honor special needs or reasonable requests from customers. If one is not sure of the preparation method, ask the waitstaff. Many restaurants willingly serve the sauce, gravy, or dressing on the side; then children can add these higher-fat toppings to the food in moderate amounts. Some restaurants will even accommodate requests to reduce salt in preparing the food or to eliminate chopped eggs from salads. Simply ask if modifications can be made.

Encourage children to taste the food before picking up the salt shaker. Children will not acquire a strong taste for salt if they are not exposed to large quantities of it constantly (see chapter 3). When dressing or sauces are ordered on the side,

TABLE 39.3

Guide to Fast Food Choices

Food	Choose more	Choose less
Fish	Baked fish, remove batter or bread coating	Fried fish
Chicken	Skinless pieces, remove fried coating	Nuggets (usually contain ground chicken skin)
Hamburger	Burgers that have only one patty	Burgers that come with sauce and fatty toppings like bacon and cheese
Deli sandwiches (including grinders and submarines)	Slices of turkey or chicken breast, lean roast beef or ham, vegetables (lettuce, tomatoes, sprouts, onions), whole-grain breads	Cheese, bologna, chicken salad, tuna salad, seafood salad (and other salads that contain mayonnaise)
Pizza	Vegetable toppings (peppers, onions, mushrooms, broccoli, spinach)	Sausage, extra cheese, pepperoni, bacon
Breakfast foods	Bagels with fruit spreads or jams, small whole-grain muffins, half of a large muffin	Regular cream cheese, doughnuts, Danish pastries, hash brown potatoes, bacon, sausage
Beverages	Juices, low-fat milk, water	Soft drinks, milk shakes, malted milks
Desserts	Low- or nonfat frozen yogurt, sherbet	Cookies, ice cream, fruit pies (these are often fried, and, in any case, the crust is high in fat)
Condiments	Mustard, low-calorie dressings and sauces, small amounts of regular dressings and sauces	Creamy sauces (mayonnaise, tartar), regular salad dressings, ketchup (high in sodium)

use only small to moderate amounts. It is difficult to taste the real flavor of the dish if it is swimming in dressing or sauce. Help children learn to use a small amount of butter, margarine, and sour cream on rolls, bread, and baked potatoes.

Do not force children to finish everything on their plate; restaurant portions may well be too big for them. Some restaurants may allow two children to share one dish, and uneaten portions can always be taken home, even in fancy restaurants.

The main concerns with dessert are usually the high fat content and the absence of other nutrients. With a little attention, the ending of a meal can be both sweet and healthy. When it comes to desserts, angel food cake is a better choice than regular cake with frosting. Frozen yogurt, ice milk, fruit ice, and sorbet are lower in fat and calories than ice cream. Fresh fruits and gelatins are preferable to pastries and cheesecakes. If a higher-fat dessert is chosen, children can be encouraged to share with another person.

Finding the Way among Different Cuisines

AMERICAN Typical American foods are actually a combination and evolution of northern European cooking: for example, English, Irish, and

German. Dinners from these countries usually include some kind of roast meat, potatoes, and vegetables. A typical English breakfast consists of eggs; bacon, ham, or sausage; and toast. American Northerners have added hash brown potatoes, and Southerners have added grits. Protein and fat are abundant in these meals, but they lack fiber, vegetables, and fruits. One can improve the balance by choosing a smaller portion of meat and ordering more carbohydrates, such as rice, pasta, or broiled/baked potatoes.

Many restaurants have a salad bar. Children should be encouraged to choose fresh raw vegetables and fruits. Beans are also good choices. Mayonnaise-based items like coleslaw, potato salad, and some pasta salads are high in fat and should only be used in small amounts. Avoid adding a large amount of cheese, chopped eggs, and bacon bits. Noncreamy dressings are, of course, healthier than the creamy ones, but the do-it-yourself oil and vinegar dressing is also a good choice if more vinegar than oil is used.

ITALIAN Italian cuisine can be divided into northern and southern styles. Northern Italian dishes contain more animal products like meat, butter, cheese, and eggs. Southern Italian foods contain more pastas and vegetables, such as artichokes, eggplant, peppers, and tomatoes, and olive oil is used. Antipasto, a popular appetizer, is high in both fat and salt. A better choice for starting the meal would be minestrone soup. Many Italian restaurants offer garlic bread, which is usually high in fat (butter) and salt. Plain warm bread or bread sticks would be a healthier choice, with a little Parmesan or Romano cheese sprinkled on for added flavor. Italian cuisine is famous for its vast array of sauces. Marinara and plain tomato sauce are low in fat but contain a lot of sodium. Alfredo and pesto sauces, on the other hand, are rather high in fat. Cheese and sausage are also common in Italian cooking. Dishes with large amounts of sausage or cheese—like lasagna, veal parmigiana, and cannelloni—should be ordered only occasionally. Pizza can be a wise choice, if it is a vegetable pizza without extra cheese.

MEXICAN Common ingredients in authentic day-to-day Mexican food are tortillas, eggs, a mixture of beans and rice, stew, and cooked vegetables. The popular ingredients in Mexican restaurants—refried beans, sour cream, guacamole, salsa—are more like special occasion foods for Mexicans.

The first thing one usually sees upon being seated in a Mexican restaurant is a basket of chips and a bowl of salsa. Unfortunately, children may fill up on chips, which are high in fat and sodium, before the main meal arrives. The Mexican names of food on the menu can be confusing, so do not hesitate to ask about the ingredients and how the dishes are prepared. Dishes that include fried tortillas, refried beans, sour cream, and high-fat ground beef should be chosen only occasionally. Other high-fat items include nachos, beef and cheese enchiladas, and chimichangas. Fajitas are made with marinated lean beef or chicken and vegetables that are grilled in a small amount of oil and served with soft tortillas. It is a great choice, for it is a balanced and reasonably lean dish, but the condiments that accompany it (sour cream and guacamole) should be used sparingly. Guacamole, a popular dip, is made with avocado and garlic. Avocado is high in fat, but it is mainly monounsaturated fat, and the avocado does provide additional nutrients, so it is acceptable when used in moderation. Mexican rice, made of rice and tomatoes, is a healthy side dish, as are plain beans, but the refried beans will provide too much fat. Other healthy choices include soft tacos and vegetable quesadillas.

CHINESE AND JAPANESE In general, Asian cuisines use very little oil in cooking except for deep-fried dishes, but they can be high in sodium because of the extensive use of soy sauce. Obtaining a balanced meal at an Asian restaurant can be easy because most dishes combine meat, poultry, or fish with vegetables. These dishes are often served with steamed rice, which is prepared without added salt. Common seasonings include ginger root, scallions, garlic, and soy sauce. Foods are prepared in bite-size pieces, which allow for rapid cooking and minimize the loss of nutrients. Vegetables are stir-fried or steamed rather than boiled, which also minimizes nutrient loss into cooking water.

Sashimi is a popular Japanese dish, but it uses uncooked fish, which can cause food-borne infections if it has been contaminated. Tofu (steamed bean curd) is high in protein and common in Asian cuisines. Although about 50 percent of the calories come from fat, the fats in tofu are primarily polyunsaturated and monounsaturated fats. Fresh fruits are typical desserts in Asian restaurants, and fortune cookies contain only 25 calories each.

To limit your fat intake, avoid items like fried rice, fried wonton, egg rolls, tempura, egg foo yung, batter-dipped items, and spareribs. Soy sauce and teriyaki sauce are high in sodium and should be added only sparingly at the table. Miso soup is also high in sodium.

FRENCH Although a number of French dishes contain quite a large amount of cream and cheese, there are a lot of healthy choices as well. Healthy choices include poached or broiled fish, salad niçoise (if the dressing is used sparingly), coq au vin, bouillabaisse (fish soup), and ratatouille. Menu items are sometimes in French and one should not feel embarrassed to ask for additional information on ingredients and cooking method. Less healthy items to watch for are quiche (a cheese and egg pie), duck or goose (they are naturally high in fat), fondue, croissants, rich pastries, béarnaise and hollandaise sauce, and vegetables prepared "au gratin" (with added cheese).

Resources

AICR Information Series III, Cook's Day Off: A Handbook for Eating Out and Following the Dietary Guidelines to Lower Cancer Risk. Washington, DC: American Institute for Cancer Research, 1990.

Warshaw, H. *The Restaurant Companion.* Chicago, IL: Surrey Books, 1990.

PART SIX

Recipes

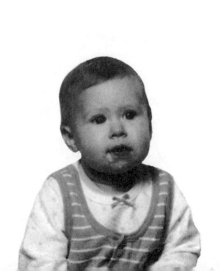

These recipes were submitted by some of the most respected chefs in the United States. The recipes were chosen for their tastiness, ease of preparation, and healthful ingredients. Most are easy to prepare, and some are intended to be prepared by children themselves.

Each recipe has been tested professionally, and, when necessary, adaptations have been made to assure recipe success. Approximate preparation times are listed for added convenience, and a nutrient analysis has also been calculated for each recipe.

Some recipes showcase special ingredients and gourmet techniques. To save time or to cater to a child's picky eating habits or special needs, use shortcuts or encourage the child to participate in the cooking process. For example, open a can of beans instead of preparing dried beans from scratch, or skip the skinning and seeding of fresh tomatoes; allow the child to wash the fruit and stir ingredients.

Serving sizes represent typical restaurant portions; therefore, depending on a child's age, the actual portion size served may need to be adjusted. Although the recipes use only quality ingredients, the dishes are not necessarily low in fat or calories. As stressed throughout the book, the whole diet, not just individual foods, should be considered when developing a healthy meal plan. Balance, variety, and moderation are the best guides to food choices. Most important, the entire family should enjoy the majority of the recipes that follow.

Foods for Infants
Carrot and Potato Puree
French Green Lentil and Rice Puree
Pea Puree

Squash and Apple Puree

Breakfast Foods

Banana Carrot Bread

Banana-Split Pancakes

Cantaloupe Soup

Corn Pancakes with Maple Fruit Compote

Muesli and Yogurt

Whole-Wheat Blueberry Muffins

Lunch Box Treats

Cherry Tomatoes and Olives

Garlic Toast

Herb Cheese

Strawberry Compote

Waldorf Tuna Salad

Snacks

Cheese Potato Crisp

Flatbread with Monterey Jack Cheese

Parsnip Chips

Peanut Butter Bread

Pita Snacks

Trail Mix

Meat, Poultry, and Fish Entrées

Alsatian Baekeofa

Arizona Turkey

Beef and Vegetable Burritos

Cajun-Style Chicken Fingers

Curried Chicken and Rice

Foolproof Roast Chicken

Healthy Twist Meatloaf

Raspberry-Ginger Chicken

Soft Teriyaki Chicken Tacos

Summer Salad with Tuna Fish Dressing
and Croutons

Whole-Wheat Turkey Pizzas

Carbohydrate-Dense Dishes

Baked Elbow Pasta with Shrimp and Zucchini

Black-Eyed Pea Salsa

Fava Bean Puree

My Favorite Fried Rice

Rice à l'Orange

Rice and Potato Minestra

Spaetzle with Fromage Blanc and Herbs

Twisted Cornmeal Breadsticks

White Bean–Vegetable Casserole

Vegetarian Selections

Angel Hair Pasta
with Roasted Red Pepper–Tomato Sauce

Cream of Spinach with Soft-Cooked Eggs

Eggplant Sauce

Green Risotto with Vegetables

Lentil Stew

Pasta with Peanut Sauce

Pizza Presto

Sweet Corn Ravioli

Vegetable Lasagna

Vegetable Side Dishes

Gingered Carrots

Mashed Parsnips and Potatoes

Mashed Yellow Turnips with Crispy Shallots

Oven French Fries

Roasted Root Vegetables

Sautéed Spinach with Garlic

Spinach-Mushroom Pudding

Desserts

Chocolate Cake with Raspberry Sauce

Cocoa Brownies

Crepes for Kids

Maple-Glazed Tropical Fruit Salad

Oatmeal Cookies

Poached Pears

Rice Pudding

Strawberries with Balsamic Vinegar

Super Cherry Tiramisu

Tabbouleh with Fresh Fruit Ratatouille

....

Foods for Infants

Carrot and Potato Puree
French Green Lentil and Rice Puree
Pea Puree
Squash and Apple Puree

· · · · · · · ·

Carrot and Potato Puree

Serves 8
Preparation time: 18 minutes
Cooking time: 15 minutes

From: Roxsand Scocos, Roxsand Restaurant and Bar, Phoenix, Arizona

2 cups peeled, diced carrots
1½ cups peeled, diced all-purpose potatoes
¼ cup milk
2 tablespoons butter, softened

1. Put carrots and potatoes in a steamer. Cover and steam over simmering water until very tender, about 15 minutes.

2. Transfer to a food processor. Add milk and butter and process until pureed.

Nutrient analysis per ¼-cup serving
Calories 67; Protein 1 g; Carbohydrates 9 g; Fat—total 3 g; Saturated fat 2 g; Cholesterol 9 mg; Dietary fiber 1 g; Calcium 20 mg; Iron 0 mg; Sodium 44 mg

......

French Green Lentil and Rice Puree

Serves 8
Preparation time: 15 minutes
Cooking time: 70–80 minutes

From: Roxsand Scocos, Roxsand Restaurant and Bar, Phoenix, Arizona

Look for dark green French lentils in specialty food shops or health food stores. If you substitute ordinary green lentils, be sure to cover the lentils with at least 3 cups of water in step 2, and cook them for an additional 10 minutes.

½ cup short-grain brown rice
1 cup water
½ cup French green lentils, picked over and
  rinsed
¼ cup chopped carrots
¼ cup chopped celery
¼ cup milk
2 tablespoons butter, softened
2 tablespoons chopped fresh parsley (optional)

1. In a medium saucepan, combine rice and 1 cup of water. Cover and bring to a boil. Reduce heat and simmer, covered, for 50 minutes. Remove from heat and let stand, covered, for 15 to 20 minutes or until rice is tender and liquid is absorbed.

2. Meanwhile put lentils in a small saucepan and cover generously with water. Bring to a boil, reduce heat, and simmer, uncovered, for 20 to 30 minutes or until tender. Drain well.

3. Put carrots and celery in a steamer. Cover and steam over simmering water until tender, 10 to 15 minutes.

4. Transfer rice, lentils, and vegetables to a food processor or blender. Add milk, butter, and parsley and process until pureed.

Nutrient analysis per ¼-cup serving
Calories 122; Protein 4 g; Carbohydrates 18 g; Fat—total 4 g; Saturated fat 2 g; Cholesterol 7 mg; Dietary fiber 2 g; Calcium 25 mg; Iron 1 mg; Sodium 40 mg

. . . .

Pea Puree

Serves 6
Preparation time: 10 minutes
Cooking time: 10 minutes

From: Kathy Cary, Lilly's la Pêche, Louisville, Kentucky

Adding ripe pear to this puree gives it a sweet and refreshing flavor.

1 10-ounce package frozen peas
1 medium-size ripe pear, peeled, cored, and
    chopped
⅛ teaspoon grated nutmeg

1. Cook peas according to package directions. Drain well.

2. Transfer peas to a food processor. Add pear and nutmeg and process until pureed.

Nutrient analysis per ¼-cup serving
Calories 53; Protein 3 g; Carbohydrates 11 g; Fat—total 0 g; Saturated fat 0 g; Cholesterol 0 mg; Dietary fiber 3 g; Calcium 15 mg; Iron 1 mg; Sodium 41 mg

· · · · · · · ·

Squash and Apple Puree

Serves 8
Preparation time: 20 minutes
Cooking time: 20 minutes

From: Roxsand Scocos, Roxsand Restaurant and Bar, Phoenix, Arizona

Cut the squash and apple into ½-inch pieces for quick cooking.

2 cups peeled, diced butternut squash (1 medium squash)
1½ cups peeled, diced Granny Smith apples (about 2 medium apples)
¼ teaspoon ground cinnamon
½ teaspoon vanilla extract

1. Place squash and apples in a steamer. Cover and steam over simmering water until very tender, about 20 minutes.

2. Transfer squash and apples to a food processor or blender. Add cinnamon and vanilla and process until pureed.

Nutrient analysis per ¼-cup serving
Calories 25; Protein 0 g; Carbohydrates 7 g; Fat—total 0 g; Saturated fat 0 g; Cholesterol 0 mg; Dietary fiber 1 g; Calcium 17 mg; Iron 0 mg; Sodium 31 mg

. . . .

Breakfast Foods

Banana Carrot Bread
Banana-Split Pancakes
Cantaloupe Soup
Corn Pancakes with Maple Fruit Compote
Muesli and Yogurt
Whole-Wheat Blueberry Muffins

· · · · · · · ·

Banana Carrot Bread

Makes 1 loaf (12 slices)
Preparation time: 15 minutes
Baking time: 1 hour

From: Elizabeth Terry, Elizabeth on 37th,
Savannah, Georgia

This not-too-sweet bread is perfect to slice for breakfast, serve as an after-school snack, or pack in a lunch box.

1¾ cups unbleached all-purpose flour
¼ cup wheat germ
2 teaspoons baking powder
½ teaspoon baking soda
½ teaspoon salt
2 tablespoons unsalted butter, softened
2 tablespoons vegetable oil
¼ cup packed light brown sugar
2 large eggs
2 medium-size ripe bananas, mashed
1 cup shredded carrots
½ cup buttermilk

1. Preheat oven to 350°F. Grease a 9-×-5-inch loaf pan.

2. In a medium bowl, mix flour, wheat germ, baking powder, baking soda, and salt. Set aside.

3. In a medium bowl, beat butter, oil, and sugar with an electric mixer until smooth and blended. Beat in eggs one at a time, beating well after each addition. Beat in bananas and carrots.

4. To banana-carrot mixture, alternately add flour mixture and buttermilk in small batches. Stir in each batch with a rubber spatula just until blended.

5. Scrape batter into prepared pan. Bake for 1 hour or until a toothpick inserted into the center comes out clean. Set pan on a wire rack to cool for 10 minutes. Turn bread out onto rack and let cool completely before slicing.

Nutrient analysis per slice
Calories 159; Protein 4 g; Carbohydrates 24 g; Fat—total 6 g; Saturated fat 2 g; Cholesterol 41 mg; Dietary fiber 1 g; Calcium 71 mg; Iron 1 mg; Sodium 196 mg

· · · · · · · ·

Banana-Split Pancakes

Serves 6 (12 pancakes)
Preparation time: 20 minutes
Cooking time: 10 minutes

From: Kathy Farrell-Kingsley, Newtown, Connecticut

These breakfast splits are colorful and fun to make. If you set out the topping ingredients, children can build their own. Substitute any berry that is in season, or offer a combination of berries.

Pancakes
1 cup all-purpose flour
¾ cup whole-wheat flour
1 tablespoon sugar (optional)
2 teaspoons baking powder
½ teaspoon salt
1 teaspoon ground cinnamon
½ teaspoon ground nutmeg
2 large eggs
3 tablespoons vegetable oil
1¼ cups milk

Topping
3 medium-size ripe bananas
8 ounces frozen vanilla yogurt
8 ounces frozen strawberry yogurt
1 8-ounce can crushed unsweetened pineapple, drained
¾ cup fresh sliced strawberries (or any other berry)
¾ cup granola
whole strawberries, hulled, for garnish

1. Preheat oven to 200°F.
2. In a small bowl, mix all-purpose flour, whole-wheat flour, sugar, baking powder, salt, cinnamon, and nutmeg.
3. In a medium bowl, whisk together eggs, oil, and milk. Add flour mixture and stir just until combined.
4. Heat a lightly greased griddle or large skillet over medium-high heat until hot enough for a few drops of water to dance on the surface. For each pancake pour about ¼ cup of the batter onto the hot griddle. Cook until bubbles appear on the surface, and edges are lightly browned, about 1½ minutes. Flip pancakes and cook about 1 minute or until undersides are golden brown. Transfer pancakes to a plate and keep warm in oven while cooking remaining batter.
5. *To assemble:* Peel each banana and cut in half lengthwise, then crosswise. Place 2 pancakes on each serving plate. Top each serving with 2 banana pieces and a scoop each of vanilla and strawberry yogurt. Spoon pineapple and berries over yogurt and sprinkle with some granola. Garnish with a whole strawberry and serve right away.

Nutrient analysis per 2-pancake serving
Calories 488; Protein 14 g; Carbohydrates 76 g; Fat—total 16 g; Saturated fat 4 g; Cholesterol 82 mg; Dietary fiber 6 g; Calcium 313 mg; Iron 3 mg; Sodium 436 mg

Cantaloupe Soup

Serves 4
Preparation time: 15 minutes plus
at least 4 hours to chill

From: Odessa Piper, L'Etoile, Madison, Wisconsin

This chilled fruit soup can be served for breakfast, lunch, or dessert. You can buy plastic squeeze bottles in kitchen supply shops, or you can recycle a ketchup squeeze bottle.

1 large ripe cantaloupe, seeded, with the flesh cut
    into chunks
1 to 3 teaspoons sugar
1 to 3 teaspoons fresh lemon juice
1 cup plain nonfat yogurt
1 teaspoon peeled, minced fresh ginger root
fresh mint leaves, for garnish
fresh berries, for garnish

1. Put cantaloupe in a food processor or blender and puree. Transfer to a medium bowl. Stir in sugar and lemon juice to taste. Cover and refrigerate for 4 hours or until thoroughly chilled.

2. In a small bowl, mix yogurt and ginger. Pass through a fine sieve into a squeeze bottle.

3. Ladle chilled soup into serving bowls. Let children write their names or make designs by squeezing yogurt onto soup. Garnish with fresh mint and berries, if desired.

Nutrient analysis per 1-cup serving
Calories 90; Protein 5 g; Carbohydrates 18 g; Fat—total 0.5 g; Saturated fat 0 g; Cholesterol 1 mg; Dietary fiber 1 g; Calcium 137 mg; Iron 0 mg; Sodium 39 mg

....

Corn Pancakes with Maple Fruit Compote

Serves 6 (12 pancakes)
Preparation time: 10 minutes plus 1 hour to stand
Cooking time: 10 minutes

From: Mary Sue Milliken and Susan Feniger,
Border Grille, Santa Monica, California

This is a wonderful way to add grains to your child's diet. Use whatever fruits are seasonally available for the compote—such as plums, pears, peaches, strawberries, or raspberries—and chop them up before tossing them with maple syrup.

Maple Fruit Compote
2 cups cut-up fresh fruits or whole small berries
1 cup pure maple syrup

Corn Pancakes
1 cup yellow cornmeal, preferably organic
¼ cup unbleached all-purpose flour
¾ teaspoon baking soda
¾ teaspoon salt
1 cup buttermilk
½ cup milk
2 tablespoons butter, melted

1. *To make compote:* In a medium bowl, combine fruit and maple syrup. Toss gently and let stand for 1 hour at room temperature. Transfer to a medium saucepan and warm just before serving.

2. Preheat oven to 200°F.

3. In a medium bowl, mix cornmeal, flour, baking soda, and salt.

4. In a small bowl, mix buttermilk, milk, and butter. Add to cornmeal mixture, stirring just until blended. Stir again before pouring batter onto the griddle.

5. Heat a lightly greased griddle or large heavy skillet over medium-high heat until hot enough for a few drops of water to dance on the surface.

6. For each pancake pour about ¼ cup of the batter onto the hot griddle. Cook for 1 to 1½ minutes on each side or until golden brown on both sides. Transfer pancakes to a plate and keep warm in oven while cooking remaining batter.

7. Serve right away with warm fruit compote.

Nutrient analysis per 2-pancake serving
Calories 331; Protein 5 g; Carbohydrates 67 g; Fat—total 6 g; Saturated fat 3 g; Cholesterol 15 mg; Dietary fiber 3 g; Calcium 115 mg; Iron 2 mg; Sodium 521 mg

. . . .

Muesli and Yogurt

Serves 6
Preparation time: 10 minutes

From: Roxsand Scocos, Roxsand Restaurant and Bar, Phoenix, Arizona

Use your favorite store-bought muesli for this recipe. The apple can be unpeeled or peeled, depending on your preference.

3 cups muesli
3 cups vanilla nonfat yogurt
2 medium-size ripe bananas
1 medium Granny Smith apple

1. Put muesli in a large bowl and add yogurt. Toss until blended.

2. Dice banana and apple and add to muesli mixture. Stir gently until blended. Serve right away.

Nutrient analysis per 1-cup serving
Calories 299; Protein 10 g; Carbohydrates 65 g; Fat—total 2 g; Saturated fat 0.5 g; Cholesterol 2 mg; Dietary fiber 5 g; Calcium 241 mg; Iron 5 mg; Sodium 138 mg

. . . .

Whole-Wheat Blueberry Muffins

Makes 12 muffins
Preparation time: 15 minutes
Baking time: 25 minutes

From: Kathy Farrell-Kingsley, Newtown, Connecticut

These muffins are also delicious when made with raspberries, strawberries, diced peaches, or other fresh fruit.

1⅓ cups whole-wheat flour
1 cup unbleached all-purpose flour
½ cup sugar
1 teaspoon baking soda
1 teaspoon baking powder
½ teaspoon salt
¼ teaspoon ground allspice
1 cup buttermilk
2 tablespoons vegetable oil
1 large egg white (2 tablespoons)
1¼ cups fresh or thawed frozen blueberries

1. Preheat oven to 375°F. Line 12 standard-size muffin pan cups with foil muffin cups.
2. In a small bowl, combine whole-wheat flour, all-purpose flour, sugar, baking soda, baking powder, salt, and allspice.
3. In a medium bowl, whisk together buttermilk, oil, and egg white. Add dry ingredients to buttermilk mixture, stirring just until moistened. Gently fold in blueberries.
4. Spoon batter into muffin cups, filling each about two-thirds full. Bake for 20 to 25 minutes or until tops are lightly golden. Set pan on a wire rack for 5 minutes. Turn muffins out onto rack and cool completely.

Nutrient analysis per muffin
Calories 154; Protein 4 g; Carbohydrates 29 g; Fat—total 3 g; Saturated fat 0.5 g; Cholesterol 1 mg; Dietary fiber 2 g; Calcium 54 mg; Iron 1 mg; Sodium 261 mg

....

Lunch Box Treats

Cherry Tomatoes and Olives
Garlic Toast
Herb Cheese
Strawberry Compote
Waldorf Tuna Salad

. . . .

Cherry Tomatoes and Olives

Serves 1
Preparation time: 10 minutes

From: Alice Waters, Chez Panisse, Berkeley, California

Here is a good recipe for late summer, when sweet ripe cherry tomatoes are abundant. Any variety of tomato will taste good, but cherry tomatoes are an appealing size for children.

½ cup ripe cherry tomatoes, stemmed and cut in half
2 teaspoons olive oil
pinch of salt
6 ripe pitted olives, any variety

1. In a small bowl, mix tomatoes, oil, and salt.
2. Stir in olives.

Nutrient analysis per serving
Calories 125; Protein 1 g; Carbohydrates 6 g; Fat—total 11 g; Saturated fat 1.8 g; Cholesterol 0 mg; Dietary fiber 2 g; Calcium 23 mg; Iron 1 mg; Sodium 711 mg

. . . .

Garlic Toast

Serves 1
Preparation time: 10 minutes

From: Alice Waters, Chez Panisse, Berkeley,
California

Garlic toast is delicious served with Herb Cheese
(page 311) and Cherry Tomatoes and Olives
(page 309). Use a flavorful sturdy bread, like
sourdough bread or a baguette.

2, ½-inch-thick slices good bread
1 clove garlic, peeled
1 tablespoon olive oil

1. Toast bread slices.
2. Brush toasted bread with olive oil. Gently
rub surface of bread with garlic clove. Cut each
slice of bread into 2- or 3-inch pieces.

Nutrient analysis per serving
Calories 261; Protein 5 g; Carbohydrates 27 g; Fat—
total 15 g; Saturated fat 2 g; Cholesterol 0 mg; Dietary
fiber 1 g; Calcium 43 mg; Iron 1 mg; Sodium 305 mg

. . . .

Herb Cheese

Serves 4
Preparation time: 10 minutes plus time to chill

From: Alice Waters, Chez Panisse, Berkeley, California

This recipe calls for fresh parsley and chervil, but you can use any fresh herbs that you have on hand. Herbed cream cheese can be served as a spread or dip.

1 8-ounce package cream cheese, softened
2 tablespoons chopped fresh parsley
1 tablespoon chopped fresh chervil

1. In a small bowl, mix cream cheese and herbs with a wooden spoon until well blended.

2. *To serve as a lunch box treat:* Divide the mixture into 4 equal portions. Wrap each portion in plastic. Pack one portion in a lunch box. Refrigerate remaining portions up to 1 week.

Nutrient analysis per ¼-cup serving
Calories 199; Protein 4 g; Carbohydrates 2 g; Fat—total 20 g; Saturated fat 13 g; Cholesterol 62 mg; Dietary fiber 0 g; Calcium 51 mg; Iron 1 mg; Sodium 169 mg

. . . .

Strawberry Compote

Serves 1
Preparation time: 5 minutes plus 20 minutes to stand

From: Alice Waters, Chez Panisse, Berkeley, California

Cold storage can create a refreshingly chilled compote for a child's school dessert. Put the compote in a plastic container, place a sealed plastic sandwich bag containing 4 ice cubes on top of the compote, then put the lid on the container—the compote will be cool by lunchtime. Or you can chill the compote ahead of time and put it in a thermos.

5 to 8 medium-size ripe strawberries, hulled
¼ cup orange juice
4 ice cubes (optional)

1. Cut strawberries in quarters or halves depending on their size.

2. In a small bowl, combine strawberries and orange juice. Let stand at room temperature for 20 minutes before chilling.

Nutrient analysis per serving
Calories 86; Protein 2 g; Carbohydrates 20 g; Fat—total 1 g; Saturated fat 0 g; Cholesterol 0 mg; Dietary fiber 3 g; Calcium 34 mg; Iron 1 mg; Sodium 3 mg

· · · · · · · ·

Waldorf Tuna Salad

Serves 3
Preparation time: 10 minutes

From: Lucie Costa, North Plank Road Tavern, Newburgh, New York

Fill pita pockets with this tuna salad, or spread it on your favorite bread.

1 6-ounce can albacore white tuna packed in
   water, drained
2 tablespoons Neufchâtel cheese (light cream
   cheese), softened
⅓ cup white raisins, chopped
1 tablespoon apple juice

1. In a medium bowl, mix tuna, cream cheese, raisins, and apple juice until well blended. Or put tuna in a food processor or blender and pulse on and off until finely chopped; add cream cheese and apple juice and process just until blended; then stir in raisins.

Nutrient analysis per ⅓-cup serving
Calories 160; Protein 17 g; Carbohydrates 15 g; Fat—total 4 g; Saturated fat 2 g; Cholesterol 32 mg; Dietary fiber 1 g; Calcium 19 mg; Iron 1 mg; Sodium 266 mg

. . . .

Snacks

Cheese Potato Crisp
Flatbread with Monterey Jack Cheese
Parsnip Chips
Peanut Butter Bread
Pita Snacks
Trail Mix

. . . .

Cheese Potato Crisp

Serves 4
Preparation time: 10 minutes plus time to cool
Cooking time: 50 minutes

From: Lidia Bastianich, Felidia Restaurant, New York, New York

½ pound Idaho potatoes (2 to 3 medium), scrubbed
1 tablespoon olive oil
1 small yellow onion, thinly sliced (¼ cup)
salt and freshly ground black pepper to taste
12 ounces Montasio, Asiago, or Parmesan cheese, thinly sliced and divided into fourths

1. Put potatoes in a medium saucepan, add enough water to cover, and boil for 15 to 20 minutes or until tender. Drain and cool.

2. When potatoes are cool enough to handle, peel them and cut them into thin slices.

3. In a large skillet, heat oil over medium heat. Add onion and sauté until golden, 3 to 4 minutes. Add sliced potatoes and season mixture lightly with salt and pepper. Cook, stirring often, until potatoes are golden, 5 to 10 minutes.

4. Heat a 7½-inch skillet (preferably nonstick) over medium-high heat. Cover bottom of skillet with one-fourth of the sliced cheese. Spread one-half of the potato mixture over the cheese and press into place. Cover with slices of cheese—use another fourth of the original amount. Cook for 5 minutes. Turn the crisps, using a spatula, and cook for an additional 5 minutes. Remove to paper towels to drain. Repeat with the remaining cheese and potatoes.

5. Cut each crisp into 4 wedges and serve warm.

Nutrient analysis per 2-wedge serving
Calories 443; Protein 32 g; Carbohydrates 21 g; Fat—total 25.5 g; Saturated fat 14 g; Cholesterol 58 mg; Dietary fiber 1 g; Calcium 1,018 mg; Iron 1 mg; Sodium 1,367 mg

· · · · · · · ·

Flatbread with Monterey Jack Cheese

Serves 12
Preparation time: 20 minutes plus 1 hour 5 minutes to rise
Baking time: 20 minutes

From: Cory Schreiber, Wildwood Restaurant and Bar, Portland, Oregon

You can make this recipe with a pizza pan in place of a pizza stone, but the stone enhances the crust quality.

1 cup warm water (105° to 110°F)
1 tablespoon active dry yeast
1 teaspoon sugar
1 cup plain low-fat yogurt
1 teaspoon salt
3¾ cups white bread flour
1 cup whole-wheat flour
olive oil
cornmeal
12 slices low-fat Monterey Jack cheese (about
   8 ounces)

1. In a large bowl, combine water, yeast, and sugar. Let stand until foamy, about 5 minutes. Add yogurt and salt and whisk until blended.

2. In a small bowl, mix bread flour and whole-wheat flour. Using a wooden spoon, stir enough of the flour mixture into the yogurt mixture to form a soft dough. Turn dough out onto a lightly floured work surface and knead about 5 minutes, until smooth and elastic. Transfer dough to a large oiled bowl, turning the dough to coat it with oil. Cover the bowl with plastic wrap and let dough rise in a warm, draft-free place about 45 minutes or until doubled in volume.

3. Preheat oven to 450°F. Preheat pizza stone (if used) according to manufacturer's directions.

4. Punch down dough and turn out onto a lightly floured work surface. Divide dough into 12 equal pieces. Shape each piece into a ball and place balls on an oiled baking sheet. Cover loosely with plastic wrap and let rise about 20 minutes or until doubled in volume.

5. On a lightly floured work surface, pat and stretch each piece of dough into an oblong about 6 inches long. Lightly coat each oblong with olive oil (use a spray if you wish). Put 3 to 4 oblongs on the pizza stone or pan. Set the rest aside on a baking sheet dusted with cornmeal.

6. Bake flatbreads on the pizza stone or pan for 4 to 5 minutes or until golden brown. Place a slice of cheese on each flatbread and bake bread for 1 minute more or until cheese is melted. Remove from oven, cut each oblong into 2 wedges, and serve warm. Bake the remaining flatbreads the same way.

Nutrient analysis per 2-wedge serving
Calories 125; Protein 9 g; Carbohydrates 14 g; Fat—total 4 g; Saturated fat 2 g; Cholesterol 11 mg; Dietary fiber 2 g; Calcium 181 mg; Iron 1 mg; Sodium 294 mg

. . . .

Parsnip Chips

Serves 10
Preparation time: 10 minutes
Cooking time: 15 minutes

*From: Cory Schreiber, Wildwood Restaurant and
Bar, Portland, Oregon*

Look for large parsnips for this recipe; they are
easier to peel than small ones.

2 pounds parsnips
canola oil, for frying
salt (optional)

1. Using a vegetable peeler, peel outside skin
from parsnips; discard skin. Continue to peel
parsnips into long, somewhat even strips.
(Discard inner core if you cannot peel it into
strips.)

2. Fill a heavy medium saucepan with 3 inches
of oil, and heat oil to 350°F. Test temperature
with a thermometer or by placing a parsnip strip
in the oil. If it crisps and the oil bubbles, the
temperature is right.

3. Fry parsnips in small batches. Fry each
batch for 45 to 60 seconds or until light brown.
Using a slotted spoon, remove chips to paper
towels to drain. (They will seem soft at first but
will crisp up in 1 to 2 minutes while draining.)
Allow oil to return to 350°F before adding next
batch.

4. Season with salt, if desired. Serve at room
temperature. The chips will stay crisp up to
6 hours at room temperature.

Nutrient analysis per 1-cup serving (excludes optional
salt)
Calories 135; Protein 1 g; Carbohydrates 13 g; Fat—
total 9 g; Saturated fat 1 g; Cholesterol 0 mg; Dietary
fiber 3 g; Calcium 25 mg; Iron 0 mg; Sodium 7 mg

. . . .

Peanut Butter Bread

Makes 1 loaf (16 slices)
Preparation time: 15 minutes
Baking time: 45 minutes

From: Lucie Costa, North Plank Road Tavern, Newburgh, New York

This nutritious quick bread is delicious spread with jam. For a variation, stir mini-semisweet chocolate chips into the batter before baking.

1 cup all-purpose flour
1 cup whole-wheat flour
2 tablespoons wheat or bran germ
4 teaspoons baking powder
⅔ cup smooth peanut butter
¼ cup sugar or honey
1¼ cups milk
½ cup mini-semisweet chocolate chips (optional)

1. Preheat oven to 350°F. Grease a 9-×-5-inch loaf pan or use a nonstick loaf pan.

2. In a small bowl, mix all-purpose flour, whole-wheat flour, wheat germ, and baking powder.

3. In a medium bowl, cream peanut butter and sugar with an electric mixer. Alternately beat in batches of flour mixture and milk just until blended. Stir in chocolate chips, if desired.

4. Scrape batter into prepared pan and spread evenly. Bake for 45 minutes or until a cake tester inserted into the center comes out clean.

5. Set pan on a wire rack to cool for 10 minutes. Turn bread out onto rack and cool completely. Store in an airtight container or plastic wrap at room temperature up to 3 days.

Nutrient analysis per slice (without added chocolate chips)
Calories 142; Protein 5 g; Carbohydrates 18 g; Fat—total 6 g; Saturated fat 1.5 g; Cholesterol 3 mg; Dietary fiber 2 g; Calcium 98 mg; Iron 1 mg; Sodium 183 mg

. . . .

Pita Snacks

Serves 4
Preparation time: 15 minutes
Cooking time: 3 minutes

From: Kathy Farrell-Kingsley, Newtown, Connecticut

4 whole-wheat pita breads
1 tablespoon olive oil
2 tablespoons chopped fresh basil or 1 teaspoon dried basil
¼ teaspoon dried thyme
⅛ teaspoon garlic powder
36 ripe cherry tomatoes, stemmed and sliced
2 tablespoons grated Parmesan cheese

1. Preheat broiler.

2. Cut pita breads into quarters. Lightly brush each quarter with olive oil.

3. In a small cup, mix basil, thyme, and garlic powder and sprinkle mixture evenly over the bread.

4. Put 2 to 3 slices of tomato on each pita quarter and sprinkle with Parmesan cheese.

5. Broil until cheese is slightly brown, about 3 minutes. Serve right away.

Nutrient analysis per 4 wedges
Calories 131; Protein 5 g; Carbohydrates 22 g; Fat—total 4 g; Saturated fat 1 g; Cholesterol 2 mg; Dietary fiber 3 g; Calcium 41 mg; Iron 1 mg; Sodium 207 mg

· · · · · · · ·

Trail Mix

Serves 4
Preparation time: 10 minutes

From: Lucie Costa, North Plank Road Tavern, Newburgh, New York

1 cup toasted whole-grain oat cereal (like
    Cheerios)
¼ cup chopped dates
¼ cup raisins
¼ cup unsalted cashews
¼ cup shredded unsweetened coconut

1. In a medium bowl, mix all ingredients.
Store in an airtight container at room
temperature up to 1 week.

Nutrient analysis per ½-cup serving
Calories 165; Protein 3 g; Carbohydrates 24 g; Fat—
total 8 g; Saturated fat 4 g; Cholesterol 0 mg; Dietary
fiber 3 g; Calcium 23 mg; Iron 2 mg; Sodium 66 mg

········

Meat, Poultry, and Fish Entrées

Alsatian Baekeofa
Arizona Turkey
Beef and Vegetable Burritos
Cajun-Style Chicken Fingers
Curried Chicken and Rice
Foolproof Roast Chicken
Healthy Twist Meatloaf
Raspberry-Ginger Chicken
Soft Teriyaki Chicken Tacos
Summer Salad with Tuna Fish Dressing and Croutons
Whole-Wheat Turkey Pizzas

· · · · · · · ·

Alsatian Baekeofa

Serves 6
Preparation time: 15 minutes
Baking time: 2½ hours

From: Thomas Henkelmann, Greenwich,
Connecticut

An easy-to-prepare beef stew that can also be
made with lamb, pork, or chicken.

4 medium all-purpose potatoes, peeled and thinly
sliced
4 medium carrots, peeled and sliced into 1-inch
rounds
2 medium leeks (white part and 1 inch of the
green), well rinsed and sliced into ½-inch
rounds
2 medium-size yellow onions, sliced
3 stalks celery, cut into 1-inch pieces
salt and freshly ground black pepper to taste
1½ pounds boneless beef chuck, well trimmed
and cut into 1-inch pieces
3 large cloves garlic, peeled and thinly sliced
1 sprig fresh thyme or ½ teaspoon dried thyme
leaves, crumbled
1 sprig fresh rosemary or ½ teaspoon dried
rosemary leaves, crumbled
1 10½-ounce can low-sodium chicken broth
3 tablespoons fresh lemon juice (1 lemon)

1. Preheat oven to 350°F.
2. Layer potatoes over bottom of a deep
2-quart casserole with a lid.
3. Set aside one-third of the carrots, leeks,
onions, and celery. Layer the rest of the
vegetables in order (carrots, leeks, onion, and
celery) over the potatoes. Season with salt and
pepper.
4. Arrange the meat evenly over the
vegetables. Sprinkle with garlic, salt, and pepper.
Place sprigs of fresh thyme and rosemary over
the meat or sprinkle it with dried herbs.
5. Spread reserved vegetables over the meat in
one layer.
6. In a small bowl, mix broth and lemon juice.
Pour mixture into casserole.
7. Cover casserole and bake for 2 to 2½ hours
or until meat and vegetables are tender. Serve
right away.

Nutrient analysis per approximately 1⅔-cup serving
Calories 353; Protein 31 g; Carbohydrates 33 g; Fat—
total 11.5 g; Saturated fat 4 g; Cholesterol 90 mg;
Dietary fiber 4 g; Calcium 74 mg; Iron 5 mg; Sodium
141 mg

. . . .

Arizona Turkey

Serves 6
Preparation time: 15 minutes
Baking time: 30 minutes

From: Lucie Costa, North Plank Road Tavern, Newburgh, New York

This dish can also be made with skinless, boneless chicken breast halves that have been pounded ¼ inch thick. Serve it warm with rice and complement it with fresh orange sections for dessert.

6 turkey breast cutlets (about 1½ pounds)
1 medium-size yellow onion, sliced
1 medium-size green bell pepper, seeded and
   sliced
Barbecue Sauce (makes 2 cups)
2 tablespoons white vinegar
1 tablespoon prepared mustard
1 cup canned chicken broth
1 cup canned tomato sauce
1 tablespoon Worcestershire sauce
2 teaspoons chili powder
1 teaspoon garlic powder
1 teaspoon onion powder
½ teaspoon hot pepper sauce, or to taste
½ teaspoon ground oregano
½ teaspoon salt
⅛ teaspoon cayenne pepper, or to taste

1. Preheat oven to 350°F.

2. *To make barbecue sauce:* In a medium glass, plastic, stainless steel, or ceramic bowl, mix all sauce ingredients until well blended.

3. Place turkey cutlets in a baking dish large enough to hold them in a single layer. Top with onion and bell pepper slices. Pour barbecue sauce over the meat and vegetables.

4. Cover dish with lid or foil and bake for 30 minutes or until turkey is cooked through.

Nutrient analysis per serving
Calories 201; Protein 25 g; Carbohydrates 7 g; Fat—total 8 g; Saturated fat 2 g; Cholesterol 60 mg; Dietary fiber 2 g; Calcium 40 mg; Iron 2 mg; Sodium 709 mg

· · · · · · · ·

Beef and Vegetable Burritos

Serves 6
Preparation time: 25 minutes
Cooking time: 30 minutes

From: Lucie Costa, North Plank Road Tavern, Newburgh, New York

To keep these burritos on hand for a quick lunch or dinner, omit the lettuce and wrap each assembled burrito in foil or waxed paper. Place the burritos in a zipper-lock plastic bag and freeze them for up to 3 months. Thaw in the refrigerator and reheat in the oven at 350°F for 10 to 15 minutes or until they are heated through and the cheese is melted. Serve with celery sticks and corn on the cob.

6 10-inch flour tortillas
1 teaspoon olive oil
1 cup finely chopped onion
1 cup finely chopped green bell pepper
¼ cup finely chopped carrot
¼ cup finely chopped celery
12 ounces lean ground beef
2 teaspoons chili powder
1 teaspoon garlic powder
1 teaspoon onion powder
1 teaspoon ground oregano
1 cup canned crushed tomatoes
½ cup canned red kidney beans, drained and
    rinsed
salt and ground black pepper to taste

1 cup shredded cheddar cheese
½ cup shredded lettuce

1. Preheat oven to 325°F. Stack tortillas and wrap in foil. Put the wrapped tortillas in the oven for 8 to 10 minutes. Turn oven off and keep tortillas in oven until ready to use.

2. In a large skillet (preferably nonstick), heat oil over medium heat. Add onion and bell pepper and cook, stirring often, until soft, about 5 minutes. Add carrot and celery and cook, stirring often, until soft, about 5 minutes.

3. Add ground beef and stir with a wooden spoon to break it up.

4. Add chili powder, garlic powder, onion powder, oregano, tomatoes, beans, salt, and pepper. Cook, uncovered, about 15 minutes, stirring occasionally, until all liquid is gone and beef is no longer pink.

5. *To assemble burritos:* Spoon about ¾ cup of the beef mixture slightly below the center of each tortilla. Top with shredded cheese and lettuce. Fold the bottom of tortilla to cover the filling. Fold the sides toward the center, then roll up the tortilla from the bottom. Serve right away.

Nutrient analysis per burrito
Calories 344; Protein 23 g; Carbohydrates 27 g; Fat—total 16 g; Saturated fat 7 g; Cholesterol 65 mg; Dietary fiber 4 g; Calcium 179 mg; Iron 3 mg; Sodium 380 mg

· · · · · · · ·

Cajun-Style Chicken Fingers
Serves 4
Preparation time: 15 minutes
Baking time: 10 minutes

From: Priscilla Martel, Chester, Connecticut

Cajun Spice imparts a fine flavor to meats and vegetables. Add it before baking or cooking.

1 pound boneless, skinless chicken breasts,
    rinsed and patted dry
1 tablespoon soy sauce
1 recipe Cajun Spice (recipe follows) or
    1 tablespoon purchased Cajun seasoning mix
2 tablespoons chopped peanuts
½ cup plain dry bread crumbs
1 lemon, cut in wedges

1. Preheat oven to 375°F.
2. Cut chicken breasts into finger-length ¾-inch-wide strips. Put chicken strips into a medium bowl. Add soy sauce and toss to coat.
3. Put Cajun Spice into a small paper or plastic bag. Add chicken strips and shake to coat.
4. Into another paper or plastic bag, put peanuts and bread crumbs; shake to mix.

Transfer chicken to bag with bread crumbs and shake to coat. Press gently to make crumbs adhere to chicken.
5. Spread chicken in a single layer on a baking sheet. Lightly coat chicken with nonstick cooking spray. Bake for 8 to 10 minutes or until chicken is cooked through and peanut-crumb coating is crisp. Serve with lemon wedges.

Cajun Spice (makes about 1 tablespoon)
1 teaspoon garlic powder
½ teaspoon ground oregano
½ teaspoon ground black pepper
½ teaspoon paprika
¼ teaspoon cayenne pepper

1. In a small bowl, mix all ingredients until well blended.

Nutrient analysis per serving
Calories 235; Protein 30 g; Carbohydrates 13 g; Fat—total 7 g; Saturated fat 1 g; Cholesterol 72 mg; Dietary fiber 2 g; Calcium 54 mg; Iron 2 mg; Sodium 429 mg

· · · · · · · ·

Curried Chicken and Rice

Serves 4
Preparation time: 10 minutes
Cooking time: 48 minutes plus 10 minutes to stand

From: Elizabeth Terry, Elizabeth on 37th, Savannah, Georgia

Curry powder and oranges flavor this healthful chicken dish. It is delicious with steamed broccoli.

1 tablespoon vegetable oil
4 skinless chicken thighs (about 1½ pounds), rinsed and patted dry
salt and freshly ground black pepper
1 cup long-grain brown rice
1 tablespoon curry powder
2 teaspoons grated orange zest
2¼ cups water
2 peeled, diced navel oranges
2 tablespoons toasted slivered almonds

1. In a large skillet (preferably nonstick), heat oil over medium-high heat. Add chicken and cook until browned, 2 to 3 minutes on each side. Sprinkle with salt and pepper and remove to a plate with a slotted spoon.

2. Add rice, curry powder, and orange zest to skillet. Cook, stirring often, for 2 minutes.

3. Add water and bring to a boil. Return chicken to skillet. Reduce heat, cover, and simmer for 30 minutes or until rice is tender and liquid is absorbed. Turn off heat and let stand for 10 minutes.

4. Top each serving with chopped oranges and toasted almonds.

Nutrient analysis per chicken thigh
Calories 415; Protein 36 g; Carbohydrates 22 g; Fat—total 20 g; Saturated fat 5 g; Cholesterol 121 mg; Dietary fiber 3 g; Calcium 70 mg; Iron 3 mg; Sodium 117 mg

. . . .

Foolproof Roast Chicken

Serves 4
Preparation time: 20 minutes
Cooking time: 40 minutes

From: Charles van Over, Chester, Connecticut

This method of roasting chicken assures even cooking throughout.

1 whole roasting chicken
2 tablespoons olive oil or vegetable oil
1 teaspoon salt
2 teaspoons cayenne pepper

1. *To prepare chicken:* Remove neck and gizzard. Cut off wings at first joint, if desired. Hold chicken tail-side up. With a sharp knife, cut downward and along the backbone on both sides. Remove backbone, split chicken open, and place breast-side down. Remove breastbone to help chicken lie flat and cook evenly. Rinse chicken and pat dry. (Freeze chicken bones, gizzard, and neck to make stock for other recipes.)

2. Preheat oven to 450°F.

3. Coat chicken with 1 tablespoon of the oil and season with salt and cayenne pepper. (The cayenne enhances the flavor of the chicken. After the chicken is roasted you will not taste the pepper.)

4. In a large heavy ovenproof skillet (preferably nonstick), heat 1 tablespoon of the oil over medium-high heat. Add chicken, skin side down, and cook until skin is browned and crisp.

5. Turn chicken skin-side up in skillet and place skillet in oven. Reduce oven temperature to 400°F. Roast about 30 minutes or until skin is crispy and juices run clear when a thigh joint is pierced. (If you are not serving the chicken right away, it can be held in a 200°F oven for 20 minutes.)

6. Transfer chicken to a cutting board and cut into serving pieces.

Nutrient analysis per quarter chicken
Calories 420; Protein 41 g; Carbohydrates 0 g; Fat—total 27 g; Saturated fat 7 g; Cholesterol 132 mg; Dietary fiber 0 g; Calcium 24 mg; Iron 2 mg; Sodium 656 mg

·······

Healthy Twist Meatloaf

Serves 8
Preparation time: 15 minutes plus 10 minutes to stand
Baking time: 45 minutes

From: Priscilla Martel, Chester, Connecticut

1 pound lean ground beef
2 cups finely chopped onion
1 cup shredded carrots
2 slices whole-wheat bread, ground into bread
   crumbs
½ cup wheat bran
1 teaspoon chopped fresh basil or ¼ teaspoon
   dried basil, crumbled
1 teaspoon chopped fresh thyme or ¼ teaspoon
   dried thyme, crumbled
1 teaspoon chopped fresh rosemary or ¼
   teaspoon dried rosemary, crumbled
⅛ teaspoon cayenne pepper
salt and freshly ground black pepper to taste
dash of soy sauce
3 tablespoons tomato paste plus 3 or
   4 tablespoons for glaze (optional)
⅓ cup water
3 large egg whites

1. Preheat oven to 350°F.

2. In a large bowl, mix beef, onion, carrots, bread crumbs, wheat bran, basil, thyme, rosemary, cayenne, salt, pepper, and soy sauce.

3. In a small cup, mix 3 tablespoons of tomato paste and the water until well blended. Add tomato mixture and egg whites to beef mixture and blend thoroughly.

4. Transfer mixture to a 9-x-5-inch loaf pan. Coat top with additional tomato paste, if desired. Cover pan with foil and bake for 45 minutes or until juices run clear or a meat thermometer registers 170°F.

5. Remove meatloaf from oven. Leave foil on and let stand for 10 minutes. Drain off any juices before slicing.

Nutrient analysis per serving
Calories 185; Protein 16 g; Carbohydrates 12 g; Fat—total 8 g; Saturated fat 3 g; Cholesterol 42 mg; Dietary fiber 3 g; Calcium 32 mg; Iron 2 mg; Sodium 153 mg

. . . .

Raspberry-Ginger Chicken

Serves 4
Preparation time: 10 minutes plus 30 minutes to marinate
Cooking time: 12 minutes

Adapted from: Todd Weisz, Turnberry Isle and Resort Club, Aventura, Florida

½ cup chicken broth
½ cup raspberry vinegar
¼ cup low-sodium soy sauce
3 tablespoons Dijon mustard
2 tablespoons honey
1 teaspoon peeled, minced fresh ginger
2 tablespoons chopped fresh cilantro
2 tablespoons chopped fresh mint
4 skinless, boneless chicken breast halves, rinsed and patted dry
fresh mint leaves, for garnish

1. In a shallow glass, plastic, stainless steel, or ceramic bowl, combine broth, vinegar, soy sauce, mustard, honey, ginger, cilantro, and mint. Add chicken breast halves and turn to coat. Marinate at room temperature for 30 minutes, turning occasionally.

2. Meanwhile, prepare a charcoal grill, or preheat a gas grill or broiler. Remove chicken from marinade; reserve marinade. Grill or broil chicken 4 to 6 inches from heat source for 5 to 6 minutes on each side or until no longer pink in the center. Transfer chicken to a serving platter.

3. Put marinade in a small saucepan, bring it to a boil over medium-high heat, and boil for 5 minutes.

4. Spoon marinade over chicken. Garnish with fresh mint leaves and serve right away.

Nutrient analysis per chicken breast half
Calories 209; Protein 29 g; Carbohydrates 13 g; Fat—total 4 g; Saturated fat 1 g; Cholesterol 73 mg; Dietary fiber 0 g; Calcium 33 mg; Iron 2 mg; Sodium 924 mg

········

Soft Teriyaki Chicken Tacos

Serves 6
Preparation time: 20 minutes
Cooking time: 23 minutes

From: Lucie Costa, North Plank Road Tavern, Newburgh, New York

These tacos can also be made with strips of boneless turkey breast. Serve them warm with steamed broccoli and fresh grapes.

6 7-inch flour tortillas
2 tablespoons canola oil
½ cup finely chopped onion
12 ounces skinless, boneless chicken breast
    halves, cut crosswise into thin strips
1 cup canned chicken broth
½ cup orange juice
1 tablespoon soy sauce
2 tablespoons tomato paste
1 teaspoon garlic powder
1 teaspoon ground ginger
1 tablespoon cornstarch dissolved in
    2 tablespoons water
2 cups shredded carrots
1 cup shredded lettuce
¾ cup shredded cheddar cheese

1. Preheat oven to 325°F. Stack tortillas and wrap in foil. Put the wrapped tortillas in the oven for 8 to 10 minutes. Turn oven off and keep tortillas in oven until ready to use.

2. Meanwhile, in a large skillet, heat oil over medium heat. Add onion and cook, stirring often, until soft, about 5 minutes. Add chicken and cook, stirring, for 2 minutes. Add broth, orange juice, soy sauce, tomato paste, garlic powder, and ginger. Simmer, uncovered, for 10 minutes or until chicken is cooked through.

3. With a slotted spoon, remove chicken and onions to a plate and set aside. Stir cornstarch mixture and add it to skillet. Cook sauce in skillet, stirring often, until it has thickened. Return chicken and onions to skillet.

4. *To assemble tacos:* Spread about ½ cup of the chicken mixture over the center of each tortilla. Top with shredded carrots, lettuce, and cheese and roll it up.

Nutrient analysis per taco
Calories 307; Protein 22 g; Carbohydrates 26 g; Fat—total 13 g; Saturated fat 4 g; Cholesterol 51 mg; Dietary fiber 2 g; Calcium 141 mg; Iron 2 mg; Sodium 697 mg

········

Summer Salad with Tuna Fish Dressing and Croutons

Serves 6
Preparation time: 10 minutes
Cooking time: 20 minutes

From: Mary Sue Milliken and Susan Feniger, Border Grille, Santa Monica, California

This is a big hit with tuna lovers of any age. Add any other cold leftover vegetables your child likes, and serve it on a hot summer night.

half of a small baguette or other country-style
　bread, cut into ¾-inch cubes, crust intact
3 tablespoons olive oil
salt and freshly ground black pepper to taste
¾ pound green beans, ends snapped off and
　discarded
1 medium head romaine lettuce, rinsed and torn
　into bite-size pieces
1 medium cucumber, peeled and sliced
8 ounces cherry tomatoes, stemmed and cut in
　half

Tuna Fish Dressing (makes 1 cup)
1 6-ounce can white albacore tuna packed in
　water, undrained
½ cup olive oil
⅓ cup fresh lemon juice (2 lemons)
½ teaspoon salt
½ teaspoon freshly ground black pepper

1. Bring a medium saucepan of water to a boil. Blanch beans in boiling water until crisp-tender, 3 to 5 minutes. Drain and spread on a plate to cool. When beans are cool, cut into 1-inch lengths.

2. *To make croutons:* In a large skillet, heat olive oil over medium heat. Add bread cubes and toss to coat with oil. Sprinkle with salt and pepper. Cook over low heat, shaking pan occasionally, until bread is golden brown. Remove from heat and set aside.

3. *To make dressing:* In a food processor or blender, combine tuna, oil, lemon juice, salt, and pepper. Process until blended.

4. In a large serving bowl, combine lettuce, cucumber, tomatoes, and cooled green-bean pieces. Add dressing and toss salad to mix and coat vegetables. Sprinkle with croutons and serve right away.

Nutrient analysis per serving
Calories 359; Protein 12 g; Carbohydrates 21 g; Fat—total 27 g; Saturated fat 4 g; Cholesterol 12 mg; Dietary fiber 4 g; Calcium 54 mg; Iron 2 mg; Sodium 483 mg

. . . .

Whole-Wheat Turkey Pizzas

Serves 6
Preparation time: 10 minutes
Cooking time: 20 minutes
Baking time: 12 minutes

From: Lucie Costa, North Plank Road Tavern, Newburgh, New York

Everybody loves pizza. These individual pizzas are made with ground turkey and whole-wheat English muffins. With steamed green beans on the side they make a perfect meal.

Tomato Sauce
2 cups canned crushed tomatoes
1 teaspoon garlic powder
1 teaspoon onion powder
¼ teaspoon dried basil, crumbled
¼ teaspoon ground oregano
½ teaspoon ground fennel
salt and ground black pepper to taste

Turkey Topping
1 teaspoon olive oil
12 ounces ground turkey
1 teaspoon garlic powder
1 teaspoon onion powder
½ teaspoon Italian seasoning
½ teaspoon salt

6 whole-wheat English muffins, split
9 ounces shredded low-fat mozzarella cheese

1. Preheat oven to 400°F.

2. *To make sauce:* In a medium saucepan, mix crushed tomatoes, garlic powder, onion powder, basil, oregano, fennel, salt, and pepper. Cook over medium heat, uncovered, for 15 minutes, stirring occasionally.

3. *To make turkey topping:* In a large skillet (preferably nonstick), heat oil over medium heat. Add turkey, stirring with a wooden spoon to break it up. Season with garlic powder, onion powder, Italian seasoning, and salt. Cook, stirring often, about 10 minutes or until turkey is no longer pink. Optional: Transfer turkey mixture to a food processor or blender and process until finely ground.

4. Put muffin halves on a baking sheet, split side up. Spoon turkey topping over muffins and top with sauce. Sprinkle with mozzarella.

5. Bake for 10 to 12 minutes or until topping is heated through and cheese is melted.

Nutrient analysis per whole-muffin pizza (2 halves)
Calories 320; Protein 25 g; Carbohydrates 26 g; Fat—total 14 g; Saturated fat 6 g; Cholesterol 58 mg; Dietary fiber 6 g; Calcium 472 mg; Iron 3 mg; Sodium 905 mg

....

Carbohydrate-Dense Dishes

Baked Elbow Pasta with Shrimp and Zucchini
Black-Eyed Pea Salsa
Fava Bean Puree
My Favorite Fried Rice
Rice à l'Orange
Rice and Potato Minestra
Spaetzle with Fromage Blanc and Herbs
Twisted Cornmeal Breadsticks
White Bean-Vegetable Casserole

········

Baked Elbow Pasta with Shrimp and Zucchini

Serves 6
Preparation time: 20 minutes
Cooking time: 25 minutes

From: Lidia Bastianich, Felidia Restaurant, New York, New York

With this pasta dish all you need to round out the meal are a tossed salad and some crusty bread.

12 ounces elbow macaroni
2 tablespoons olive oil
1 large clove garlic, minced
1 small yellow onion, finely chopped (½ cup)
1 medium zucchini, scrubbed, trimmed, and chopped (1½ cups)
salt and freshly ground black pepper to taste
8 ounces small shrimp, peeled and deveined
1 cup canned tomato sauce
4 ounces fontina cheese, shredded (1 cup)

1. Cook macaroni according to package directions. Drain well and transfer to a large bowl.

2. Meanwhile, in a large skillet, heat oil over medium heat. Add garlic and onion and sauté until soft, about 5 minutes. Add zucchini. Season with salt and pepper. Cook, stirring often, for 3 minutes. Add shrimp and cook over medium-high heat, stirring often, for 2 minutes. Add tomato sauce and cook for 3 minutes. Pour mixture over macaroni and toss to mix.

3. Preheat broiler. Transfer mixture to a 3-quart baking dish and top with cheese. Broil 4 to 6 inches from heat source until cheese is melted and lightly browned and filling is heated through. Serve right away.

Nutrient analysis per 1½-cup serving
Calories 252; Protein 16 g; Carbohydrates 22 g; Fat—total 11 g; Saturated fat 4 g; Cholesterol 95 mg; Dietary fiber 2 g; Calcium 133 mg; Iron 3 mg; Sodium 567 mg

· · · · · · · ·

Black-Eyed Pea Salsa

Serves 6
Preparation time: 15 minutes

From: Lucie Costa, North Plank Road Tavern,
Newburgh, New York

This salsa tastes great with Arizona Turkey (page 326) or Soft Teriyaki Chicken Tacos (page 333).

1 15-ounce can black beans, rinsed and drained
1 15-ounce can black-eyed peas, rinsed and
   drained
1 cup chopped yellow or red onion
1 cup chopped green bell pepper
1 cup frozen corn kernels, thawed
2 tablespoons chopped fresh parsley
2 tablespoons extra-virgin olive oil
1 teaspoon red wine vinegar
¼ teaspoon salt, or to taste

1. In a medium bowl, mix all ingredients until well blended. Serve chilled or at room temperature.

Nutrient analysis per serving
Calories 260; Protein 13 g; Carbohydrates 43 g; Fat—total 5 g; Saturated fat 1 g; Cholesterol 0 mg; Dietary fiber 12 g; Calcium 46 mg; Iron 4 mg; Sodium 96 mg

· · · · · · · ·

Fava Bean Puree

Serves 6
Preparation time: 15 minutes
Cooking time: 15 minutes
Baking time: 20 minutes

From: Waldy Malouf, The Hudson River Club, New York, New York

This puree goes well with lamb and roast chicken and makes a good filling for cooked zucchini blossoms. Fava beans must be shelled and peeled, as described below. Three pounds of fava beans yields 3 cups of shelled beans but only 2 cups of peeled beans.

3 pounds fava beans, shelled
1 clove garlic, cut
1 tablespoon Roasted Garlic Puree (recipe follows)
¼ cup chicken stock or fava bean cooking liquid
1 egg white
salt and freshly ground black pepper to taste

1. Bring a 3-quart pot half full of water to a boil. Drop shelled fava beans into the boiling water. Return water to a boil and continue to boil beans for 5 minutes. Drain, reserving ¼ cup of the cooking liquid if desired. Put beans into a large bowl of cold water.
2. Preheat oven to 350°F. Rub a 2-quart baking dish with the cut clove of garlic.

3. When beans are cool enough to handle, drain well and peel. To peel: Hold the seamed end of a bean between two fingers and nick the opposite smooth end with a fingernail. Gently squeeze the bean from the pod (it will pop right out).
4. Put peeled beans in a food processor or blender. Add Roasted Garlic Puree, chicken stock, and egg white. Process until pureed. Add salt and pepper to taste.
5. Transfer puree to prepared baking dish. Bake, uncovered, for 15 to 20 minutes. Serve right away.

Roasted Garlic Puree (makes ½ cup)
This sweet, intense garlic puree is good added to Fava Bean Puree or mashed potatoes, dabbed on rack of lamb, or stirred into vinaigrette.

3 heads garlic
6 tablespoons olive oil

1. Preheat oven to 300°F.
2. Cut heads of garlic in half crosswise. In a small saucepan, boil garlic in salted water for 5 minutes; drain.
3. Spread oil over bottom of an 8-inch baking

pan. Put garlic heads in pan, cut side down. Roast, uncovered, for 1 hour or until garlic cloves are soft.

4. Remove garlic cloves and put them (unpeeled) in a food processor or blender. Process until pureed.

5. Store puree in refrigerator, covered, up to 10 days.

Nutrient analysis per ⅓-cup serving
Calories 67; Protein 5 g; Carbohydrates 11 g; Fat—total 0.5 g; Saturated fat 0 g; Cholesterol 0 mg; Dietary fiber 3 g; Calcium 26 mg; Iron 1 mg; Sodium 493 mg

········

My Favorite Fried Rice

Serves 4 as a main course or 8 as a side dish
Preparation time: 20 minutes
Cooking time: 30 minutes plus 10 minutes to stand

From: Susannah Foo, Philadelphia, Pennsylvania

Most fried rice recipes call for long-grain rice, but the medium- or short-grain varieties have a richer, sweeter flavor. Serve this dish with grilled steak or sautéed chicken breasts, or on its own for lunch. Fresh tomato and basil give it a delightful taste. Seeding the tomato isn't mandatory, but it is easy to do: just cut the tomato in half crosswise and flick the seeds out with your fingertip.

2 cups medium- or short-grain white rice
2 cups cold water
5 tablespoons corn oil
4 large eggs, lightly beaten
½ cup diced red onion
1 cup diced Canadian bacon
½ cup cooked fresh or thawed frozen peas
½ cup fresh or thawed frozen white or yellow
   corn kernels
4 scallions (white and green parts), finely
   chopped
1 cup seeded, diced tomato (1 large)
2 teaspoons coarse or kosher salt
freshly ground black pepper to taste
½ cup chopped fresh basil

1. Rinse rice two or three times or until water runs clear. Drain well. In a heavy medium

saucepan with a tight-fitting lid, bring the 2 cups of water to a boil. Add rice and stir once to loosen any grains sticking to the bottom. Reduce heat to low and cook for 5 minutes. Cover and simmer for 15 minutes. Remove pan from heat and let stand, covered, for 10 minutes or until rice is tender and liquid is absorbed.

2. In a large skillet (preferably nonstick), heat 4 tablespoons of oil over medium-high heat. Add eggs and cook until lightly set, stirring with a wooden spoon or chopsticks to break into tiny pieces. Continue to cook, stirring, until eggs are lightly browned and their aroma is released, 4 to 5 minutes. Remove to a small bowl with a slotted spoon and set aside.

3. In the same skillet, heat the remaining tablespoon of oil. Add onion and stir-fry over high heat until soft and lightly golden, about 2 minutes. Add bacon, peas, corn, and scallions and stir-fry until heated through, about 3 minutes.

4. Add tomato and sprinkle in salt. Stir in cooked rice and egg, breaking up any lumps. Mix well and heat through. Season to taste with pepper and stir in basil. Serve right away.

Nutrient analysis per 2-cup serving
Calories 324; Protein 14 g; Carbohydrates 36 g; Fat—total 14 g; Saturated fat 3 g; Cholesterol 122 mg; Dietary fiber 2 g; Calcium 32 mg; Iron 3 mg; Sodium 1,008 mg

. . . .

Rice à l'Orange

Serves 6
Preparation time: 5 minutes
Cooking time: 33 minutes plus 15 minutes to stand

From: Lucie Costa, North Plank Road Tavern, Newburgh, New York

A fragrant and nutritious rice dish that can be served with chicken, turkey, or fish.

1 tablespoon olive oil
1 cup long-grain brown rice
3 cups water
½ cup orange juice
½ cup currants
¼ teaspoon ground allspice
1 cup couscous
¼ cup toasted slivered almonds (optional)

1. In a medium saucepan, heat oil over medium heat. Add rice and stir for 1 to 2 minutes or until well coated with oil. Add water, orange juice, currants, and allspice. Bring to a boil. Reduce heat, cover, and simmer for 30 minutes.

2. Stir in couscous. Cover pan and remove from heat. Let stand for 15 minutes or until all liquid is absorbed.

3. Fluff rice mixture with a fork and stir in almonds. Serve right away.

Nutrient analysis per 1¼-cup serving
Calories 271; Protein 7 g; Carbohydrates 43 g; Fat— total 8 g; Saturated fat 1 g; Cholesterol 0 mg; Dietary fiber 4 g; Calcium 50 mg; Iron 1 mg; Sodium 13 mg

· · · · · · · ·

Rice and Potato Minestra

Serves 6
Preparation time: 10 minutes
Cooking time: 1 hour

From: Lidia Bastianich, Felidia Restaurant, New York, New York

An easy-to-prepare hearty soup that will keep the cold at bay.

3 tablespoons olive oil
2 medium potatoes, peeled and diced
2 medium carrots, peeled and diced
2 stalks celery, coarsely chopped
2 tablespoons tomato paste
10 cups chicken stock or canned broth
2 bay leaves
salt and freshly ground black pepper to taste
1 cup long-grain white rice
grated Parmesan cheese, for topping

1. In a large saucepan, heat oil over medium heat. Add potatoes and cook, stirring often, until browned, about 5 minutes. Add carrots and celery and cook, stirring often, for 2 to 3 minutes.

2. Stir in tomato paste, stock, bay leaves, salt, and pepper. Bring to a boil. Reduce heat, cover, and simmer for 40 minutes. Add rice. Cover and simmer for 12 minutes more or until rice is tender.

3. Remove celery and bay leaves. Adjust seasoning. Sprinkle each serving with Parmesan cheese.

Nutrient analysis per approximately 2½-cup serving
Calories 251; Protein 6 g; Carbohydrates 38 g; Fat—total 8 g; Saturated fat 0.2 g; Cholesterol 3 mg; Dietary fiber 2 g; Calcium 84 mg; Iron 2 mg; Sodium 233 mg

. . . .

Spaetzle with Fromage Blanc and Herbs

Serves 6 to 8
Preparation time: 10 minutes
Cooking time: 17 minutes

From: Thomas Henkelmann, Greenwich,
Connecticut

Fromage blanc is a very soft, fresh cheese that has
a consistency similar to sour cream.

2¾ cups all-purpose flour
4 large eggs
12 ounces fromage blanc
¼ teaspoon salt
pinch of ground nutmeg
¼ cup snipped fresh chives
1 tablespoon olive oil

1. In a large bowl, mix all ingredients except
olive oil until well blended.

2. Bring a large pot of salted water to a boil.

3. Push half the batter through a spaetzle
maker or the holes of a fine colander into the
boiling water. After the cooked batter floats to
the surface and the water returns to a boil,
simmer for 30 seconds more.

4. Using a slotted spoon, remove the spaetzle
to a colander and drain. Cook the remaining
batter the same way.

5. Transfer the spaetzle to a medium saucepan
and toss with olive oil. Warm over medium-low
heat for 4 to 5 minutes, stirring often. Serve
warm.

Nutrient analysis per approximately 1-cup serving
Calories 360; Protein 10 g; Carbohydrates 40 g; Fat—
total 17 g; Saturated fat 8 g; Cholesterol 143 mg; Dietary
fiber 2 g; Calcium 80 mg; Iron 3 mg; Sodium 139 mg

· · · · · · · ·

Twisted Cornmeal Breadsticks

Makes 20 thick and soft breadsticks or 40 crisp and thin breadsticks
Preparation time: 25 minutes plus 1 hour to rise
Baking time: 10 minutes

From: Maggie Glezer, Atlanta, Georgia

This recipe produces either soft or crisp cornmeal-crusted breadsticks, depending on how thin the dough is cut. They are fun to make with children. The recipe can be completed in less than 2 hours, or the dough can be made on one day and the breadsticks the next (letting the dough rest overnight produces more flavorful breadsticks). Adventurous cooks may add chopped fresh herbs, sautéed onion, grated cheese, chopped nuts, or dried fruits to the dough, either alone or in any combination.

1⅓ cups 2 percent milk

3 cups unbleached all-purpose flour

¼ cup plus 2 tablespoons cornmeal, yellow or white, plus cornmeal for garnish

2 teaspoons salt

1 teaspoon quick-rising active yeast

2 tablespoons olive oil, vegetable oil, or softened butter

1. In a medium microwave-safe bowl, microwave milk on High (100 percent power) for 2 minutes or until the milk steams and bubbles around the edges. Cool milk until you can comfortably stick a finger in it. (You may also heat the milk in a saucepan.)

2. *To make dough by hand:* In a large bowl, mix flour, cornmeal, salt, and yeast. Make a well in the center of the flour mixture and pour in oil and cooled milk. Mix liquids together, then gradually stir in flour. Turn dough out onto a lightly floured work surface and knead about 5 minutes. The dough should feel very soft and sticky; if necessary, add water, 1 tablespoon at a time, to adjust consistency. Knead dough until smooth.

3. *To make dough in a food processor:* Add flour, cornmeal, and salt to a food processor fitted with a steel blade; process for a few seconds to mix. Add oil and cooled milk; process about 30 seconds, then feel dough. If it is not very soft, add 1 tablespoon of water and process for 5 to 10 seconds. Feel dough again and repeat procedure until dough is fairly soft. Do not process dough for too long at a time or it will become overheated. Add yeast and process dough for another 10 to 15 seconds.

4. (optional) Place the kneaded dough in a zipper-lock plastic bag and refrigerate it up to 48 hours. Resting the dough improves the flavor of the breadsticks.

5. Sprinkle a heavy layer of cornmeal on a work surface. Turn dough out onto cornmeal and pull it into a rectangle about 1 inch thick. Sprinkle top of dough with another heavy layer of cornmeal. Cover with plastic wrap and let rise for 1 hour or until dough is puffy. If dough was refrigerated earlier (step 4), let it rise for 2 hours.

6. Place oven rack in top position. Preheat oven to 475°F. Coat a baking sheet with nonstick cooking spray and set it on a second baking sheet (to prevent burning).

7. For thick, soft breadsticks, cut dough lengthwise into 20 strips. For thin, crisp breadsticks, cut dough lengthwise into 40 strips. Stretch strips to width of baking sheet, twisting them for a pretty look. Place as many breadsticks on prepared baking sheet as will fit; space them ½ inch apart. You will need to bake them in batches.

8. Bake breadsticks for 8 to 10 minutes or until golden brown. Serve them warm or remove them to a wire rack to cool.

Nutrient analysis per 1 thick stick or 2 thin sticks
Calories 104; Protein 3 g; Carbohydrates 14 g; Fat—total 2 g; Saturated fat 0 g; Cholesterol 1 mg; Dietary fiber 1 g; Calcium 23 mg; Iron 1 mg; Sodium 222 mg

. . . .

White Bean–Vegetable Casserole

Serves 8
Preparation time: 20 minutes
Cooking time: 1 hour 20 minutes
Baking time: 40 minutes

From: Kathy Cary, Lilly's la Pêche, Louisville, Kentucky

1 pound navy beans, picked over and rinsed
2 tablespoons olive oil
1 medium-size yellow onion, chopped (1 cup)
4 cloves garlic, minced
6 plum tomatoes, seeded and chopped (2 cups)
3 cups stemmed, coarsely chopped fresh spinach
1 tablespoon grated lemon zest (1 lemon)
2 tablespoons red wine vinegar
salt and freshly ground black pepper to taste
1 cup dry unseasoned bread crumbs
6 ounces shredded Gruyère cheese (1½ cups)
2 tablespoons butter

1. Preheat oven to 350°F. Butter a shallow 3-quart casserole.

2. Put beans in a large saucepan and cover with cold water. Bring to a boil; drain in a colander.

3. Return beans to pot, add 8 cups of cold water, and bring to a boil. Reduce heat and simmer, partially covered, for 1 hour or until beans are tender. Drain, reserving 1 cup of cooking liquid.

4. In a medium skillet, heat oil over medium heat. Add onion and garlic and sauté until onion is soft, about 5 minutes.

5. In a large bowl, combine half the cooked beans with the onion and garlic mixture, tomatoes, spinach, lemon zest, vinegar, salt, and pepper. Toss gently to mix.

6. In a food processor or blender, combine the remaining beans with the reserved cup of cooking liquid. Process until pureed. Add puree to vegetable mixture and stir gently to mix.

7. Transfer mixture to prepared casserole. In a small bowl, mix bread crumbs and cheese. Sprinkle evenly over casserole. Dot with butter.

8. Bake, uncovered, for 30 to 40 minutes or until top is browned and filling is heated through. Serve right away.

Nutrient analysis per serving
Calories 398; Protein 20 g; Carbohydrates 49 g; Fat—total 15 g; Saturated fat 6.5 g; Cholesterol 30 mg; Dietary fiber 14 g; Calcium 361 mg; Iron 5 mg; Sodium 302 mg

. . . .

Vegetarian Selections

Angel Hair Pasta with Roasted Red Pepper–Tomato Sauce
Cream of Spinach with Soft-Cooked Eggs
Eggplant Sauce
Green Risotto with Vegetables
Lentil Stew
Pasta with Peanut Sauce
Pizza Presto
Sweet Corn Ravioli
Vegetable Lasagna

········

Angel Hair Pasta with Roasted Red Pepper–Tomato Sauce

Serves 4 children or 2 adults
Preparation time: 15 minutes
Cooking time: 55 minutes

Adapted from: Waldy Malouf, The Hudson River Club, New York, New York

On the side serve grilled vegetables, such as zucchini, yellow squash, and onions. The sauce can be made ahead of time and gently reheated, but cook the pasta just before serving.

1 medium-size red bell pepper, roasted, peeled, seeded, and chopped
2 pounds ripe tomatoes, rough chopped (about 3 cups)
1 jalapeño pepper, seeded and chopped (2 tablespoons)
1 large shallot, minced (3 tablespoons)
⅓ cup olive oil
½ pound angel hair pasta
salt and ground black pepper to taste

1. In a large saucepan, combine roasted bell pepper, tomatoes, jalapeño, shallot, and oil. Partially cover and cook over medium heat for 35 to 40 minutes, stirring occasionally. Strain sauce through a sieve or food mill; discard solids. Return sauce to pan and keep warm.

2. In a large pot, boil pasta in plenty of salted water for 2 to 3 minutes or until al dente. Drain and toss with sauce. Season with salt and black pepper, if desired, and serve right away.

Nutrient analysis per child's serving (2 ounces of dried pasta and approximately ½ cup of sauce)
Calories 339; Protein 6 g; Carbohydrates 37 g; Fat—total 19 g; Saturated fat 2.5 g; Cholesterol 0 mg; Dietary fiber 3 g; Calcium 17 mg; Iron 2 mg; Sodium 65 mg

. . . .

Cream of Spinach with Soft-Cooked Eggs

Serves 4
Preparation time: 10 minutes
Cooking time: 35 minutes

From: Teresa Barrenchea, Marichu Restaurant,
New York, New York

1 pound fresh spinach, well rinsed and stemmed
¼ cup unsalted butter (½ stick)
1 tablespoon all-purpose flour
4 cups milk
salt and freshly ground black pepper to taste
4 large eggs

1. Place spinach leaves in a steamer and cook over simmering water just until wilted, about 5 minutes. Drain well, cool slightly, and chop.

2. In a medium saucepan, melt butter over medium heat. Add flour and whisk until smooth. Cook, whisking constantly, for 1 minute. Gradually whisk in milk. Cook, whisking almost constantly, until smooth and thickened slightly, about 20 minutes.

3. Transfer sauce to a food processor or blender. Add spinach and process to form a chunky puree. Return cream-of-spinach mixture to saucepan. Season with salt and pepper and keep warm while cooking eggs.

4. Bring a medium saucepan of water to a boil. Using a slotted spoon, lower eggs into boiling water. Reduce heat and simmer for 4 to 5 minutes.

5. Quickly cut each egg in half, shell and all, and use a spoon to scoop the soft egg white and yolk into a small serving bowl. Top each egg with 1 cup of the cream of spinach and serve right away.

Nutrient analysis per serving
Calories 311; Protein 16 g; Carbohydrates 16 g; Fat—total 21 g; Saturated fat 11.5 g; Cholesterol 236 mg; Dietary fiber 2 g; Calcium 416 mg; Iron 3 mg; Sodium 227 mg

....

Eggplant Sauce

Serves 4
Preparation time: 10 minutes
Cooking time: 40 minutes

From: Elizabeth Terry, Elizabeth on 37th, Savannah, Georgia

Serve this sauce over pasta, or use it to top pizza.

2 tablespoons olive oil
1½ cups chopped onion (1 large)
3 cups peeled, diced eggplant (1 small)
½ cup chopped red bell pepper (1 small)
½ cup peeled, chopped carrot (1 medium)
3 cloves garlic, peeled
2 cups water
salt and ground black pepper to taste

1. In a large skillet with a lid, heat oil over medium-high heat. Add onion and cook, stirring often, until lightly browned, about 5 minutes.

2. Add eggplant and cook, stirring often, until browned, about 5 minutes.

3. Add bell pepper, carrot, garlic, and water. Bring to a boil. Reduce heat, cover, and simmer for 30 minutes or until vegetables are soft. Season with salt and pepper.

4. Transfer sauce to a food processor or blender and puree. Serve right away.

Nutrient analysis per ½-cup serving
Calories 104; Protein 1 g; Carbohydrates 10 g; Fat—total 7 g; Saturated fat 1 g; Cholesterol 0 mg; Dietary fiber 3 g; Calcium 22 mg; Iron 0 mg; Sodium 16 mg

· · · · · · · ·

Green Risotto with Vegetables

Serves 6
Preparation time: 15 minutes
Cooking time: 50 minutes

From: Lidia Bastianich, Felidia Restaurant, New York, New York

Arborio rice is a short-grain rice available in most large supermarkets or specialty food shops. Its concentrated starch content makes it the best rice for risotto.

1 cup dried fava beans
½ pound broccoli
2 tablespoons olive oil
½ cup finely chopped green onions (white part and some of the green)
1 tablespoon minced shallot
1½ cups arborio or other short-grain white rice
½ cup dry white wine
4½ to 5 cups boiling chicken broth
½ cup grated Romano cheese
freshly ground black pepper to taste

1. Put shelled beans in a medium saucepan of boiling salted water and boil for 5 minutes. Drain and put in a bowl of cold water. When beans are cool enough to handle, nick smooth ends with fingernail and gently squeeze beans from pods. If you are using canned beans, drain and rinse well, then gently squeeze beans from pods.
2. Cut off broccoli florets. Place florets in a steamer and cook over simmering water just until tender, about 7 minutes. Remove from water and set aside.
3. Peel broccoli stems; cut in half lengthwise, then crosswise into ½-inch-thick slices. Bring a medium saucepan of water to a boil. Add broccoli stems and simmer until very tender, about 10 minutes. Drain, transfer to a food processor or blender, and puree. Set aside.
4. In a wide, heavy skillet, heat olive oil over medium heat. Add onion and shallot and sauté until softened, about 5 minutes. Add rice and stir until well coated and lightly toasted.
5. Add wine and cook, stirring constantly, until wine is absorbed, about 2 minutes. Add ½ cup of the boiling broth. Cook, stirring constantly, until liquid is almost completely absorbed. Continue adding broth ½ cup at a time, making sure that most of the liquid is absorbed before adding more. (Timing from first to last addition of broth is about 20 minutes.)
6. Add pureed broccoli stems and fava beans and cook, stirring constantly, for 3 minutes. Add broccoli florets and cook, stirring constantly, for 2 minutes.
7. Remove pan from heat. Stir in cheese and black pepper to taste. Serve right away.

Nutrient analysis per 1½ cup serving
Calories 259; Protein 12 g; Carbohydrates 30 g; Fat—total 9 g; Saturated fat 2.5 g; Cholesterol 9 mg; Dietary fiber 4 g; Calcium 130 mg; Iron 2 mg; Sodium 887 mg

········

Lentil Stew

Serves 6
Preparation time: 15 minutes
Cooking time: 1 hour 20 minutes

From: Mary Sue Milliken and Susan Feniger,
Border Grille, Santa Monica, California

Once they've tried it, your children will love this stick-to-your-ribs stew. Serve it with a dollop of cool plain yogurt on top.

3 tablespoons olive oil
1 medium-size yellow onion, finely chopped
  (1 cup)
1 cup brown lentils, picked over and rinsed
4 cups water
2 medium carrots, peeled and diced
2 small kohlrabi, peeled and diced
1 stalk celery, diced
1 medium potato, peeled and diced
1 large tomato, cored, seeded, and diced
1 teaspoon salt
½ teaspoon freshly ground black pepper
plain low-fat yogurt (optional)

1. In a large saucepan, heat oil over medium-high heat. Add onion and sauté until lightly browned, about 5 minutes. Add lentils and cook, stirring often, for 2 to 3 minutes to develop flavor.

2. Add water, carrots, kohlrabi, celery, and potato. Bring to a boil. Reduce heat, cover, and simmer about 30 minutes.

3. Stir in tomato. Cover and simmer for 30 minutes more or until lentils and vegetables are tender. Season with salt and pepper. Serve with a dollop of yogurt on top.

Nutrient analysis per approximately 1⅓-cup serving
Calories 200; Protein 8 g; Carbohydrates 27 g; Fat—total 7 g; Saturated fat 1 g; Cholesterol 0 mg; Dietary fiber 6 g; Calcium 43 mg; Iron 3 mg; Sodium 393 mg

. . . .

Pasta with Peanut Sauce

Serves 6
Preparation time: 15 minutes
Cooking time: 30 minutes

Adapted from: Lucie Costa, North Plank Road Tavern, Newburgh, New York

1 pound dried rotelle (wagon-wheel) pasta
2 medium carrots, peeled and julienned
2 cups broccoli florets
1 cup canned chickpeas, rinsed and drained
¾ cup smooth peanut butter
1 cup vegetable stock
2 tablespoons soy sauce
2 tablespoons fresh lime juice
1 tablespoon honey
2 teaspoons garlic powder
½ teaspoon ground ginger
1 teaspoon hot pepper sauce

1. Cook pasta according to the package directions. Drain well. Transfer to a shallow serving bowl.

2. Blanch carrots and broccoli in boiling water until crisp-tender, for 2 to 3 minutes. Drain, rinse under cold running water, and drain again. Add to pasta along with chickpeas and toss gently to mix.

3. In a medium saucepan, combine peanut butter, stock, soy sauce, lime juice, honey, garlic powder, ginger, and hot pepper sauce. Cook, stirring often, over medium heat until creamy in texture and heated through. Pour sauce over pasta and toss gently to mix. Serve right away.

Nutrient analysis per serving
Calories 486; Protein 20 g; Carbohydrates 66 g; Fat—total 18 g; Saturated fat 3 g; Cholesterol 0 mg; Dietary fiber 7 g; Calcium 61 mg; Iron 4 mg; Sodium 517 mg

. . . .

Pizza Presto

Serves 4
Preparation time: 10 minutes
Baking time: 17 minutes

From: Priscilla Martel, Chester, Connecticut

4 English muffins or pita breads, split in half
1 cup prepared spaghetti sauce
1 cup thinly sliced green bell peppers, onions, or
    mushrooms (optional)
1 cup part-skim ricotta cheese
1 cup shredded mozzarella, Swiss, or mild
    cheddar cheese

1. Preheat oven to 375°F. Put muffins split side up on a baking sheet. Toast in oven for 5 minutes.

2. Top each muffin half with 2 tablespoons of sauce, a few sliced vegetables, 1 tablespoon of ricotta, and 2 tablespoons of shredded cheese.

3. Bake for 8 to 12 minutes or until cheese is melted and tops are golden brown. Serve right away.

Nutrient analysis per whole-muffin pizza (2 halves)
Calories 377; Protein 18 g; Carbohydrates 42 g; Fat—total 15 g; Saturated fat 7 g; Cholesterol 41 mg; Dietary fiber 4 g; Calcium 435 mg; Iron 2 mg; Sodium 756 mg

. . . .

Sweet Corn Ravioli

Serves 8 (makes about 80 small ravioli)
Preparation time: 40 minutes plus 2 hours to chill
Cooking time: 20 minutes

From: Jimmy Schmidt, Rattlesnake Club, Detroit, Michigan

Many specialty food shops sell fresh pasta—a real time-saver for making ravioli or any other stuffed pasta dish. This recipe is wonderful with fresh sweet corn, but frozen corn kernels can be substituted.

4 cups fresh corn kernels, cut from the cob
   (about 8 medium ears), or 28 ounces frozen
   corn kernels, thawed
½ cup fresh bread crumbs
5 large egg whites (¾ cup)
1 cup shredded low-fat mozzarella cheese
   (4 ounces)
salt and freshly ground black pepper to taste
1 pound fresh pasta, rolled into 8 thin sheets,
   each 2½ × 25 inches
¾ cup milk
butter, for topping
grated Parmesan cheese, for topping

1. Preheat oven to 375°F. Dust a baking sheet generously with flour.

2. In a large bowl, mix corn, bread crumbs, 4 egg whites (½ cup), and mozzarella cheese until blended. Season with salt and pepper.

3. In a small bowl, beat remaining egg white and milk.

4. Lay one sheet of pasta flat on a lightly floured work surface. Spoon small heaps of corn filling down the center of the sheet, putting about 2 teaspoonful every 2½ inches. Brush milk mixture on pasta around filling. Cover prepared sheet of pasta with another sheet of pasta, pressing sheets together to seal edges. Using a crinkle-edged ravioli cutter, cut filled pasta into square ravioli. Transfer to the baking sheet. Make the rest of the ravioli the same way. Cover ravioli with plastic wrap and refrigerate for 2 hours.

5. Bring a large pot of salted water to a boil. Add ravioli and boil gently for 6 to 10 minutes or until al dente. (To test: Taste a small section from the side of a cooked ravioli.) Drain in colander and serve right away topped with butter and Parmesan cheese.

Nutrient analysis per 10-ravioli serving
Calories 258; Protein 13 g; Carbohydrates 45 g; Fat—total 5 g; Saturated fat 2 g; Cholesterol 9 mg; Dietary fiber 4 g; Calcium 141 mg; Iron 2 mg; Sodium 213 mg

. . . .

Vegetable Lasagna

Serves 8
Preparation time: 1½ hours
Baking time: 1 hour 20 minutes plus 15 minutes to stand

From: Danny Meyer and Michael Romano, Union Square Cafe, New York, New York

This lasagna takes a while to prepare, but the results are worth the effort.

Tomato-Vegetable Sauce
3 tablespoons extra-virgin olive oil
1½ cups thinly sliced zucchini
1 cup sliced yellow onion
1 cup sliced red bell pepper
2 teaspoons minced garlic
pinch of crushed hot red pepper flakes
4 medium-size ripe tomatoes (2 pounds)
1 cup canned plum tomatoes
1 tablespoon chopped fresh basil
salt and freshly ground black pepper to taste

1 medium eggplant (1¼ pounds), peeled and
   sliced into rounds ⅛ inch thick
9 tablespoons extra-virgin olive oil
1 tablespoon coarse salt
¼ teaspoon freshly ground black pepper
1 medium zucchini (8 ounces), trimmed and
   sliced into rounds ⅛ inch thick
1 medium-size yellow squash (8 ounces),
   trimmed and sliced into rounds ⅛ inch thick
½ pound dried lasagna noodles

1 pound soft goat cheese, at room temperature
3 large eggs
2 teaspoons minced garlic
½ cup chopped fresh basil
1½ cups sun-dried tomatoes packed in oil,
   drained
¼ cup grated Parmesan cheese

To make sauce:

1. In a large saucepan, heat oil over medium heat. Add zucchini, onion, bell pepper, garlic, and red pepper flakes. Cook, stirring occasionally, for 25 minutes or until vegetables are very tender but not browned.

2. In a large saucepan, bring 2 quarts of water to a boil. Core tomatoes with a paring knife. Prepare a bowl of ice water large enough to hold the tomatoes. Plunge the tomatoes into the boiling water for 30 seconds. Using a slotted spoon, transfer them to the bowl of ice water. Using the tip of a paring knife, remove and discard peels. Cut tomatoes in half crosswise and gently squeeze them over a small bowl to remove seeds and excess juice. Flatten tomato halves on a cutting board with the palm of your hand and chop them into 1-inch pieces. Strain the bowlful of tomato juice through a fine sieve into the pot with vegetables; discard seeds.

3. Add chopped tomatoes, plum tomatoes, basil, salt, and pepper to the pot. Bring to a boil. Reduce heat and simmer, partially covered, for 1 hour.

4. Meanwhile, preheat oven to 375°F. Put eggplant in a medium bowl, drizzle with 1 tablespoon of olive oil, and toss with some of the salt and pepper. Spread eggplant in a single layer on a baking sheet. Cover with foil and bake for 20 minutes or until soft.

5. Put zucchini in a medium bowl, drizzle with 1 tablespoon of olive oil, and toss with some of the salt and pepper. Spread zucchini in a single layer on a baking sheet. Bake, uncovered, for 10 minutes or until soft. Repeat the step with yellow squash.

6. Cook lasagna noodles according to package directions; drain and brush with olive oil to prevent sticking.

7. In a medium bowl, mix goat cheese, eggs, garlic, ¼ cup of the olive oil, and the remaining salt and pepper until smooth and blended. Stir in basil and set aside.

8. Transfer tomato-vegetable sauce to a food processor and puree, in batches if necessary.

9. *To assemble lasagna:* Lightly brush a 9-x-9-inch pan with olive oil. Cover the bottom with a layer of lasagna noodles. Spread on enough tomato-vegetable sauce, about ⅔ cup, to cover the noodles. Layer eggplant, then zucchini, over sauce. Spread half the goat cheese mixture over the vegetables. Arrange half the sun-dried tomatoes over the cheese. Beginning with noodles, repeat the layers but use yellow squash instead of zucchini. Finish with a layer of noodles and ⅔ cup of the sauce. Top with Parmesan cheese. Reserve any remaining sauce.

10. Cover lasagna with foil and bake for 1 hour. Uncover and bake for 15 to 20 minutes more or until cheese browns. Remove from oven and let stand for 15 minutes before cutting into squares and serving. Warm any remaining sauce and serve it with the lasagna.

Nutrient analysis per serving
Calories 530; Protein 20 g; Carbohydrates 33 g; Fat—total 37 g; Saturated fat 13 g; Cholesterol 108 mg; Dietary fiber 5 g; Calcium 177 mg; Iron 3 mg; Sodium 1,404 mg

. . . .

Vegetable Side Dishes

Gingered Carrots
Mashed Parsnips and Potatoes
Mashed Yellow Turnips with Crispy Shallots
Oven French Fries
Roasted Root Vegetables
Sautéed Spinach with Garlic
Spinach-Mushroom Pudding

. . . .

Gingered Carrots

Serves 4
Preparation time: 25 minutes
Cooking time: 20 minutes

*From: Kathy Cary, Lilly's la Pêche, Louisville,
Kentucky*

3 cups chicken broth or water
1 pound peeled baby carrots
2 tablespoons frozen orange juice concentrate
1 tablespoon butter
1 tablespoon light brown sugar
¼ teaspoon ground ginger
salt and freshly ground black pepper to taste
2 tablespoons finely chopped fresh parsley

1. In a medium saucepan, bring broth to a
boil. Add carrots and simmer, uncovered, until
tender, about 15 minutes. Drain in a colander.

2. In the same saucepan, mix orange juice
concentrate, butter, brown sugar, ginger, salt, and
pepper. Cook over medium heat, stirring often,
until smooth and blended.

3. Add carrots and parsley and toss gently to
coat. Serve right away.

Nutrient analysis per approximately ¾-cup serving
Calories 92; Protein 1 g; Carbohydrates 15 g; Fat—total
3.5 g; Saturated fat 2 g; Cholesterol 8 mg; Dietary fiber
4 g; Calcium 34 mg; Iron 1 mg; Sodium 71 mg

· · · · · · · ·

Mashed Parsnips and Potatoes

Serves 4
Preparation time: 15 minutes
Cooking time: 30 minutes

From: Jimmy Schmidt, Rattlesnake Club, Detroit, Michigan

These mashed vegetables complement roast meats and poultry. Do not use a food processor to puree the potato, or it will become gluey.

1 pound parsnips, peeled and cut into large chunks
1 medium russet potato, peeled and cut into large chunks
½ cup plain nonfat yogurt
salt and ground black pepper to taste
pinch of nutmeg (optional)

1. Add parsnips and potato to a large pot of cold water. Bring water to a gentle boil over medium heat and cook vegetables until very tender, about 20 minutes. Drain in a colander and transfer to a large bowl.

2. Using an electric mixer or a masher, mash the parsnip and potato chunks until almost smooth. Add yogurt, salt, pepper, and nutmeg and continue mashing until smooth and well blended. If consistency is too thick, add a little more yogurt. Serve right away.

Nutrient analysis per approximately ½-cup serving
Calories 120; Protein 4 g; Carbohydrates 27 g; Fat—total 0 g; Saturated fat 0 g; Cholesterol 0 mg; Dietary fiber 4 g; Calcium 94 mg; Iron 1 mg; Sodium 33 mg

・ ・ ・ ・ ・ ・ ・ ・

Mashed Yellow Turnips with Crispy Shallots

Serves 6
Preparation time: 15 minutes
Cooking time: 1 hour 40 minutes

From: Danny Meyer and Michael Romano, Union Square Cafe, New York, New York

Danny fondly remembers eating his grandmother's mashed potatoes topped with fried onion crisps. She served them with barbecued St. Louis baby back ribs, and even after all the meat was cleaned from the bones, the family would dip the ribs into a second or third helping of mashed potatoes, enjoying the trace flavor of barbecue sauce with the potatoes. The idea of substituting turnips for the potatoes, and shallots for the onions, came to Danny while strolling through the Greenmarket one day just before the Union Square Cafe opened. Mashed turnips have become one of the cafe's signature dishes, and the only person who has never been convinced to try them is Danny's grandmother.

6 shallots
1½ cups light olive oil or vegetable oil
3 tablespoons butter
2 medium-size yellow turnips (about 4 pounds)
1 teaspoon salt plus salt to taste
1 cup milk
6 tablespoons butter
freshly ground black pepper to taste

1. Peel and slice shallots crosswise into very thin slices, then separate the slices into rings.

2. In a medium saucepan, heat oil and butter over medium heat until mixture begins to boil. Add shallots and cook over very low heat, stirring occasionally, until rich golden brown, 30 to 40 minutes.

3. Using a slotted spoon, remove shallots to paper towels to drain. Let dry about 15 minutes or until crisp. (They can be stored airtight for several days.)

4. Peel turnips to remove their waxy skins, and cut them into generous 1-inch chunks. Put them in a large saucepan with water to cover them and 1 teaspoon of salt. Bring to a boil. Cover and simmer for 45 to 50 minutes or until tender. Drain.

5. In a medium saucepan, bring milk and butter to a simmer over medium heat.

6. Puree turnips in a food processor or blender, in batches if necessary. With the motor running, add the milk mixture through the feed tube in a steady stream and process until turnips are smooth and mixture is well blended.

7. Before serving, reheat turnip puree and season with salt and pepper. Sprinkle crispy shallots on top.

Nutrient analysis per approximately ¾-cup serving
Calories 197; Protein 4 g; Carbohydrates 19 g; Fat—total 14 g; Saturated fat 8 g; Cholesterol 34 mg; Dietary fiber 5 g; Calcium 115 mg; Iron 1 mg; Sodium 638 mg

Oven French Fries

Serves 6
Preparation time: 15 minutes plus 15 minutes to stand
Cooking time: 25 minutes

From: Charles van Over, Chester, Connecticut

2 pounds baking potatoes, peeled
1 tablespoon salt
2 tablespoons butter
2 tablespoons olive oil

1. Preheat oven to 350°F.
2. Cut potatoes into thin sticks and put them in a medium bowl. Toss with salt and let stand for 15 minutes. Pat potatoes dry with a paper towel.

3. In an ovenproof skillet, heat butter and oil over medium heat. Add potatoes and cook, stirring often, for 10 minutes or until they begin to brown.
4. Transfer skillet to oven and bake potatoes for 10 to 15 minutes or until golden brown and crisp. Serve right away or hold potatoes in a 200°F oven up to 30 minutes.

Nutrient analysis per serving
Calories 197; Protein 3 g; Carbohydrates 29 g; Fat—total 8 g; Saturated fat 3 g; Cholesterol 10 mg; Dietary fiber 2 g; Calcium 8 mg; Iron 0 mg; Sodium 1,112 mg

. . . .

Roasted Root Vegetables

Serves 6
Preparation time: 15 minutes
Cooking time: 1 hour 45 minutes

From: Waldy Malouf, Hudson River Club, New York, New York

Root vegetables combine harmoniously with each other and with many meat and fish dishes. Choose the ones your family likes best but remember that variety lends both complex flavor and appealing color. The vegetables also make a very good puree (step 4). One pound of diced vegetables yields 4 cups, enough to serve 6.

1 pound peeled root vegetables, cut into ½-inch
    pieces:
   2 parsnips
   3 carrots
   1 celery root
   ½ yellow turnip
   1 white turnip
olive oil
1 cup hot chicken broth
2 tablespoons unsalted butter, cut into pieces
    (optional)

Puree (optional)
3 tablespoons unsalted butter
¼ cup heavy cream
pinch of nutmeg

1. Preheat oven to 350°F.

2. Choose a roasting pan or casserole that is large enough to hold the vegetables in a 1½-inch layer. Oil the pan. Add the vegetables and toss to coat lightly with the oil. Roast vegetables, turning once or twice, for 30 minutes.

3. Pour the hot broth over the vegetables and dot with butter. Cover pan with foil or lid, raise temperature to 375°F, and roast vegetables until soft, about 1 hour. Uncover pan and continue to cook until all liquid has evaporated. Serve right away.

4. (optional). *To puree vegetables:* Instead of serving vegetables right away, put them in a food processor or blender with butter, heavy cream, and nutmeg. Process until smooth and blended. Pour the puree into a casserole and reheat in a 350°F oven.

Nutrient analysis per ⅔-cup serving
Calories 95; Protein 3 g; Carbohydrates 11 g; Fat—total 5 g; Saturated fat 2.5 g; Cholesterol 10 mg; Dietary fiber 4 g; Calcium 46 mg; Iron 1 mg; Sodium 179 mg

········

Sautéed Spinach with Garlic

Serves 4
Preparation time: 10 minutes
Cooking time: 7 minutes

From: Danny Meyer and Michael Romano, Union Square Cafe, New York, New York

With this quick-stir method of cooking, spinach does not have to be drained, and it keeps most of its bright green color and vitamins. You'll be surprised at how much flavor the garlic gives. Enjoy the spinach on its own or with steak, chicken, or lamb. If you have leftover spinach, you can chop it up and make a sandwich on good bread with olive oil and mozzarella.

2 pounds fresh spinach
1 large clove garlic, peeled
3 tablespoons olive oil
salt and freshly ground black pepper to taste
1 lemon, quartered (optional)

1. Remove stems from spinach leaves. Discard any leaves that are discolored or overly tough. Soak spinach in a large bowl of cold water to clean it. Change the water two or three times to ensure that the spinach is free of dirt and grit.

(Hint: With each change of water, lift the spinach out of the bowl with your hands rather than dumping the bowlful of spinach and water into a colander. That way you won't pour the sandy water back into the spinach.) Thoroughly dry the spinach in a salad spinner or with absorbent paper towels.

2. Spear the garlic clove with a fork.

3. In a sauté pan or saucepan large enough to hold all the spinach, heat oil over medium heat. Add spinach and stir quickly and constantly with the garlic on the fork until spinach is wilted, 3 to 4 minutes.

4. Season with salt and pepper and cook for 1 to 2 minutes more or until spinach is tender but not overcooked. Serve hot or at room temperature. If desired, add a generous squeeze of lemon just before serving.

Nutrient analysis per ½-cup serving
Calories 132; Protein 5 g; Carbohydrates 8 g; Fat—total 11 g; Saturated fat 1.5 g; Cholesterol 0 mg; Dietary fiber 5 g; Calcium 173 mg; Iron 5 mg; Sodium 135 mg

. . . .

Spinach-Mushroom Pudding

Serves 6
Preparation time: 10 minutes
Cooking time: 15 minutes
Baking time: 30 minutes

From: Kathy Cary, Lilly's la Pêche, Louisville, Kentucky

Serve this easy-to-make pudding as a side dish for dinner or as a main dish for lunch, with a salad on the side.

2 cups cubed fresh bread (½-×-1-inch cubes)
1 10-ounce package frozen chopped spinach
1 tablespoon olive oil
¼ cup finely chopped yellow onion
2 cups sliced button mushrooms (6 ounces)
3 large eggs
1 cup milk
⅛ teaspoon ground nutmeg (optional)
salt and ground black pepper to taste
½ cup grated Parmesan cheese (2 ounces)

1. Preheat oven to 375°F. Grease an 11-×-9-inch baking dish. Spread bread cubes evenly over the bottom.

2. Cook spinach according to package directions, drain, and squeeze dry. Arrange spinach evenly over bread cubes.

3. In a medium skillet, heat oil over medium heat. Add the onion and sauté until soft, about 5 minutes. Add mushrooms and sauté until slightly golden, about 5 minutes. Spoon mushroom mixture evenly over spinach.

4. In a medium bowl, whisk together eggs, milk, nutmeg, salt, and pepper until well blended. Pour mixture over mushrooms. Sprinkle Parmesan cheese evenly over top.

5. Bake, uncovered, for 30 minutes or until puffed and lightly golden. Serve right away.

Nutrient analysis per approximately 3-×-4-inch piece
Calories 148; Protein 9 g; Carbohydrates 12 g; Fat—total 7 g; Saturated fat 3 g; Cholesterol 48 mg; Dietary fiber 2 g; Calcium 239 mg; Iron 2 mg; Sodium 283 mg

. . . .

Desserts

Chocolate Cake with Raspberry Sauce
Cocoa Brownies
Crepes for Kids
Maple-Glazed Tropical Fruit Salad
Oatmeal Cookies
Poached Pears
Rice Pudding
Strawberries with Balsamic Vinegar
Super Cherry Tiramisu
Tabbouleh with Fresh Fruit Ratatouille

. . . .

Chocolate Cake with Raspberry Sauce

Serves 8
Preparation time: 25 minutes plus time to cool
Baking time: 25 minutes

Adapted from: Todd Weisz, Turnberry Isle and Resort Club, Aventura, Florida

6 ounces semisweet chocolate, chopped
3 tablespoons milk
1 cup sugar
2 tablespoons butter
2 cups all-purpose flour
2 teaspoons baking powder
1 cup brewed coffee, chilled
¼ cup water
3 large eggs
fresh raspberries, for garnish

Raspberry Sauce
1 pint fresh raspberries
½ teaspoon lemon juice
1 tablespoon superfine sugar

1. Preheat oven to 350°F. Lightly grease and flour an 8-inch-square baking pan.

2. In top of a double boiler, combine chocolate, milk, sugar, and butter. Heat over simmering (not boiling) water until chocolate and butter are melted and mixture is smooth. Remove pan from water.

3. In a small bowl, mix flour and baking powder.

4. In a small bowl or 2-cup measure, mix coffee and water.

5. In a large bowl, beat eggs with an electric mixer until fluffy. Beat in chocolate mixture until blended. Beat in flour mixture and coffee mixture in alternate batches until blended.

6. Scrape batter into prepared pan. Bake for 20 to 25 minutes or until a cake tester inserted in the center comes out clean. Set pan on wire rack for 10 minutes. Turn cake out onto rack and cool slightly.

7. *To make sauce:* In a food processor or blender, combine raspberries and lemon juice. Process until pureed. Strain mixture through a fine sieve into a small bowl; discard seeds. Add sugar to taste.

8. Place about 3 tablespoons of sauce onto each serving plate. Place a piece of cake over the sauce (cake can be served warm). Garnish with fresh berries.

Nutrient analysis per 4-×-2-inch slice of cake with 3 tablespoons of sauce
Calories 426; Protein 7 g; Carbohydrates 72 g; Fat—total 12 g; Saturated fat 3 g; Cholesterol 88 mg; Dietary fiber 2 g; Calcium 106 mg; Iron 3 mg; Sodium 180 mg

· · · · · · · ·

Cocoa Brownies

Makes 12 brownies
Preparation time: 15 minutes
Baking time: 30 minutes

From: Lucie Costa, North Plank Road Tavern,
Newburgh, New York

⅔ cup all-purpose flour
⅓ cup unsweetened cocoa powder
1 tablespoon baking powder
¾ cup unsweetened applesauce
½ cup sugar
¼ cup light corn syrup
1 tablespoon vegetable oil, such as canola oil
1 teaspoon vanilla extract
⅛ teaspoon salt
1 large egg white, slightly beaten

1. Preheat oven to 350°F. Lightly grease a 9-inch-square baking pan.

2. In a small bowl, mix flour, cocoa powder, and baking powder.

3. In a medium bowl, mix applesauce, sugar, corn syrup, oil, vanilla, and salt until blended. Beat in egg white until blended. Beat in flour mixture just until blended.

4. Scrape batter into prepared pan and spread evenly. Bake for 30 minutes or until a cake tester inserted into the center comes out almost clean.

5. Set pan on a wire rack and cool completely before cutting into bars. Store airtight at room temperature up to 3 days.

Nutrient analysis per brownie
Calories 107; Protein 2 g; Carbohydrates 22 g; Fat—total 2 g; Saturated fat 0.5 g; Cholesterol 18 mg; Dietary fiber 1 g; Calcium 74 mg; Iron 1 mg; Sodium 158 mg

. . . .

Crepes for Kids

Makes 15 crepes
Preparation time: 15 minutes
Cooking time: 25 minutes

From: Michael Romano and Danny Meyer, Union Square Cafe, New York, New York

These crepes can be eaten plain or stuffed with fruit or jam and topped with frozen yogurt or ice cream. Make a big batch, refrigerate or even freeze the leftovers, and reheat as many as you want. Serve them for dessert, breakfast, or brunch.

3 large eggs
1½ teaspoons vegetable oil
1 cup all-purpose flour
pinch of salt
2 tablespoons fresh orange juice
2 teaspoons grated orange zest
1½ cups milk
2 tablespoons butter, softened

1. In a medium bowl, mix eggs, oil, flour, and salt with an electric mixer until well blended. (Batter will be thick at this point.)

2. With mixer off, add orange juice and zest. With mixer at a slow speed, beat in milk until batter is smooth and thick enough to lightly coat the back of a spoon.

3. In a small saucepan, melt 1 tablespoon of the butter and cook just until it begins to brown. Add browned butter to batter, stirring to blend.

4. Heat a crepe pan or 7-inch skillet (preferably nonstick) over medium heat. Put in a small amount of the remaining butter and spread it over the bottom of the pan. Ladle in enough batter (a scant ¼ cup) to thinly and evenly coat the bottom of the pan. Cook crepe until edges begin to brown and crepe appears dry, about 35 seconds. Flip crepe with a small spatula and cook for 20 to 30 seconds more or until set. Put the cooked crepes on a baking sheet lined with parchment paper or waxed paper. Cook crepes with the remaining batter, and as they're done, pile them on top of each other, layering them between more pieces of paper. Serve warm.

5. *To store crepes:* Take the stack of crepes layered with paper and wrap it airtight in foil. Refrigerate crepes up to 5 days or freeze them up to 2 months. *To reheat:* Place wrapped crepes in a 200°F oven until warmed through.

Nutrient analysis per 7-inch crepe
Calories 76; Protein 3 g; Carbohydrates 8 g; Fat—total 4 g; Saturated fat 2 g; Cholesterol 49 mg; Dietary fiber 0 g; Calcium 36 mg; Iron 1 mg; Sodium 54 mg

· · · · · · · ·

Maple-Glazed Tropical Fruit Salad

Serves 6
Preparation time: 10 minutes
Cooking time: 10 minutes

From: Lucie Costa, North Plank Road Tavern, Newburgh, New York

1 20-ounce can pineapple chunks, packed in
   juice
3 tablespoons maple syrup
1 tablespoon cornstarch
¼ cup seedless raisins
2 medium navel oranges, peeled and sectioned,
   with white pith removed

1. Drain the juice from the pineapple can. In a medium saucepan, combine the juice with the maple syrup, cornstarch, and raisins. Heat over medium heat, stirring often, until thickened slightly.

2. Spoon pineapple chunks and orange sections into serving dishes. Spoon warm sauce over fruit and serve right away.

Nutrient analysis per approximately ¾-cup serving
Calories 122; Protein 1 g; Carbohydrates 32 g; Fat—total 0 g; Saturated fat 0 g; Cholesterol 0 mg; Dietary fiber 2 g; Calcium 40 mg; Iron 1 mg; Sodium 3 mg

········

Oatmeal Cookies

Makes 12 cookies
Preparation time: 15 minutes
Baking time: 10 minutes per batch

From: Lucie Costa, North Plank Road Tavern, Newburgh, New York

⅔ cup old-fashioned rolled oats
½ cup all-purpose flour
¼ teaspoon baking powder
¼ teaspoon baking soda
⅛ teaspoon salt
¼ cup unsalted butter, softened (½ stick)
½ cup packed light brown sugar
1 large egg white
¼ teaspoon vanilla extract
¼ cup currants

1. Preheat oven to 375°F.

2. In a small bowl, mix oats, flour, baking powder, baking soda, and salt.

3. In a medium bowl, cream butter and sugar with an electric mixer. Beat in egg white and vanilla until blended. Stir in currants.

4. Add dry ingredients and mix just until blended.

5. Drop heaping tablespoons of dough onto an ungreased cookie sheet, spacing them about 2 inches apart. Bake for 9 to 10 minutes.

6. Set cookie sheet on a wire rack to cool for 5 minutes. Transfer cookies to rack and cool completely. Store airtight at room temperature up to 3 days.

Nutrient analysis per cookie
Calories 103; Protein 2 g; Carbohydrates 15 g; Fat—total 4 g; Saturated fat 2.5 g; Cholesterol 10 mg; Dietary fiber 1 g; Calcium 18 mg; Iron 1 mg; Sodium 66 mg

. . . .

Poached Pears

Serves 4
Preparation time: 15 minutes
Cooking time: 15 minutes

From: Nick Morfogen, Ajax Tavern, Aspen, Colorado

Top each poached pear with a scoop of vanilla ice cream or a mound of whipped cream for an even richer dessert. Look for star anise in large supermarkets or Asian food shops.

1½ cups water
¾ cup sugar or ⅓ cup honey
1 cinnamon stick, broken in half
2 whole cloves
2 star anise
1 vanilla bean, split
grated rind from 1 lemon
1 ounce pear brandy (optional)
4 ripe Bartlett pears, peeled

1. In a medium stainless steel or enamel saucepan, combine water, sugar, cinnamon stick, cloves, star anise, vanilla bean, lemon rind, and brandy. Bring to a boil.

2. Add pears. Reduce heat, cover, and simmer just until tender, about 8 to 10 minutes.

3. With a slotted spoon, remove pears. Halve pears and remove core. Serve pears warm with ¼ cup of the poaching liquid spooned over each.

Nutrient analysis per pear with sauce
Calories 201; Protein 1 g; Carbohydrates 49 g; Fat—total 1 g; Saturated fat 0 g; Cholesterol 0 mg; Dietary fiber 4 g; Calcium 27 mg; Iron 1 mg; Sodium 4 mg

· · · · · · · ·

Rice Pudding

Serves 6
Preparation time: 5 minutes plus time to cool and chill
Cooking time: 60 minutes

From: Kathy Farrell-Kingsley, Newtown, Connecticut

2½ cups cold water
¼ teaspoon salt
1 cup long-grain white rice
2½ cups skim milk
½ cup sugar, or to taste
⅛ teaspoon ground cinnamon
2 large eggs
2 teaspoons vanilla extract
⅓ cup raisins (optional)

1. Bring water to a boil over high heat. Add salt, then stir in rice. Reduce heat, cover, and simmer for 35 minutes or until rice is very tender.

2. Add milk, sugar, and cinnamon. Simmer, uncovered, for 20 minutes or until most of the milk has been absorbed but the rice is still slightly liquid.

3. Beat eggs in a small bowl. Stir about 1 cup of the hot rice mixture into the eggs, then return the mixture to the pan. Stir vigorously over low heat for 1 minute. Remove from heat. Stir in vanilla and raisins.

4. Transfer mixture to a large bowl or individual serving dishes. Cool to room temperature, then refrigerate until set. Serve chilled.

Nutrient analysis per approximately 1-cup serving
Calories 268; Protein 8 g; Carbohydrates 54 g; Fat—total 2 g; Saturated fat 1 g; Cholesterol 73 mg; Dietary fiber 1 g; Calcium 149 mg; Iron 2 mg; Sodium 168 mg

········

Strawberries with Balsamic Vinegar

Serves 8
Preparation time: 10 minutes plus 20 minutes to stand

From: Lidia Bastianich, Felidia Restaurant, New York, New York

3 pints fresh strawberries, hulled, rinsed, and sliced
1 tablespoon fresh lemon juice
2 tablespoons balsamic vinegar
2 tablespoons fresh orange juice
2 tablespoons superfine sugar

1. In a large glass, plastic, ceramic, or stainless steel bowl, mix strawberries, lemon juice, and vinegar. Let stand for 15 to 20 minutes.
2. Mix in orange juice and sugar and serve.

Nutrient analysis per approximately ¾-cup serving
Calories 38; Protein 0 g; Carbohydrates 9.5 g; Fat—total 0 g; Saturated fat 0 g; Cholesterol 0 mg; Dietary fiber 1 g; Calcium 12 mg; Iron 0 mg; Sodium 1 mg

Super Cherry Tiramisu

Serves 12
Preparation time: 15 minutes plus at least 30 minutes to chill
Cooking time: 10 minutes
Baking time: 15–20 minutes

From: Lucie Costa, North Plank Road Tavern, Newburgh, New York

1 6.2-ounce package angel-food cake mix
1 cup nondairy creamer, hazelnut or amaretto flavor (liquid)
1 cup skim milk
2 tablespoons cornstarch
1 16-ounce can pitted tart cherries, drained
½ teaspoon ground cinnamon (optional)
½ teaspoon cocoa powder (optional)

1. Make cake according to package directions but bake in a standard cupcake pan (15–20 minutes). Set on a wire rack to cool. When cupcakes are cool, remove them from the pan and slice each in half crosswise.

2. In a medium saucepan, combine nondairy creamer, milk, and cornstarch. Heat over medium heat, whisking constantly, until thickened to consistency of pudding, about 10 minutes.

3. *To assemble:* Place cupcake bottoms, bottom side down, into individual serving cups or ramekins. Spoon a heaping tablespoon of cherries over each cupcake, then spoon about 2 tablespoons of pudding mixture over the cherries. Cover with a cupcake top. Set cups on a cookie sheet and refrigerate for at least 30 minutes or up to 2 hours. Just before serving, mix cinnamon and cocoa and sprinkle over each tiramisu.

Nutrient analysis per serving
Calories 106; Protein 2 g; Carbohydrates 20 g; Fat—total 2 g; Saturated fat 0.5 g; Cholesterol 0 mg; Dietary fiber 0.5 g; Calcium 49 mg; Iron 1 mg; Sodium 131 mg

········

Tabbouleh with Fresh Fruit Ratatouille

Serves 6
Preparation time: 30 minutes plus 2½ hours to stand

From: Joachim Spichal, Patina Restaurant, Los Angeles, California

Tabbouleh (makes 3 cups)
¾ cup instant couscous
1 cup guava nectar or passion fruit juice, at room
     temperature
2 tablespoons superfine sugar, or to taste
¼ cup fresh orange juice
½ teaspoon grated orange zest

Mango and Raspberry Coulis (makes ⅔ cup
     mango coulis and ¼ cup raspberry coulis)
1 ripe mango, peeled, pitted, and cut up
3½ tablespoons granulated sugar
2 tablespoons plus 1 teaspoon fresh lemon juice
½ cup fresh or thawed frozen raspberries

Fruit Ratatouille (makes 4 cups)
1 cup diced cantaloupe
1 cup peeled, diced kiwifruit (4 kiwifruits)
1 cup peeled, diced fresh pineapple
1 cup hulled, diced strawberries (½ pint)

1. *To make tabbouleh:* In a medium bowl, mix couscous, guava nectar, and sugar. Cover and let stand about 2 hours or until the couscous has absorbed all the juice. Stir in orange juice and zest and let stand for 30 minutes more or until juice is absorbed.

2. *To make coulis:* In a food processor or blender, combine mango with 2 tablespoons of the sugar and 2 tablespoons of the lemon juice. Process until pureed. Strain mixture through a fine sieve into a small bowl; set aside. Clean the work bowl of the food processor, then puree raspberries with the remaining 1½ tablespoons of sugar and 1 teaspoon of the lemon juice. Strain through a fine sieve into another small bowl; set aside.

3. *To make fruit ratatouille:* In a medium bowl, gently mix cantaloupe, kiwifruits, pineapple, and strawberries.

4. *To assemble:* In parfait glasses, alternately layer fruit ratatouille and tabbouleh. End with a layer of fresh fruit. Drizzle with mango coulis, then drizzle with raspberry coulis. Serve chilled or at room temperature.

Nutrient analysis per serving
Calories 188; Protein 2 g; Carbohydrates 46 g; Fat— total 0.5 g; Saturated fat 0 g; Cholesterol 0 mg; Dietary fiber 4 g; Calcium 3 mg; Iron 1 mg; Sodium 9 mg

. . . .

Appendixes

Growth Charts
Recommended Dietary Allowances
Recipe Conversion Table

BOYS: BIRTH TO 36 MONTHS
PHYSICAL GROWTH
NCHS PERCENTILES*

NAME _____ RECORD # _____

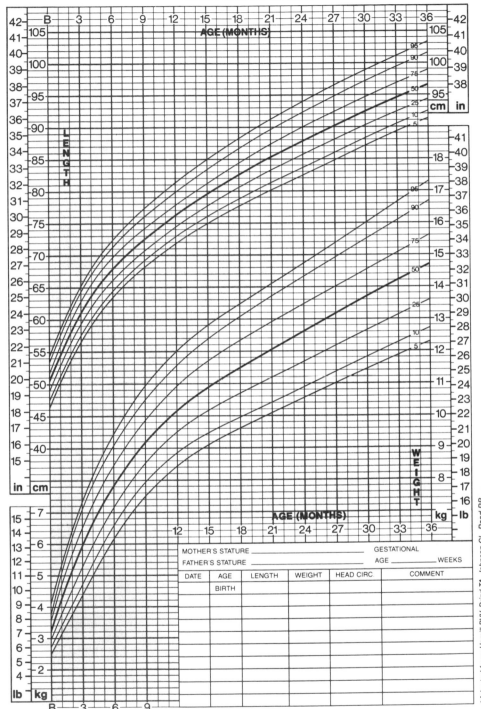

*Adapted from: Hamill PVV, Drizd TA, Johnson CL, Reed RB, Roche AF, Moore WM: Physical growth: National Center for Health Statistics percentiles. AM J CLIN NUTR 32:607-629, 1979. Data from the Fels Longitudinal Study, Wright State University School of Medicine, Yellow Springs, Ohio.

© 1982 Ross Laboratories

MOTHER'S STATURE _____ GESTATIONAL
FATHER'S STATURE _____ AGE _____ WEEKS

DATE	AGE	LENGTH	WEIGHT	HEAD CIRC	COMMENT
	BIRTH				

APPENDIX

NAME_____ _____ RECORD #_____

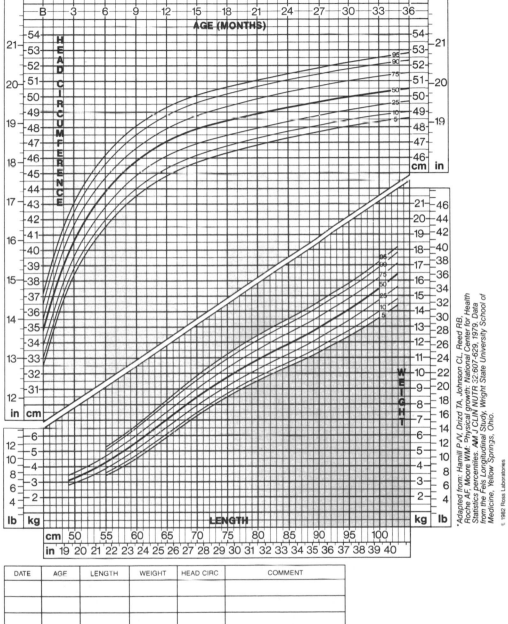

*Adapted from: Hamill P/V, Drizd TA, Johnson CL, Reed RB, Roche AF, Moore WM: Physical growth: National Center for Health Statistics percentiles. AM J CLIN NUTR 32:607-629, 1979. Data from the Fels Longitudinal Study, Wright State University School of Medicine, Yellow Springs, Ohio.

© 1982 Ross Laboratories

DATE	AGE	LENGTH	WEIGHT	HEAD CIRC	COMMENT

Reprinted with permission
of Ross Laboratories

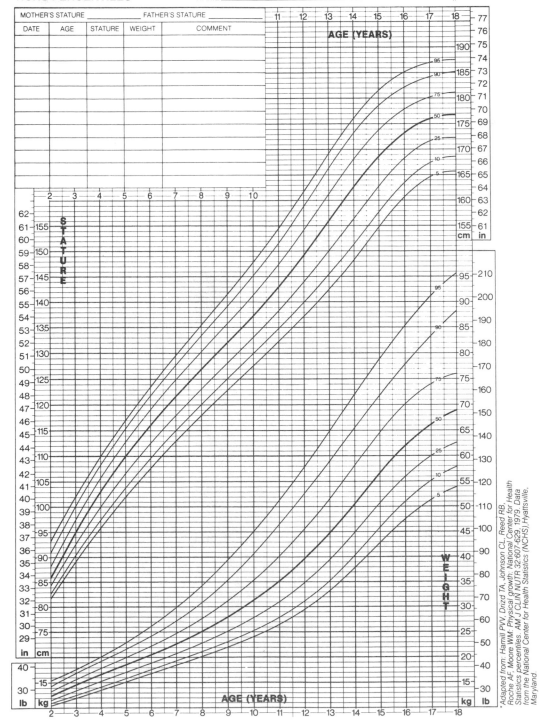

BOYS: 2 TO 18 YEARS
PHYSICAL GROWTH
NCHS PERCENTILES*

NAME _____ RECORD # _____

*Adapted from: Hamill PVV, Drizd TA, Johnson CL, Reed RB, Roche AF, Moore WM: Physical growth: National Center for Health Statistics percentiles. AM J CLIN NUTR 32:607-629, 1979. Data from the National Center for Health Statistics (NCHS), Hyattsville, Maryland.

© 1982 Ross Laboratories

**BOYS: PREPUBESCENT
PHYSICAL GROWTH
NCHS PERCENTILES***

NAME _____ RECORD # _____

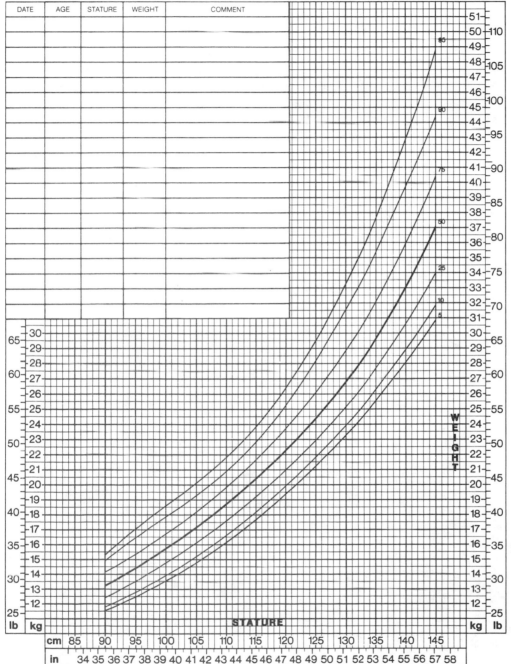

DATE	AGE	STATURE	WEIGHT	COMMENT

STATURE

cm 85 90 95 100 105 110 115 120 125 130 135 140 145

in 34 35 36 37 38 39 40 41 42 43 44 45 46 47 48 49 50 51 52 53 54 55 56 57 58

*Adapted from: Hamill PVV, Drizd TA, Johnson CL, Reed RB, Roche AF, Moore WM. Physical growth: National Center for Health Statistics percentiles. AM J CLIN NUTR 32:607-629, 1979. Data from the National Center for Health Statistics (NCHS), Hyattsville, Maryland.

c 1982 Ross Laboratories

Reprinted with permission
of Ross Laboratories

GIRLS: BIRTH TO 36 MONTHS
PHYSICAL GROWTH
NCHS PERCENTILES*

NAME _____ RECORD # _____

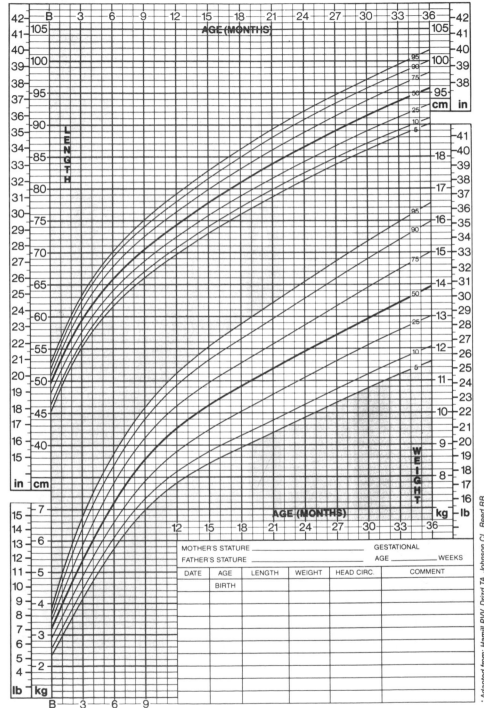

* Adapted from: Hamill PVV, Drizd TA, Johnson CL, Reed RB, Roche AF, Moore WM: Physical growth: National Center for Health Statistics percentiles. AM J CLIN NUTR 32:607-629, 1979. Data from the Fels Longitudinal Study, Wright State University School of Medicine, Yellow Springs, Ohio.

© 1982 Ross Laboratories

MOTHER'S STATURE _____ GESTATIONAL
FATHER'S STATURE _____ AGE _____ WEEKS

DATE	AGE	LENGTH	WEIGHT	HEAD CIRC.	COMMENT
	BIRTH				

NAME _____ RECORD # _____

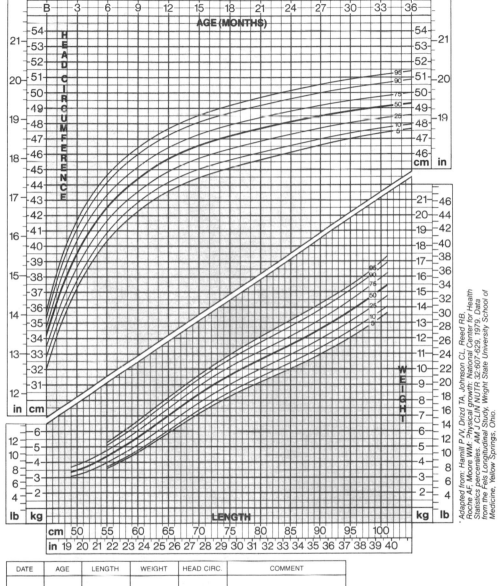

DATE	AGE	LENGTH	WEIGHT	HEAD CIRC.	COMMENT

* Adapted from: Hamill P√V, Drizd TA, Johnson CL, Reed RB, Roche AF, Moore WM: Physical growth: National Center for Health Statistics percentiles. AM J CLIN NUTR 32:607-629, 1979. Data from the Fels Longitudinal Study, Wright State University School of Medicine, Yellow Springs, Ohio.

© 1982 Ross Laboratories

Reprinted with permission
of Ross Laboratories

GROWTH CHARTS

GIRLS: 2 TO 18 YEARS
PHYSICAL GROWTH
NCHS PERCENTILES*

NAME _____ RECORD # _____

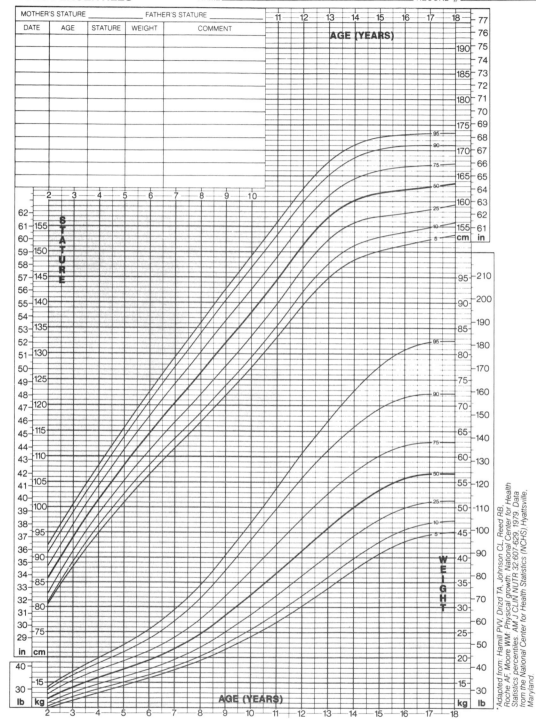

*Adapted from: Hamill PVV, Drizd TA, Johnson CL, Reed RB, Roche AF, Moore WM: Physical growth: National Center for Health Statistics percentiles. AM J CLIN NUTR 32:607-629, 1979. Data from the National Center for Health Statistics (NCHS), Hyattsville, Maryland.

© 1982 Ross Laboratories

GIRLS: PREPUBESCENT
PHYSICAL GROWTH
NCHS PERCENTILES*

NAME _____ RECORD # _____

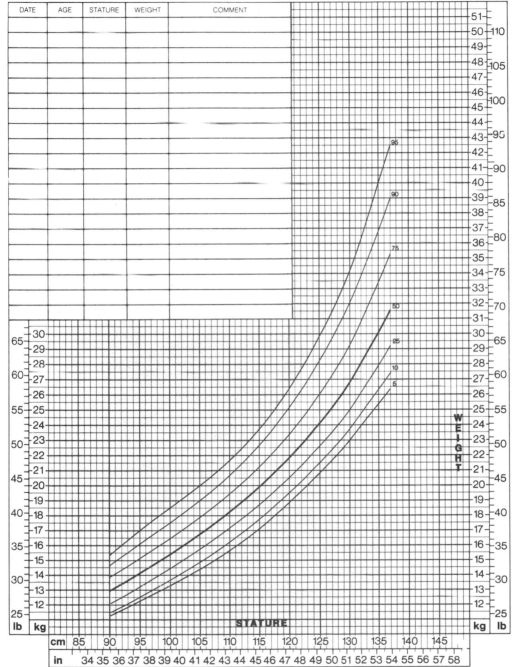

DATE	AGE	STATURE	WEIGHT	COMMENT

*Adapted from: Hamill PVV, Drizd TA, Johnson CL, Reed RB,
Roche AF, Moore WM: Physical growth: National Center for Health
Statistics percentiles. AM J CLIN NUTR 32:607-629, 1979. Data
from the National Center for Health Statistics (NCHS), Hyattsville,
Maryland.

© 1982 Ross Laboratories

GROWTH CHARTS

393

Recommended Dietary Allowances
Revised 1989

Category	Age (years) or condition	Weight[a] (kg)	Weight[a] (lb)	Height[a] (cm)	Height[a] (in)	Protein (g)	Fat-soluble vitamins Vitamin A (μg RE)[b]	Vitamin D (μg)[c]	Vitamin E (mg α-TE)[d]	Vitamin K (μg)
Infants	0.0–0.5	6	13	60	24	13	375	7.5	3	5
	0.5–1.0	9	20	71	28	14	375	10	4	10
Children	1–3	13	29	90	35	16	400	10	6	15
	4–6	20	44	112	44	24	500	10	7	20
	7–10	28	62	132	52	28	700	10	7	30
Males	11–14	45	99	157	62	45	1,000	10	10	45
	15–18	66	145	176	69	59	1,000	10	10	65
	19–24	72	160	177	70	58	1,000	10	10	70
	25–50	79	174	176	70	63	1,000	5	10	80
	51 +	77	170	173	68	63	1,000	5	10	80
Females	11–14	46	101	157	62	46	800	10	8	45
	15–18	55	120	163	64	44	800	10	8	55
	19–24	58	128	164	65	46	800	10	8	60
	25–50	63	138	163	64	50	800	5	8	65
	51 +	65	143	160	63	50	800	5	8	65
Pregnant						60	800	10	10	65
Lactating	1st 6 months					65	1,300	10	12	65
	2nd 6 months					62	1,200	10	11	65

Source: Food and Nutrition Board, National Academy of Sciences–National Research Council. Reprinted with permission from *Recommended Dietary Allowances,* 10th ed. Copyright © 1989 by the National Academy of Sciences. Courtesy of the National Academy Press, Washington, DC.

Note: The allowances, expressed as average daily intakes over time, are intended to provide for individual variations among most normal persons as they live in the United States under usual environmental stresses. Diets should be based on a variety of common foods in order to provide other nutrients for which human requirements have been less well defined.

Water-soluble vitamins							Minerals						
Vita-min C (mg)	Thia-mine (mg)	Ribo-flavin (mg)	Nia-cin (mg NE)[e]	Vita-min B$_6$ (mg)	Folate (μg)	Vita-min B$_{12}$ (μg)	Cal-cium (mg)	Phos-phorus (mg)	Mag-nesium (mg)	Iron (mg)	Zinc (mg)	Iodine (μg)	Sele-nium (μg)
30	0.3	0.4	5	0.3	25	0.3	400	300	40	6	5	40	10
35	0.4	0.5	6	0.6	35	0.5	600	500	60	10	5	50	15
40	0.7	0.8	9	1.0	50	0.7	800	800	80	10	10	70	20
45	0.9	1.1	12	1.1	75	1.0	800	800	120	10	10	90	20
45	1.0	1.2	13	1.4	100	1.4	800	800	170	10	10	120	30
50	1.3	1.5	17	1.7	150	2.0	1,200	1,200	270	12	15	150	40
60	1.5	1.8	20	2.0	200	2.0	1,200	1,200	400	12	15	150	50
60	1.5	1.7	19	2.0	200	2.0	1,200	1,200	350	10	15	150	70
60	1.5	1.7	19	2.0	200	2.0	800	800	350	10	15	150	70
60	1.2	1.4	15	2.0	200	2.0	800	800	350	10	15	150	70
50	1.1	1.3	15	1.4	150	2.0	1,200	1,200	280	15	12	150	45
60	1.1	1.3	15	1.5	180	2.0	1,200	1,200	300	15	12	150	50
60	1.1	1.3	15	1.6	180	2.0	1,200	1,200	280	15	12	150	55
60	1.1	1.3	15	1.6	180	2.0	800	800	280	15	12	150	55
60	1.0	1.2	13	1.6	180	2.0	800	800	280	10	12	150	55
70	1.5	1.6	17	2.2	400	2.2	1,200	1,200	320	30	15	175	65
95	1.6	1.8	20	2.1	280	2.6	1,200	1,200	355	15	19	200	75
90	1.6	1.7	20	2.1	260	2.6	1,200	1,200	340	15	16	200	75

[a] Weights and heights of Reference Adults are actual medians for the U.S. population of the designated age, as reported by NHANES II. The median weights and heights of those under 19 years of age were taken from Hamill, P. V. V., and Drizd, C. L., et al., Physical growth: National Center for Health Statistics percentiles, *American Journal of Clinical Nutrition* 32, no. 16, 1979. The use of these figures does not imply that the height-to-weight ratios are ideal.

[b] Retinol equivalents. 1 retinol equivalent = 1 μg retinol or 6 μg β-carotene.

[c] As cholecalciferol. 10 μg cholecalciferol = 400 IU of vitamin D.

[d] α-Tocopherol equivalents. 1 mg d-α tocopherol = 1 α-TE.

[e] 1 NE (niacin equivalent) is equal to 1 mg of niacin or 60 mg of dietary tryptophan.

Estimated Safe and Adequate Daily Dietary Intakes of Selected Vitamins and Minerals

Category	Age (years)	Vitamins		Trace Elements[a]				
		Biotin (μg)	Pantothenic acid (mg)	Copper (mg)	Manganese (mg)	Fluoride (mg)	Chromium (μg)	Molybdenum (μg)
Infants	0–0.5	10	2	0.4–0.6	0.3–0.6	0.1–0.5	10–40	15–30
	0.5–1	15	3	0.6–0.7	0.6–1.0	0.2–1.0	20–60	20–40
Children and	1–3	20	3	0.7–1.0	1.0–1.5	0.5–1.5	20–80	25–50
adolescents	4–6	25	3–4	1.0–1.5	1.5–2.0	1.0–2.5	30–120	30–75
	7–10	30	4–5	1.0–2.0	2.0–3.0	1.5–2.5	50–200	50–150
	11 +	30–100	4–7	1.5–2.5	2.0–5.0	1.5–2.5	50–200	75–250
Adults		30–100	4–7	1.5–3.0	2.0–5.0	1.5–4.0	50–200	75–250

Source: Food and Nutrition Board, National Academy of Sciences–National Research Council. Reprinted with permission from *Recommended Dietary Allowances,* 10th ed. Copyright © 1989 by the National Academy of Sciences. Courtesy of the National Academy Press, Washington, DC.

Note: Because there is less information on which to base allowances, these figures are not given in the main table of RDA and are provided here in the form of ranges of recommended intakes.

[a] Since the toxic levels for many trace elements may be only several times usual intakes, the upper levels for the trace elements given in this table should not be habitually exceeded.

Recipe Conversion Table

U.S. Weights and Measures
1 pinch = less than ⅛ teaspoon (dry)
1 dash = 3 drops to ¼ teaspoon (liquid)
3 teaspoons = 1 tablespoon = ½ ounce (liquid and dry)
2 tablespoons = 1 ounce (liquid and dry)
4 tablespoons = 2 ounces (liquid and dry) = ¼ cup
5⅓ tablespoons = ⅓ cup
16 tablespoons = 8 ounces = 1 cup = ½ pound
16 tablespoons = 48 teaspoons
32 tablespoons = 16 ounces = 2 cups = 1 pound
64 tablespoons = 32 ounces = 1 quart = 2 pounds
1 cup = 8 ounces (liquid) = ½ pint
2 cups = 16 ounces (liquid) = 1 pint
4 cups = 32 ounces (liquid) = 2 pints = 1 quart
16 cups = 128 ounces (liquid) = 4 quarts = 1 gallon
1 quart = 2 pints (dry)
8 quarts = 1 peck (dry)
4 pecks = 1 bushel (dry)

Temperatures: °Fahrenheit (F) to °Celsius (C)
–10°F = –23.3°C (freezer storage)
  0°F = –17.7°C
 32°F = 0°C (water freezes)
 50°F = 10°C
 68°F = 20°C (room temperature)
100°F = 37.7°C
150°F = 65.5°C
205°F = 96.1°C (water simmers)
212°F = 100°C (water boils)
300°F = 148.8°C
325°F = 162.8°C
350°F = 177°C (baking)
375°F = 190.5°C
400°F = 204.4°C (hot oven)
425°F = 218.3°C
450°F = 232°C (very hot oven)
475°F = 246.1°C
500°F = 260°C (broiling)

Conversion Factors
If you need to convert measurements into their equivalents in another system, here's how to do it.

ounces to grams: multiply ounce figure by 28.3 to get number of grams

grams to ounces: multiply gram figure by .0353 to get number of ounces

pounds to grams: multiply pound figure by 453.59 to get number of grams

pounds to kilograms: multiply pound figure by 0.45 to get number of kilograms

ounces to milliliters: multiply ounce figure by 30 to get number of milliliters

cups to liters: multiply cup figure by 0.24 to get number of liters

Fahrenheit to Celsius: subtract 32 from the Fahrenheit figure, multiply by 5, then divide by 9 to get Celsius figure

Celsius to Fahrenheit: multiply Celsius figure by 9, divide by 5, then add 32 to get Fahrenheit figure

inches to centimeters: multiply inch figure by 2.54 to get number of centimeters

centimeters to inches: multiply centimeter figure by .39 to get number of inches

Adapted from the conversion table that appeared in *All Around the World Cookbook* by Sheila Lukins. © 1994 by Sheila Lukins. Reprinted by permission of Workman Publishing Company, Inc. All rights reserved.

CONTRIBUTORS

. . . .

Barbara Ackerman, R.N., I.B.C.L.C.
Yale–New Haven Children's Hospital

Ronald Angoff, M.D.*
Associate Clinical Professor of Pediatrics
Child Study Center
Yale University School of Medicine

Walter R. Anyan, Jr., M.D.*
Professor of Pediatrics
Section Chief, Adolescent Medicine
Yale University School of Medicine

Robert S. Baltimore, M.D.*
Professor of Pediatrics (Infectious Disease) and
    Epidemiology and Public Health
Yale University School of Medicine

Linda M. Bartoshuk, Ph.D.*
Professor of Psychology
Professor of Surgery (Otolaryngology)
Yale University School of Medicine

Susan Boulware, M.D.*
Assistant Clinical Professor of Pediatrics
    (Endocrinology)
Yale University School of Medicine

Jane E. Brody
Author, *New York Times*
    Personal Health Columnist

Sonia Caprio, M.D.*
Associate Professor of Pediatrics
    (Endocrinology)
Yale University School of Medicine

*Denotes affiliation with Yale–New Haven Children's Hospital

Thomas Carpenter, M.D.*
Associate Professor of Pediatrics
  (Endocrinology)
Yale University School of Medicine

Donna Caseria, M.S., R.D.
Clinical Nutrition Research Coordinator
Yale–New Haven Children's Hospital

Lisa Devine, R.D.
Clinical Nutrition Specialist
Yale–New Haven Children's Hospital

Valerie B. Duffy, Ph.D., R.D.
Assistant Professor
University of Connecticut
School of Allied Health Professions
Lecturer, Surgery (Otolarngology)
Yale University School of Medicine

Marie Egan, M.D.*
Assistant Professor of Pediatrics
  (Respiratory Medicine)
Yale University School of Medicine

Brian Forsyth, M.D, Ch.B, F.R.C.P.(C.)*
Associate Professor of Pediatrics
Child Study Center
Yale University School of Medicine

Kathy French, M.S., R.D.
Pediatric Nutrition Specialist
Yale–New Haven Children's Hospital

Teresa Fung, M.S., R.D., C.N.S.D.
Clinical Nutrition Specialist
Yale–New Haven Children's Hospital

Linda Gay, M.S., R.D., C.D.E.
Ambulatory Nutrition Specialist
Yale–New Haven Children's Hospital

Barry Goldberg, M.D.
Clinical Professor of Pediatrics
Yale University School of Medicine

Frank Gruskay, M.D.*
Associate Clinical Professor of Pediatrics
Yale University School of Medicine

Nancy A. Held, M.S., R.D., C.D.E.
Pediatric Endocrine Nutrition Specialist
Yale University School of Medicine

Rosa Hendler, M.D.
Research Scientist in Internal Medicine
  (Endocrinology)
Yale University School of Medicine

Jane Kerstetter, Ph.D., R.D.
Associate Professor
University of Connecticut
School of Allied Health Professions
Lecturer, Internal Medicine
Yale University School of Medicine

Donald Kohn, D.D.S.*
Clinical Professor Surgery (Dental) and
  Pediatrics
Yale University School of Medicine

Mary Kuras, M.Ed., C.C.C.-S.L.P.
Lecturer, Surgery (Otolaryngology)
Yale University School of Medicine

Sylvia J. Lavietes, M.S.W., L.C.S.W.
Assistant Clinical Professor of Pediatrics
  (Social Work)
Yale University School of Medicine

John M. Leventhal, M.D.*
Professor of Pediatrics
Child Study Center
Yale University School of Medicine

Erica L. Liebelt, M.D.*
Assistant Professor of Pediatrics
   (Emergency Department)
Yale University School of Medicine

Ellen Liskov, M.P.H., R.D.
Ambulatory Nutrition Specialist
Yale-New Haven Children's Hospital

Tara Prather Liskov, M.S., R.D.
Lead Ambulatory Nutrition Specialist
Yale-New Haven Children's Hospital

Linda C. Mayes, M.D.*
Arnold Gesell Associate Professor
Child Study Center and Pediatrics and
   Psychology
Yale University School of Medicine

Mary E. McDonnell, M.S., R.D.
Clinical Nutrition Specialist
Yale-New Haven Children's Hospital

Colston F. McEvoy, M.D.*
Assistant Professor of Pediatrics
   (Gastroenterology/Hepatology)
Yale University School of Medicine

Ellen B. Milstone, M.D.*
Associate Clinical Professor of Dermatology
Yale University School of Medicine

Leonard M. Milstone, M.D.*
Professor of Dermatology
Yale University School of Medicine
Chief of Dermatology
Veterans Affairs Connecticut Health Care System

M. Susan Moyer, M.D.*
Associate Professor of Pediatrics
   (Gastroenterology/Hepatology)
Yale University School of Medicine

Elahna Paul, M.D., Ph.D.
Resident in Pediatrics
Yale-New Haven Children's Hospital

John A. Persing, M.D.*
Professor of Surgery and Neurosurgery
Section Chief of Plastic Surgery
Yale University School of Medicine

Crystal Reil, R.D.
Genetic Nutrition Specialist
Yale-New Haven Children's Hospital

Elisabeth A. Reilly, P.N.P., A.P.R.N.
Program Instructor
Pediatric Nurse Practitioner Program
Yale University School of Medicine

Margretta Reed Seashore, M.D.*
Professor of Genetics and Pediatrics
Yale University School of Medicine

Bennett Shaywitz, M.D.*
Professor of Pediatrics
Section Chief, Pediatric Neurology
Professor, Child Study Center
Yale University School of Medicine

Sally Shaywitz, M.D.*
Professor of Pediatrics (Neurology)
Child Study Center
Yale University School of Medicine

Norman Siegel, M.D.
Professor of Pediatrics and Medicine
Section Chief, Pediatric Nephrology
Yale University School of Medicine

Ed Strenkowski, M.A., R.D.
Clinical Nutrition Specialist
Yale-New Haven Children's Hospital

Ruth H. Striegel-Moore, Ph.D.
Professor and Chair
Department of Psychology
Wesleyan University

William V. Tamborlane, M.D.*
Professor of Pediatrics
Section Chief, Pediatric Endocrinology
Yale University School of Medicine

Lisa Tartamella, R.D.
Clinical Nutrition Specialist
Yale-New Haven Children's Hospital

Charles van Over
Board of Directors
Friends of the Children's Hospital
    at Yale-New Haven

Scott Van Why, M.D.*
Assistant Professor of Pediatrics (Nephrology)
Yale University School of Medicine

Janet Z. Weiswasser
Executive Director
Friends of the Children's Hospital
    at Yale-New Haven
Program Development and Community
    Relations
Yale University School of Medicine
Department of Pediatrics

Ruth Whittemore, M.D.*
Clinical Professor of Pediatrics (Cardiology)
Yale University School of Medicine

Joseph Woolston, M.D.*
Associate Professor of Psychiatry
Child Study Center and Psychiatry
Yale University School of Medicine

INDEX
....

Absorption, of food and nutrients, 9–11, 13–15

Accent (seasoning), 262

Acclimatization, 102

Acesulfame-K (acesulfame potassium), 168, 214, 261, 263

Acidosis, 162, 186

Acne, 108–11

Addiction, to alcohol, 116–17

Additives, 257, 260–64

ADHA (attention deficit hyperactivity disorder), 195–98, 260

Adolescence, 64–73, 78, 79; dairy consumption in, 28; acne during, 108; obesity risk during, 135

Adrenal hyperplasia, 183

Adrenaline surge, 212

Advertising, 71, 78, 81, 134, 283

Alar, 259

Albumen, 145

Alcohol: palatability of, 21–22; adolescent abuse of, 23, 112–17; corn

allergy and, 146; peptic disease and, 178; caloric content of, 201

Algae, 86

Alimentum, 142, 144, 146

Allergies, 140–47; taste perception and, 18; to proteins, 31; breast milk as protection against, 33; in infants, 39, 41, 42; protein deficiency and, 53; to milk, 56; to sulfites, 261–62

Almonds, 69, 217

Amenorrhea, 126, 127

American food, 286–87

Amino acids, 87; proteins made up of, 14, 86, 164, 205; supplementation of, 99, 105

Amylase, 13

Anabolic steroids, 105

Anaphylaxis, 141, 142, 143

Androgens, 5

Anemia, 171, 179, 235–37; postpartum, 33; in toddlers, 53–54; in

adolescents, 70; alcohol-induced, 115

Angel food cake, 72, 222, 286

Anorexia nervosa, 72, 101, 102, 125–31

Antibodies, 206; in breast milk, 32; allergy, 140, 141

Antioxidants, 21, 106

Antrum, 10–11, 12

Anus, 13

Anxiety, 73; alcohol used in response to, 116; in treatment of eating disorders, 127

Apnea, 136, 177

Apple juice. See Juice

Apples, 28, 211, 218, 252, 255, 259

Applesauce, 90, 222, 279

Appliances, kitchen, 273–74

Arginine, 105

Arrhythmias, cardiac, 115

Artificial coloring, 261, 263

Ascites, 114

Ascorbic acid (vitamin C): water-solubility of, 15, 229; in fruits and vegetables, 62; iron absorption aided by, 70, 87; excess intake of, 106; sources of, 233, 234; as nitrosamine retardant, 261; in fast food, 284, 285

Asian food, 262, 288

Asparagus, 27, 70, 211

Aspartame, 168, 184, 197, 214, 257, 261, 262–63

Aspartic acid, 105, 262

Asthma, 31, 142, 261, 262

Atherosclerosis, 148, 149, 160, 215, 253

Athletics, 97–107. *See also* Exercise

Atopic dermatitis, 141, 142

Attention deficit hyperactivity disorder (ADHD), 195–98

Aversions, 23

Avocados, 223, 287

Baby bottle tooth decay, 121–22

Baby foods, 42

Baby-sitters, 81

Bacon, 217, 225, 260, 261

Bagels, 27, 41, 98, 104, 105, 131, 248

Baking soda, 245

Bananas, 28, 34, 91, 120, 255

Barley, 145, 178, 212, 218, 248, 252

Barley malt, 212

Basal metabolic rate (BMR), 202

Beans, 28, 34, 101, 252; in child's diet, 56–57; folate content of, 70; protein and zinc content of, 86, 99, 205

Bedwetting, 136, 162

Beef, 28, 34, 153, 216, 217

Beer, 112

Benzoic acid, 261

Benzoyl peroxide, 261

Beta-carotene, 230

β-galactosidase, 179

BHA (butylated hydroxyanisole), 261, 262

BHT (butylated hydroxytoluene), 261, 262

Bicarbonate, absorption by colon of, 11

Bickel, Horst, 183

Bile, 11, 14–15, 180

Bile acid, 159

Bile salts, 218, 254

Biliary atresia, 180

Binge eating disorder, 125, 127, 128, 129, 130

Biotin, 231, 233

Biotinidase deficiency, 183

Birch, Leann, 23

Bitterness, 16, 17; sex differences and, 21

Blackheads, 109

Bloating: in lactose intolerance, 14; sweeteners as cause of, 168, 211; in peptic disease, 177, 178; fiber intake and, 256

Blood alcohol level, 113–14

Blood cells, red. *See* Hemoglobin

Blood pressure, high. *See* Hypertension

Blood-sugar level, 19, 114, 162, 167

Body fat, in puberty, 5–6

Body image, in adolescence, 72, 125, 126–27

Body Mass Index, 94–95, 135

Body proportions, 4–5

Body temperature, 89, 91, 114

Body weight: at birth, 4; during adolescence, 66; of athletes, 100–101; eating disorders and, 125–32

Bologna, 28, 153, 220, 225, 249

Bolus, 10, 11, 12

Bones: growth of, 66; calcium needed for, 234–35

Booth, David, 23

Bottle-feeding, 35–36, 56, 121, 122, 190, 191–92. *See also* Formula, infant

Botulism, 42, 214, 260

Bran, 145, 253, 255

Branched chain ketonuria. *See* Maple syrup urine disease

BRAT diet, 91

Bread, 27, 70; in child's diet, 54–55; protein content of, 34, 86; iron content of, 86; carbohydrate content of, 98; before athletic event, 104; cholesterol content of, 155, 156; in low-fat diet, 222–23; water content of, 241; sodium content of, 248; fiber content of, 255

Breakfast, 51; in school-age child's diet, 61; skipping of, 72; recipes for, 301–6

Breast cancer, 33, 70

Breastfeeding, 31–39, 56; food acceptance and, 23; vitamin C intake and, 70; parental roles and, 79; vegetarian diet and, 87; food allergies and, 142, 144; cystic fibrosis and, 174; of child with cleft lip or palate, 190–91; protein intake and, 207; sodium and, 248

Breasts, development of, 5, 65–66

Brewer's yeast, 106

Broccoli, 34, 69, 70, 72, 146, 202, 255

Brown sugar, 212

Buckwheat, 178

Bulimia nervosa, 72, 101, 102, 125, 128–32

Bulking agents, 214

Butter, 28, 57, 144, 216, 217, 226, 248

Buttermilk, 144

Butylated hydroxyanisole (BHA), 261, 262

Butylated hydroxytoluene (BHT), 261, 262

Cabbage, 27, 146

Caffeine, 73, 104, 106, 197–98, 202. *See also* Coffee; Soda; Tea

Cake, 145, 217, 226, 249

Calcium: in dietary guidelines, 28; in breastfeeding mother's diet, 34; in child's diet, 54, 62, 220; in adolescent's diet, 66, 69, 87; in vegetarian diet, 86, 87; pregnancy and, 87; in athlete's diet, 99–100, 106; milk allergy and, 144; vitamin toxicity and, 230, 231; bone health and, 234–35, 236; zinc absorption decreased by, 237; in fast food, 284, 285

Calcium caseinate, 144

Calcium chloride, 21

Calories, caloric intake: regulation of, 19; in dietary guidelines, 26, 28, 218; in infancy, 31; in breast milk, 32; in breastfeeding mother's diet, 35; in childhood, 53; in school-age child's diet, 61; in adolescent's diet, 68; fast food as source of, 73; during illness, 89; in athlete's diet, 100–2; eating disorders and, 130–31; childhood obesity and, 133–34; cystic fibrosis and, 172–74; as nutritional building block, 201–4; effect of fiber on, 254; in fast food, 284, 285

Calories Plus, 174

Cancer, 26; food aversions and, 23; vegetables as protection against, 27; fats as cause of, 28, 70, 216; breast, 33; ovarian, 33; low incidence among vegetarians of, 85; alcohol abuse and, 115; fiber as protection against, 253

Candy. See Sweets

Canned goods, 274

Canola oil, 156, 217, 222, 226

Caramel color, 146, 261

Carbohydrate loading, 98

Carbohydrates: protein eaten with, 9; digestion of, 11, 12, 13–14; in dietary guidelines, 25–27; simple vs. complex, 69; in athlete's diet, 98, 104; acne and, 110; tooth decay and, 119–20; diabetes treatment and, 166–69; malabsorption of, 178; caloric content of, 201; as

nutritional building block, 209–14; types of, 210; recipes dense in, 339–49

Carbonation, of alcoholic beverages, 115

Cardiac arrhythmias, 115

Cardiovascular disease. See Atherosclerosis; Heart disease; Stroke

Carnitine, 106, 182

Carotene, 229, 261

Carrot oil, 261

Carrots, 27, 42, 72, 98, 211, 229, 254

Casein, 144, 176

Casein hydrolysate formula, 144

Cataracts, 186

Cauliflower, 27, 34, 211

Celery, 27, 72, 120, 254

Celiac sprue, 145, 178

Cellulose, 212, 253

Cereal, 27, 34, 87, 101; in infant's diet, 41; in child's diet, 54–55; iron content of, 70, 86; before athletic event, 104; calcium content of, 144; cholesterol content of, 155, 156; in low-fat diet, 222–23; zinc content of, 237; sodium content of, 248, 249; fiber content of, 254

Cerebral palsy, 184

Cheese, 28, 221; in breastfeeding mother's diet, 34; in infant's diet, 43; in toddler's and preschooler's diet, 55, 56; in athlete's diet, 99; tooth decay prevented by, 120; allergy to, 144; cholesterol content of, 153, 154; lactose content of, 179; saturated fats in, 217; in low-fat diet, 224–25; sodium content of, 248, 249

Cheeseburgers, 284, 285

Chemotherapy, 23

Cherries, 28, 211

Chewing, 10, 46–47

Chewing gum, 120, 214

Chicken, 28, 34, 61, 73, 86, 153, 285, 286

Chicken noodle soup, 89

Childhood, growth and development in, 4–6

Chili, 156, 223

Chinese food, 288

Chloride, 11, 234

Chlorine, 261

Chocolate, 42, 73, 108, 110, 217, 223, 225, 279

Choking hazards, 41, 42, 47, 59

Cholestasis, 180

Cholesterol: metabolizing by liver of, 11; low level in vegetarian diet of, 85; "good," 135; hazards of, 148–49; defined, 149–50; types of disorder, 150–51; treatment of disorders, 151–60; as nutritional building block, 215–28; fiber as reducer of, 254; in fast food, 284, 285

Cholestipol Hcl, 160

Cholestyramine, 159, 160

Choline, 106

Chromium, 106, 237, 238

Chymotrypsin, 13

Cirrhosis, 114, 171

Citrus fruits, 42, 142, 146–47, 178, 218, 252

Cleft lip and palate, 188–93

Clotting of blood, 171, 186, 231

Cocoa butter, 216–17

Cocoa powder, 223

Coconut, 105, 226

Coconut oil, 156, 217, 226

Cod-liver oil, 229

Coercion, and child's food acceptance, 23, 40, 43, 47, 55

Coffee: child's growth and, 3; social role of, 20; iron absorption decreased by, 70; in adolescent's diet, 73; peptic disease and, 178

Cola, 104, 145

Colds: taste perception and, 18; vitamin C and, 234

Colic, 43, 142

Colitis, 179
Collagen, 234
Collard greens, 27
Colon. *See* Large intestine
Coloring, artificial, 261, 263
Colostrum, 32
Comedo, 109
Complex carbohydrates. *See* Poly-
saccharides
Condensed milk, 144
Conditioning, of aversions and
preferences, 23
Constipation, 13, 43, 175–76; in
school-age child, 62; low inci-
dence among vegetarians of, 85;
in peptic disease, 177; iron sup-
plementation as cause of, 237;
fiber as protection against, 253
Contamination of food, 59
Contracting, in dieting, 138
Cookies, 28, 145, 156, 217, 226, 251,
279
Cook Like a Peasant, Live Like a King
(Scott), 22
Copper, 106, 237, 238
Corn, 98, 212; allergy to, 146
Corn chips, 28
Corned beef, 245
Corn oil, 156, 217, 226
Corn syrup, 120, 146, 168, 211, 212
Cortisone, 109, 136
Cottage cheese, 34, 144, 153, 154,
217, 224, 249
Cottonseed oil, 156, 217
Coughing, 89, 171, 192
Cow's milk, 28, 40, 43
Crab, 34, 86, 143
Crackers, 27, 54, 72, 90, 120, 221,
222, 248, 251
Cranberry juice. *See* Juice
Cream, 144, 217, 224, 225
Cream cheese, 131, 224, 251
Cream sauces, 223, 249
Crohn's disease, 179–80
Croissants, 222, 288
Cromolyn sodium, 143

Crying, in infancy, 43
Cured meat, 245, 249
Cushing's disease, 109, 136
Cystic fibrosis, 102, 170–74, 183, 231,
246

Daminozide, 259
Day care, 81
Defecation, 13
Defrosting of food, 276
Dehydration, 15, 241, 242–43; from
diarrhea, 90, 91, 176; during
exercise, 98, 99, 102–3, 104;
from alcohol consumption, 114;
ketones as cause of, 162; from salt
loss, 174; skim milk as cause of,
219
Demands for food, by toddlers, 46
Dementia, alcohol-associated, 114
Dessert: toddler's eating habits and,
46; recipes for, 375–84
Development: defined, 3; of children,
4–6; neurobehavioral, of infants,
31; physiological, of infants, 31;
physical, of toddlers, 46–48, 52–
54; of preschoolers, 50; cognitive,
of adolescents, 68
Dextrin, 146, 212, 214
Dextrose. *See* Glucose
DHA (docosahexaenoic), 33
Diabetes, 33, 114, 135, 150; defined, 161–62; causes of, 162–63;
treatment of, 163–69; cystic
fibrosis–related, 171
Diabetic ketoacidosis, 162
Diarrhea, 12, 15, 41, 90–91, 176; in
lactose intolerance, 14, 140, 142,
144; breast milk as protection
against, 33; in school-age child,
63; fluid intake and, 88, 89; in
gluten allergy, 145; peptic disease
and, 177, 178; intestinal disorders
and, 179, 180; sugar alcohols as
cause of, 211; water lost through,
243; salt lost through, 245, 246;
fiber as protection against, 253

Dietary Guidelines for Americans
(1990), 26
Digestion, 9–15
Dilatation of blood vessels, 114
Dinner, as family ritual, 62, 80
Dipeptides, 14
Disaccharides, 14, 210, 211–12
Discipline: of school-age child, 63;
food as improper tool of, 80. *See
also* Coercion, and child's food
acceptance
Diverticular disease, 85
Doughnuts, 28, 57, 217, 226
Dried beans, 28, 237, 248, 254, 255
Dried fruits, 28, 70, 120, 251, 278
Drug abuse, 128
Dumping syndrome, 12
Duodenum, 11, 12–13, 179
Dust mites, 142
Dyes (food coloring), 261, 263

Ear infections, 33, 190
Early satiety, 11
Eating disorders, 125–32
Eczema, 141, 262
Edema, 241
Eggplant, 28
Eggs, 28, 34, 42; amino acid and iron
content of, 86; protein content
of, 99; salmonella risk and, 102;
allergy to, 141, 142, 145; cholesterol content of, 153, 154, 156,
216, 225; protein content of, 205;
sodium content of, 248
Electrolytes: absorption by colon of,
11–12; loss during illness of, 88,
242; in athlete's diet, 102, 103,
105; loss from diarrhea of, 176;
function of, 234
Emulsifiers, 146
Endogenous opiates, 19
Energy: needs in adolescence, 67;
needs of athletes, 100; intake of,
201–2, 203–4; expenditure of,
202–4; vitamins and, 229. *See also*
Calories, caloric intake

English muffins, 27, 54, 104, 222, 278

Ensure, 174

Enzymes, 10, 11, 13, 14, 31, 178, 206, 234

Enzyme supplements, 172

Eosinophilia-myalgia syndrome, 239

Epinephrine kits, 143

Equal (sweetener), 184, 257, 262-63

Ergogenic aids, 105-6

Erythrosine (Red Dye No. 3), 261

Esophagitis, 177

Esophagus, 10, 12, 114

Estrogen, 5, 106

Eustachian tube, 190

Evaporated milk, 144

Exceed (sports drink), 104

Exercise: salt regulation and, 20; by school-age child, 62; eating disorders and, 127, 128; obesity and, 138-39; in diabetes treatment, 165; thirst increased by, 241-42. *See also* Athletics

Exocrine glands, 170, 171

Familial combined hyperlipidemia, 150-51

Familial hypercholesterolemia, 150

Family meals, 50-51, 77-83

Farina, 145

Fast food, 283-85; early exposure to, 49-50; in adolescent's diet, 73, 81; cholesterol content of, 156, 226; salt content of, 244, 249, 251. *See also individual kinds of fast food*

Fasting, 138, 206

Fats: digestion of, 11, 12, 14-15; children's taste for, 23; in dietary guidelines, 26, 28-29; in breast milk, 32; in child's diet, 49-50, 53, 57; in adolescent's diet, 69; as cancer risk, 28, 70; in fast food, 73; in athlete's diet, 99; acne and, 110; obesity risk and, 135; cholesterol content of, 154, 156; cystic fibrosis and, 172-73; malabsorption of, 180; caloric content of,

201, 209; as nutritional building block, 215-28; in lunch planning, 279; in fast food, 284, 285. *See also* Triglycerides

Fatty acid disorders, 182

Fatty acid oxidation, 187

FD&C Yellow No. 5, 263, 265

Feces. *See* Stool

Feingold, Benjamen, 196

Ferrulates, 106

Fertilizers, 260

Ferulic acid, 106

Fever, 89, 91, 179, 202, 242

Fiber, 252-56; in digestion, 12, 13-14, 218; in dietary guidelines, 27, 28; in child's diet, 55, 63, 70; in vegetarian diet, 85; gluten allergy and, 145; diabetes and, 167; constipation and, 176; diarrhea and, 176-77; polysaccharide, 212; zinc absorption decreased by, 237; soluble vs. insoluble, 252-53

Figs, 28, 34, 222

Filiform papillae, 20

Finesse (fat substitute), 221

Fish, 34, 42; in dietary guidelines, 28; in child's diet, 56-57, 60; iron content of, 70; zinc content of, 86, 237; allergy to, 141, 142, 143; cholesterol content of, 153, 216; protein content of, 205; fat content of, 217, 225-26; sodium content of, 248, 249; as fast food, 286

Flatulence, 168, 211. *See also* Gas

Flavor, 17

Flour, wheat, 145

Fluid intake, 240-43: during illness, 88-89; in athlete's diet, 102, 103-4. *See also* Dehydration

Fluoride, 32, 40, 118, 119, 121, 213

Fluorosis, 119

Folate, 70, 115, 179

Folic acid, 34, 179, 231, 232, 235

Fölling, Asbjörn, 183

Food groups, 25-26

Food Guide Pyramid, 26-29, 43, 54, 70, 97-98, 222-27, 277

Food intake, regulation of, 18-19

"Food jags," 19

Food processors, 273

Formula, infant, 39-40; breast milk vs., 31-32; colicky infant and, 43; milk allergy and, 142, 144; cystic fibrosis and, 174; gastro-esophageal reflux and, 177; fluid intake and, 242; salt content of, 248; heating of, 273-74. *See also* Bottle-feeding

Fox, A. L., 20

Free radicals, 106

Freezing of food, 273, 275, 276

French food, 288

French fries, 73, 105, 223, 226, 284, 285

French toast, 145, 156, 249

Fried foods, 108, 178, 223, 226, 285

From Fish to Philosopher (Smith), 243

Frozen yogurt, 28, 72, 286

Fructose, 120, 121, 211; in digestion, 14; supertasters' perceptions of, 21; in sports drinks, 104; corn allergy and, 146; diabetes treatment and, 168; diarrhea aggravated by, 176; intolerance toward, 182, 187; as alternative to sucrose, 213-14

Fruit: in dietary guidelines, 28; in infant's diet, 41; in toddler's and preschooler's diet, 55-56; tooth decay and, 120; monosaccharide content of, 211; fat content of, 223-24; water content of, 241; sodium content of, 248, 251; fiber content of, 253, 254; in lunch planning, 278

Fruitarian diet, 85

Fruit juices, 28, 41, 55-56, 72, 120; after athletic event, 105; diabetes and, 167; as sweetener, 168, 213-14; diarrhea aggravated by, 176; sodium content of, 248; metha-

Fruit juices (continued)
nol content of, 262; in lunch
planning, 278. *See also* Juice
Fullness, in digestion, 12
Fundus, 10, 12
Fungiform papillae, 20–21

Galactose, 14, 182, 187–88, 211
Galactosemia, 182, 183, 187–88, 211
Gallbladder, 11, 14
Gas: in lactose intolerance, 14; in
peptic disease, 178; fiber intake
and, 256. *See also* Flatulence
Gastric juices, 11
Gastritis, 177
Gastroenteritis, 243
Gastroesophageal reflux, 12, 171, 177
Gastrointestinal (GI) tract, 9;
anatomy of, 10–12; motility of,
12–13; infections of, 33, 113;
effect of alcohol on, 114; allergic
symptoms and, 142; disorders of,
175–80; water lost through, 243
Gatorade, 104
Gelatin, 72, 89, 106, 214
Gemfibrozil, 160
Ginseng, 106
Gliadin, 178
Globulin, 145
Glucose, 120, 146, 168, 178, 211,
212; control by liver of, 11; in
digestion, 14; used in exercise, 98,
103–4; obesity and, 136; diabetes
and, 161–67; diarrhea and, 176;
amino acids converted to, 206;
zinc absorption aided by, 237
Glutamate, 105
Gluten, 144–45, 178
Glycerol, 216
Glycine, 105
Glycogen, 14, 98, 105, 106, 212
Goal setting, 138
"Good cholesterol." *See* High-density
lipoprotein (HDL)
Graham crackers, 145, 222, 251
Grains, 86, 156, 205, 241, 248

Granola bars, 61, 222, 251
Grapefruit, 28
Grape juice. *See* Juice
Grapes, 28, 42
GRAS (generally recognized as safe)
designation, 261
Gravies, 226
"Grazing," 130
Green beans, 28
Ground beef, 153, 225
Growth: defined, 3; in infancy, 4; in
childhood, 4–6, 52; measurement
of, 6–8; caloric requirements and,
61; vegetarian diet and, 87; of
athletes, 100
Growth charts, 7–8, 52, 66, 93, 204,
387–93
Growth hormone, 105
Growth spurts, 34–35, 53, 62, 213;
sexual maturation and, 64–67
Gums, edible, 212, 252
Guthrie, Robert, 182

Ham, 28, 220, 245, 260
Hamburger, 57, 73, 226, 286
Hard palate, 188
Hay fever, 142
Head: size of, 4; measurement of, 7
Health claims, 267, 269
Hearing loss, 190
Heartburn, 12, 171, 177
Heart disease, 26; fats as cause of, 28,
70, 215–16; low incidence among
vegetarians of, 85; resistance to
heat and, 102; effect of cholesterol
and saturated fats on, 105, 148,
160; obesity and risk of, 133; salt
as cause of, 244, 247–48; fiber as
protection against, 253
Heart rate, 102–3
Heat-related illness, 102, 103
Heat stroke, 103
Height, 6–8, 136, 138
Helicobater pylori, 177
"Heme" iron, 69–70, 236
Hemicellulose, 212, 252, 253

Hemoglobin, 53, 66–67, 206, 235
High-density lipoprotein (HDL),
135, 149, 150, 151, 160, 216,
217–18
High-fructose corn syrup (HFCS),
211
Histamine, 143
Hives, 142, 143
HMG-Co-A reductase inhibitor, 160
Holiday meals, 50–51
Homocystinuria, 182, 183, 186
Honey, 42, 120, 168, 213, 214
Hormones, 5, 206
Hot dogs, 28, 42, 56–57, 105, 153,
216, 217, 249
Humidity, 102, 103
Hydrogenated oils, 156, 218
Hydrogenated starch hydrolysate
(HSH), 168, 221
Hyperactivity, 183, 195–98
Hyperammonemia, 186
Hypercholesterolemia, 148
Hyperinsulinemia, 136, 150
Hyperlipidemia, 148, 149, 150–51
Hyperphenylalaninemias, 183
Hypertension: excessive salt intake
and, 20, 70, 244, 247–48; alcohol
abuse and, 114, 115; obesity and,
135, 136
Hypertriglyceridemia, 151
Hypoglycemia, 114, 117, 165, 182,
187
Hypotension, 142
Hypothyroidism, 136, 150, 183

IBD. *See* Inflammatory bowel disease
(IBD)
Ice cream: in dietary guidelines,
28; in adolescent's diet, 73; sore
throat soothed by, 89; as binge
food, 132; lactose intolerance and,
144; cholesterol content of, 154;
sugar content of, 211, 217, 224;
fat substitutes in, 221; sodium
content of, 248, 251

IgE antibody, 143
Ileum, 11, 15, 179–80
Illness, nutrition and, 88–91
Immune reactions to food, 140, 141
Immunization, breastfeeding as form of, 32
Immunosuppressive therapy, 179
Impulsivity, 195, 196
Inattention, 195, 196
Infalyte, 89
Infancy, 30–44, 78, 79; growth in, 4; digestion in, 12; taste perceptions in, 17–18; obesity risk in, 135; fat intake in, 219; labeling rules and, 268–69; recipes for, 295–98
Infant botulism, 42, 214
Inflammatory bowel disease (IBD), 177, 179
Insomnia, 73
Insulin, 136, 161–69, 212
Insulin-dependent diabetes mellitus (IDDM), 161
Intestines. *See* Large intestine; Small intestine
Invert sugar, 212
Iodides, 110
Iodine, 237, 238
Iron, 31, 220; in infant formula, 40, 43–44; in child's diet, 53–54, 62; loss during menstruation of, 66; in adolescent's diet, 69–70; in vegetarian diet, 86–87; pregnancy and, 87; in athlete's diet, 100, 106; gluten allergy and, 145; Crohn's disease and, 179; deficiency of, 235–37
Iron poisoning, 237
Irradiation of food, 263
Irritability, 41, 127, 145, 177, 178, 183, 212
Irritable bowel syndrome, 177
Isoleucine, 182, 186
Isomil, 90
Isomil DF, 91
Italian food, 287
Itching, 143, 180

Jam, 28, 211, 222
Japanese food, 288
Jaundice, 180
Jejunum, 11, 179
Jelly, 28, 57, 98, 131, 211
Juice: tomato, 22, 178; vegetable, 27, 249; apple, 63, 88, 89, 91, 98; orange, 70, 104, 144; cranberry, 89; grape, 98; lemon, 223, 227. *See also* Fruit juices
Juvenile diabetes, 162–69

Kale, 34
Kasha, 145
Kelp, 106
Ketchup, 222, 249
Ketone, 162
Kidney beans, 28, 86, 212, 255
Kidneys, animal, 216
Kidneys, human: effect of protein on, 168; metabolic disorders and, 187; fluid intake and, 241, 242, 243; salt regulated by, 245, 247
Kindercal, 90
Kitchen, stocking of, 273–76
Kiwi, 28
Kosher diet, 56, 245

Labeling of foods, 213, 222–26, 250, 265–69
Lactase, 178
Lactase-phlorizin hydrolase, 13
Lactic acid, 146
Lacto-ovo-vegetarian diet, 84–85
Lactose, 14; diarrhea aggravated by, 90–91; tooth decay caused by, 120, 121; intestinal disorders and, 178; sweetness of, 212; food labeling of, 213; zinc absorption aided by, 237
Lactose intolerance, 14, 39, 69, 140, 144, 176, 179
Lacto-vegetarian diet, 85
Lamb, 28, 34, 153, 216, 217, 225
Lard, 156, 216, 217, 226

Large intestine, 11–12, 13, 15; cancer of, 70; fiber intake and, 253
Laxatives: eating disorders and, 128
Learning disabilities, 195
Lecithin, 106, 146
Legumes: magnesium content of, 34; zinc content of, 86; protein and caloric content of, 87; cholesterol absent from, 156; carbohydrate content of, 212; fiber content of, 218, 252, 253, 255
Lemon juice. *See* Juice
Lente insulin, 164
Lentils, 255
Lettuce, 28, 278
Leucine, 182, 186
Lightheadedness, during digestion, 12
Lima beans, 27, 255
Linoleic acid, 217
Linolenic acid, 217
Lip, cleft, 188–93
Lipase, 13, 14
Lipids. *See* Fats
Lipoproteins, 135, 136, 149–50, 216
Liver, animal, 34, 153, 216, 225
Liver, human: in digestion, 11, 12, 14; effect of saturated fats on, 105; effect of alcohol on, 114; high cholesterol and, 150; transplant of, 151; cystic fibrosis and, 171; diseases of, 180; metabolic disorders and, 186, 187
Lopid, 160
Low-density lipoprotein (LDL), 149, 150, 151, 159, 160, 216, 217, 218, 254
Lower-body obesity, 135
Lower esophageal sphincter (LES), 10, 12
"Low-fat" label, 153
Low-fat milk, 28
L-trytophan, 239
Lunch, 277–82; in school-age child's diet, 61; recipes for, 309–13. *See also* School lunches

Lunch meat, 28, 56–57, 220, 278–79
Lungs: cystic fibrosis and infections of, 171; gastroesophageal reflux and diseases of, 177
Lupus, 150
Lysine, 105

Macrobiotic diet, 85
Magnesium, 34, 55, 106, 234, 236
Magnetic resonance imaging (MRI), 135
Malabsorption, 171, 172, 174, 178–79
Maldigestion, 178
Malt, 145
Maltase-glucoamylase, 13
Maltitol, 168
Maltodextrins, 146, 221
Maltose, 168, 212
Malt syrup, 145
Manganese, 237
Mannitol, 146, 211
Mannose, 211
Maple syrup, 120, 211
Maple syrup urine disease (MSUD), 182, 183, 186
Margarine, 28, 57, 131, 144, 156, 217, 218, 222, 226, 248
Marmalade, 222
Mayonnaise, 131, 217, 221, 222, 226
Meat: in dietary guidelines, 28; in infant's diet, 42; alternatives to, 54; in child's diet, 56–57; safety and, 59; iron content of, 70, 86; zinc content of, 86, 237; cholesterol content of, 153, 154; protein content of, 205; in low-fat diet, 225–26; water content of, 241; sodium content of, 248, 249; in lunch planning, 278–79
Meatloaf, 57
Meconium, 32
Medium tasters, 20–21
Melon, 28, 120
Memory loss, 114
Menstrual cycle: taste perception

and, 21; onset of, 5, 65–66, 67; basal metabolic rate and, 203
Mental retardation, 183, 184
Metabolic disorders, 181–87
Metabolic rate, 202–3
Methanol, 262
Methionine, 182, 186
Methylphenidate, 198
Mevacor, 160
Mexican food, 287
Micelles, 14–15
Microwave ovens, 273–74
Middle ear infection, 18
Milk, 23, 28, 31–39, 40, 43, 120; alternatives to, 54, 224–25; in child's diet, 56; in adolescent's diet, 64, 72; picky eaters and, 83; as source of amino acids, 86; during illness, 91; triglycerides in, 105, 217; skim vs. whole, 131, 153; allergy to, 141, 142, 143–44, 176; cholesterol content of, 154, 216; caloric content of, 202; protein content of, 205; sodium content of, 248
Milkshakes, 101–2, 251
Milk solids, 144
Millet, 145, 178, 212
Minerals: in dietary guidelines, 25, 27, 28; infants' need for, 31; in breastfeeding mother's diet, 33; in child's diet, 53–54, 62; in adolescent's diet, 66–67, 69–70; in athlete's diet, 99–100, 106; acne and, 110; in milk products, 144; facts about, 234–39; fiber intake and, 255–56
Minimal brain dysfunction (MBD), 195
Miso, 146, 288
Moderation, as value imparted to children, 50, 129
Molasses, 120, 168, 212
Molybdenum, 237
Monosaccharides, 14, 210–11
Monosodium glutamate (MSG), 249, 261, 262

Monounsaturated fat, 217, 218
Mood swings, 114
Morbid obesity, 135
Motility, of GI tract, 9, 12–13
Mouth, 10
MSG (monosodium glutamate), 249, 261, 262
MSUD. *See* Maple syrup urine disease
Mucilages, 212
Mucus, 170, 171
Muscles: growth during adolescence of, 66–67; protein intake and, 205, 206
Mustard, 145, 222, 226, 249

National Cholesterol Education Program, 218–19
National Research Council, 25
Navy beans, 28
Nephrotic syndrome, 150
Neurobehavioral development, 31
Newborns: size of, 4; digestion by, 12; taste perceptions of, 17–18
Niacin, 62, 160, 231, 232
Night blindness, 230
Nitrites, 260–61
Nitrogen, dietary, 186
Nitrogen oxides, 261
Nitrosamines, 260–61
"Non-heme" iron, 69–70, 236
Nonimmune reactions to food, 140, 141
Non-insulin-dependent diabetes mellitus (NIDDM), 162
Non-purging bulimia nervosa, 128
Nontasters, 20–21
NPH insulin, 164
Nutramigen, 142, 144, 146
Nutrasweet, 168, 184, 196, 257, 262–63
Nutrient content claims, 267, 268
Nuts, 28, 34, 42, 87, 108, 217; in child's diet, 56–57; protein content of, 86; oral hygiene and, 120; allergy to, 141, 142, 143; vitamin

E content of, 231; zinc content of, 237; fiber content of, 254

Oat bran, 62, 218, 254
Oatmeal, 145
Oats, 145, 156, 178, 212, 218, 248, 252
Obesity, 8, 28, 70, 96, 133–39; recent increases in, 26; definitions of, 95; resistance to heat and, 102; energy expenditure and, 202; effect of fiber on, 254
Octacosanol, 106
Oils, 28–29, 57, 69, 154, 248
Oleoresins, 261
Olestra, 221
Olfaction, 17
Olive oil, 156, 217, 226
Olives, 211, 223, 249
Omega-3 fatty acids, 33, 105, 217
Orange juice. See Juice
Organic foods and gardening, 260
Ornithine, 105
Ornithine transcarbamylase (OTC) deficiency, 182, 186
Orthonasal olfaction, 17
Osteoporosis, 33, 127, 235
Otitis media, 18
Ovamucin, 145
Ovarian cancer, 33
Ovaries, maturation of, 5
Oysters, 34, 86

Pacifiers, 36, 121, 122
Palatal fistula, 193
Palate, cleft, 188–93
Palm kernel oil, 156
Palm oil, 105, 156, 217, 226
Pancakes, 54, 101, 145, 222, 224, 249
Pancreas: in digestion, 11, 12, 14, 170–71; effect of alcohol on, 114; obesity and, 136; insulin produced by, 161, 162, 163, 164
Pantothenic acid, 62, 231, 233
Papillae, 20
Pasta: in dietary guidelines, 27; in

infant's diet, 43; in toddler's and preschooler's diet, 54–55; in athlete's diet, 98, 104; wheat allergy and, 145; cholesterol absent from, 156, 222, 223; salt content of, 248; fiber content of, 254
Peanut butter: in dietary guidelines, 28; in breastfeeding mother's diet, 34; as choking hazard, 42; in athlete's diet, 99; tooth decay and, 120; fat content of, 217, 225; sodium content of, 248, 251
Peanut oil, 156, 217
Peanuts, 34, 141, 142, 143; allergy to, 146, 212, 217
Peas, 27, 34, 70, 86, 248, 252, 255
Pecans, 143, 217
Pectins, 212, 252, 254
Pedialyte, 89
Pediasure, 90
Penis, enlargement of, 66
Peppers, 27, 178
Pepsin, 13, 14
Peptic disease, 177–78
Peptidases, 13
Peptide hydrolases, 13, 14
Percent Daily Values, 266–67
Period, menstrual. See Menstrual cycle
Peristalsis, 12, 13
Pesco-vegetarian diet, 84, 86
Pesticides, 257–60
Pets, 142
Phenylalanine, 182, 183, 184, 262, 263
Phenylketonuria (PKU), 181–85, 263
Phenylthiocarbimide (PTC), 20
Pheresis, 151
Phosphate, 106
Phosphorus, 234, 236
Phytates, 70, 236
Piaget, Jean, 68
Picky eaters, 81–83; alternative foods for, 54, 63
Pilosebaceous unit, 109
Pineapple, 211, 224

Pinto beans, 28, 86
Pita bread, 222, 278
Pizza, 52, 73, 156, 220, 225, 249, 286
PKU (phenylketonuria), 181–85, 263
Plaque, dental, 119, 121
Plums, 28, 211, 222
Pollen, 106
Pollo-vegetarian diet, 84
Polydextrose, 214, 221
Polypeptides, 14
Polysaccharides, 27, 210, 212–13
Polyunsaturated fat, 217–18
Popcorn, 27, 72, 251
Pork, 28, 34, 153, 216, 225
Postpartum anemia, 33
Potassium, 234, 246; absorption by colon of, 11; loss during illness of, 88; loss during exercise of, 103
Potato chips, 28, 221, 226
Potatoes: in dietary guidelines, 27; in breastfeeding mother's diet, 34; in infant's diet, 43; in sick child's diet, 90; in athlete's diet, 98; tooth decay and, 120; vitamin C content of, 146; cholesterol absent from, 156; starch content of, 212; additives used with, 262
Potato mixes, 249
Potato salad, 249
Poultry: in dietary guidelines, 28; in child's diet, 56–57; iron content of, 70; zinc content of, 86, 237; cholesterol content of, 153, 216; in low-fat diet, 225–26; sodium content of, 248, 249
Powdered milk, 144
Preadolescents, 60–63
Pregnancy: sodium craved during, 20; taste perception during, 21; dairy consumption during, 28; vitamin C needs during, 70; vegetarian diet and, 87; obesity risk and, 135
Premature birth, 37
Preschoolers, 48–59, 220
Preservatives, 261, 262

Pretzels, 27, 54, 72, 105, 120, 222, 251
Prosobee, 90
Proteins: carbohydrates eaten with, 9; digestion of, 11, 12, 14; synthesis by liver of, 11; in dietary guidelines, 26, 27, 28; in infancy, 31; in breast milk, 32; in breast-feeding mother's diet, 34; in childhood, 53; in adolescent's diet, 68–69; in vegetarian diet, 86; in athlete's diet, 98–99, 104; in low-calorie diet, 138; food allergies and, 142; in milk products, 144; diabetes treatment and, 167–68; cystic fibrosis and, 172–74; PKU treatment and, 184; caloric content of, 201, 209; as nutritional building block, 205–8; zinc absorption aided by, 237
Protrusion reflex, 31
PTC (phenylthiocarbimide), 20
Puberty, growth and development in, 4, 5–6, 64–73
Pubic hair, growth of, 65
Pudding, 72, 89, 90, 120, 214, 249
Pumpernickel bread, 255
Purging bulimia nervosa, 128
Pylorus, 11, 12
Pyridoxine (vitamin B$_6$), 34, 62, 182, 186, 231, 232

Questran, 169
Quetelet Index, 94–95
Quickkick, 104
Quinine, 21

Radio-allergosorbent test (RAST), 143
Raisins, 28, 42, 98, 120, 251
Rashes, 41, 171
Recipes: for infants, 295–98; for breakfast, 301–6; for lunch, 309–13; for snacks, 317–22; for entrées, 325–35; carbohydrate-dense, 339–49; vegetarian, 353–62; vegetable, 365–71; dessert, 375–84
Recommended Dietary Allowances (RDAs), 25, 52–53, 62, 68, 157
Rectal prolapse, 171
Rectum, 12, 13
Red blood cells. See Hemoglobin
Reflexes, in infancy, 31
Refrigeration of food, 274, 275, 276
Refusal of food, 46, 48–49, 125
Regurgitation, and heartburn, 12
Respiratory infections, 33
Restaurant meals, 51–52, 285–88
Retinoid toxicity, 230
Retinol. See Vitamin A
Retronasal olfaction, 17
Reward, food as, 137
Reye's syndrome, 187
Rhinitis, 142
Riboflavin, 56, 62, 231, 232
Rice: in dietary guidelines, 27; in infant's diet, 43; in toddler's and preschooler's diet, 54–55; in sick child's diet, 90, 91; in athlete's diet, 98; cholesterol absent from, 156, 222; carbohydrate content of, 212
Rice cakes, 27
Rice mixes, 249
Rickets, 86, 230–31
Ritalin, 198
Roast beef, 28
Role playing, in dieting, 138
Rolls, 27, 222, 248, 278
Rooting reflex, 31, 39
Roughage. See Fiber
Royal jelly, 106
Runny nose, 89
Rye, 145, 178, 212
Rye bread, 254

Saccharin, 168, 214, 261, 262
Safety: in kitchen, 51; at mealtime, 58–59
Safflower oil, 156, 217, 226
Salad dressing, 57, 145, 214, 217, 221, 222, 223, 226, 249
Salami, 225, 249
Saliva, 10, 13, 120, 170
Salivary amylase, 14
Salmonella, 102
Salsa, 222, 223, 251, 287
Salt. See Sodium
Saltiness, 16, 17
Salt pork, 245
Sandwiches, 278, 279–80, 286
Sardines, 34, 69
Sashimi, 288
Satiety, 78; early, 12; sensory-specific, 19; eating disorders and, 128; obesity and, 134, 138; fiber intake and, 253, 254
Saturated fat, 148–60, 216–17, 218
Sausage, 211, 217, 225, 260
Scandi Shakes, 174
School-age children, 60–63, 78, 79
School lunches, 61, 157, 277, 280–82. See also Lunch
Scott, Jack Denton, 22
Scurvy, 234
Seasonality of foods, 22
Sebum, 109, 110
Secondary sexual characteristics, 5
Secretory IgA, 141, 142
Seeds, 34, 70, 86
Seizure, 183
Selenium, 106, 237, 238
Self-monitoring, in dieting, 138
"Sell by" date, 274–75
Semi-vegetarian diet, 84
Sensory-specific satiety, 19
Sexual maturation, growth spurt and, 64–67
Shellfish, 34, 69, 108, 141, 143, 225, 237
Sherbet, 91, 144, 251
Shock, as allergic reaction, 142
Shopping with children, 51, 274, 275
Shortening, 146, 156, 222, 226, 262
Shredded wheat, 255

Shrimp, 34, 86, 153, 216

Sick children, 88-91

Sickle cell disease, 183

Simplesse, 221

Skim milk, 28, 99, 131, 153, 202, 219

Skin, poultry, 153

Skin-fold thickness, 95-96

Skin tests, for allergies, 143

Sleep: of infants, 30, 34, 56; effect of alcohol on, 114; calories burned during, 201, 202

Sleep apnea, 136, 177

Small intestine, 11, 12-13, 252, 253

Smell, and food preferences, 17

Smith, Homer, 245

Smoked meat, 245, 249

Smoking, 70-71, 142, 202, 247

Snacks, 57-58, 62, 72, 120; in treatment of eating disorders, 130-31, 132; in diabetes treatment, 166-67; low-salt, 251; recipes for, 317-22

Sneezing, 89

Snoring, 136

Socialization, 50-52, 77, 80

Societal influences: on feeding, 81; on alcohol use, 117

Soda, 28, 49-50, 57, 73, 108, 284

Sodium, 234, 244-51; absorption of, 11, 15; bodily need for, 19-20; hypertension linked to, 20, 70; in fast food, 73, 284, 285; loss during illness of, 88; loss during exercise of, 102, 103; cystic fibrosis and, 174; fluid intake and, 241-42

Sodium benzoate, 245

Sodium caseinate, 144, 245

Soft palate, 188, 190

Sorbitol, 146, 166, 176, 211

Sore throat, 89

Soup, 90, 145, 249

Sour cream, 221, 222, 223

Sourness, 17

Soybean oil, 156, 217, 226

Soybeans, 34, 212

Soy products: milk, 39, 87, 144, 207; zinc content of, 86; allergy to, 141, 142, 146, 176

Soy sauce, 145, 249, 285, 288

Spastic colon, 177

Spices: oral sensation and, 18; peptic disease and, 177-78

Spinach, 27, 34, 97, 144, 146

Spirulina, 86

Spitting up, by infant, 43

Spoon-feeding, of child with cleft lip or palate, 192-93

Sports drinks, 103-4, 105

Squash, 28, 229, 255

Starches, 212; digestion of, 10, 13-14, 31; young adults' taste for, 23

Steatorrhea, 171

Step-One and Step-Two diets, 152, 154-59

Steroids, 105

Stomach: in digestion, 10, 12

Stool: in digestion, 12, 13, 85; infant's, 34; cystic fibrosis and, 171, 172; fiber and, 252, 253. See also Constipation; Diarrhea

Storage of food, 274, 275, 276

Strawberries, 28, 146, 211, 252

Stress fractures, 99

Stroke, 148

Succinate, 106

Sucrase-isomaltase, 13

Sucrose, 21, 120, 121, 168, 196, 211, 213-14

Sugar: digestion of, 13-14; hungers for, 19-20; tooth decay caused by, 28, 119-21; in breast milk, 32; in preschooler's diet, 49-50; in athlete's diet, 98, 104; diabetes and, 161, 167; hyperactivity and, 195, 197; caloric content of, 209. See also individual types of sugar

Sugar beets, 211

Sugar cane, 211

Sugar intolerance, 14

Sulfites, 261-62

Sunflower oil, 156, 217, 226

Sunnette, 263

Supertasters, 20-22

Sustacal, 174

Swallowing, 10, 12

Sweating, 170, 246; during digestion, 12; during exercise, 102, 103; cystic fibrosis and, 174

Sweeteners: caloric vs. noncaloric, 168; alternative, 213-14

Sweetness, 16, 17, 19-20

Sweet 'N Low, 168

Sweet One, 168, 263

Sweet potatoes, 120, 211, 229

Sweets, 28-29, 49-50, 57, 108, 120, 132, 156, 213, 214; cholesterol content of, 155; diabetes and, 161, 167; in lunch planning, 279

Swelling: as allergic reaction, 142, 143; from cholesterol deposits, 150

Swiss Sweet, 263

Tannins, 70, 236

Tartrazine (Yellow Dye No. 5), 261, 263

Taste, 16-24

Taste buds, 20-22

Taste pores, 21

Tea, 70, 73

Teething, 41-42

Television: advertising on, 71, 78, 81, 134, 283; eating while watching, 132; sedentary lifestyle and, 134

Temperature: of toddlers' food, 46; of exercise environment, 102, 103. See also Body temperature

10K (sports drink), 104

Teriyaki sauce, 285, 288

Testes: maturation of, 5, 66

Testosterone, 5

Tetrachlorodibenzodioxin, 109

Texture of foods, 18

Thawing of food, 276

Thermogenesis, 202

Thermoregulation, 102–3
Thiamine, 62, 115, 182, 186, 231, 232
Thickening agents, 214
Thrust reflex, 31, 40
Thyroid gland, underactive, 8
Timing of meals, 47, 132, 137;
    diabetes treatment and, 166–67
Toast, 90, 91, 131
Tocopherols, 231
Tocotrienols, 231
Toddlers, 45–48, 50–59, 78, 79, 220,
    268–69
Tofu, 34, 69, 86, 146, 176, 288
Toilet training, 13
Tomatoes, 27, 42, 142, 146
Tomato juice. *See* Juice
Tomato sauce, 222, 249, 285
Tongue: anatomy of, 20–21; thrust
    reflex of, 31, 40
Tooth decay, 40, 41, 50, 56, 118–22,
    213
Tortilla chips, 221, 251
Tortillas; 222, 278
Toxoplasmosis, 183
Trailblazer, 221
Transfatty acids, 218
Triglycerides, 105, 135, 136, 149, 150,
    160, 180, 216
Tripeptides, 14
Trypsin, 13
Tryptophan, 105
Tubers, 212
Turkey, 28, 34, 57, 153, 220, 225
Turnip greens, 27
Turnips, 27
Type I diabetes, 162–69
Type II diabetes, 162
Tyrosinemia, 183

Ulcerative colitis, 179
Ulcers, 113, 115, 175, 177
Ultra-Lente insulin, 164
Ultraviolet light, 231
Underweight, 101–2
Upper-body obesity, 135
Upper respiratory illnesses, 89–90

Urine, 182, 183, 186, 241, 243, 246.
    See also Kidneys, human
Utensils, kitchen, 274

Vaginal yeast infections, 162
Valine, 182, 186
Van Over, Charles, 22
Varicose veins, 114
Variety, 19; in treatment of eating
    disorders, 131
Veal, 216
Vegan diet, 85, 86, 87, 206, 231
Vegetable juice. *See* Juice
Vegetables: palatability of, 21; in
    dietary guidelines, 27–28; in
    infant's diet, 41; alternatives to,
    54; in child's diet, 55–56; iron
    content of, 70, 86; picky eaters
    and, 83; carbohydrate content
    of, 169; caloric density of, 202;
    protein content of, 205; sucrose
    content of, 211; in low-fat diet,
    223; vitamin content of, 231,
    232, 234; water content of, 241;
    sodium content of, 248, 249; as
    healthy snack, 251; fiber content
    of, 253, 254; in lunch planning,
    278; recipes for, 365–71
Vegetarian diet, 84–87; protein de-
    ficiency and, 53; iron deficiency
    and, 54; recipes for, 353–62
Vending machines, 61
Very low-density lipoprotein
    (VLDL), 149, 160, 216
Villi, 11, 14, 178
Vinegar, 145, 178, 223
Visceral abdominal fat, 135
Vitamin A, 15, 106, 110–11, 171, 174,
    180, 229, 230
Vitamin B_6. *See* Pyridoxine
Vitamin B_{12}, 62, 85, 86, 87, 179, 180,
    231, 233, 235
Vitamin C. *See* Ascorbic acid
Vitamin D, 15, 85, 86, 87, 106, 171,
    172, 174, 180, 229, 230–31

Vitamin E, 15, 106, 171, 174, 180,
    229, 230, 231, 261
Vitamin K, 15, 106, 171, 174, 180,
    229, 230, 231
Vitamins: absorption of, 15; in
    dietary guidelines, 25, 27, 28;
    infants' need for, 31; in breast-
    feeding mother's diet, 33, 34; in
    school-age child's diet, 62; in ado-
    lescent's diet, 69–70; in athlete's
    diet, 99–100, 105–6; acne and,
    110; in milk products, 144; cystic
    fibrosis and, 171; facts about,
    229–34; fat-soluble vs. water-
    soluble, 229; fiber intake and,
    255–56; effect of pesticides on,
    260
Vitamin supplements, 62, 100, 131,
    174, 237–39
Vitellin, 145
Vomiting, 90; by newborn, 12; con-
    ditioned aversions and, 23; as
    allergic reaction, 41, 142, 144; by
    school-age child, 63; fluid intake
    and, 88, 89; intoxication and,
    113; bulimia nervosa and, 128;
    ketones as cause of, 162; from salt
    loss, 174; gastroesophageal reflux
    and, 177; peptic disease and,
    177; MSUD and, 186; metabolic
    disorders and, 187; water lost
    through, 243

Waffles, 54, 98, 145, 224, 249
Waste, 12
Water, 240–43; absorption of, 11,
    15; in infant's diet, 40; in athlete's
    diet, 102; fiber intake and, 255.
    See also Dehydration
Water intoxication, 241, 242
Weaning, 36–37, 56
Weight, 92–96; control through exer-
    cise of, 62; adolescent perceptions
    of, 68, 72; loss during illness of,
    89; of athletes, 100–1. *See also*
    Obesity

Weight curves, 93–94
Wheat, 141; allergy to, 144–45, 178; carbohydrate content of, 212; sodium content of, 248
Wheat germ, 34, 255
Wheat-germ oil, 106
Whey, 144, 176
Whiteheads, 109
Whole grains, 34, 55, 145, 253, 254
Whole milk, 28
Wine, 262

Xylitol, 211
Xylose, 211

Yale, 196–98
Yeast infections, 162
Yeasts: nutritional, 86; dry, 262
Yogurt, 221; in dietary guidelines, 28; protein and zinc content of, 34; in toddler's diet, 55, 56; in school-age child's diet, 61; in adolescent's diet, 69, 72; during illness, 89; in athlete's diet, 101, 104; as healthy snack, 120, 131, 251; milk allergy and, 144; fat content of, 153, 217, 224; cholesterol content of, 154; lactose absorption aided by, 179; sodium content of, 248; in lunch planning, 279

Zinc: sources of, 34, 55, 237; functions of, 66, 237; in vegetarian diet, 86, 87; in athlete's diet, 106; acne and, 110; in low-fat diet, 220